Demyelinating and Inflammatory Lesions of the Brain and Spine

Editors

REZA FORGHANI
ASHOK SRINIVASAN

MAGNETIC RESONANCE IMAGING CLINICS OF NORTH AMERICA

www.mri.theclinics.com

Consulting Editors
SURESH K. MUKHERJI
JENNY T. BENCARDINO

May 2024 • Volume 32 • Number 2

ELSEVIER

1600 John F. Kennedy Boulevard • Suite 1800 • Philadelphia, Pennsylvania, 19103-2899

http://www.mri.theclinics.com

MAGNETIC RESONANCE IMAGING CLINICS OF NORTH AMERICA Volume 32, Number 2
May 2024 ISSN 1064-9689, ISBN 13: 978-0-443-13169-1

Editor: John Vassallo (j.vassallo@elsevier.com)
Developmental Editor: Shivank Joshi

Magnetic Resonance Imaging Clinics of North America (ISSN 1064-9689) is published quarterly by Elsevier Inc., 360 Park Avenue South, New York, NY 10010-1710. Months of issue are February, May, August, and November. Business and Editorial Offices: 1600 John F. Kennedy Blvd., Ste. 1800, Philadelphia, PA 19103-2899. Customer Service Office: 3251 Riverport Lane, Maryland Heights, MO 63043. Periodicals postage paid at New York, NY and additional mailing offices. Subscription prices are $420.00 per year (domestic individuals), $100.00 per year (domestic students/residents), $455.00 per year (Canadian individuals), $579.00 per year (international individuals), $100.00 per year (Canadian students/residents), and $275.00 per year (international students/residents). For institutional access pricing please contact Customer Service via the contact information below. International air speed delivery is included in all *Clinics* subscription prices. All prices are subject to change without notice. **POSTMASTER:** Send address changes to *Magnetic Resonance Imaging Clinics*, Elsevier Health Sciences Division, Subscription Customer Service, 3251 Riverport Lane, Maryland Heights, MO 63043. Customer Service (orders, claims, online, change of address): Elsevier Health Sciences Division, Subscription **Customer Service, 3251 Riverport Lane, Maryland Heights, MO 63043. Tel:1-800-654-2452 (U.S. and Canada); 314-447-8871 (outside U.S. and Canada). Fax: 314-447-8029. E-mail: journalscustomerservice-usa@elsevier.com (for print support); journalsonlinesupport-usa@elsevier.com (for online support).**

Reprints. For copies of 100 or more of articles in this publication, please contact the Commercial Reprints Department, Elsevier Inc., 360 Park Avenue South, New York, NY 10010-1710. Tel.: 212-633-3874; Fax: 212-633-3820; E-mail: reprints@elsevier.com.

Magnetic Resonance Imaging Clinics of North America is covered in the *RSNA Index of Imaging Literature, MEDLINE/PubMed (Index Medicus),* and *EMBASE/Excerpta Medica*.

Contributors

CONSULTING EDITORS

SURESH K. MUKHERJI, MD, MBA, FACR
Professor of Radiology and Radiation Oncology, University of Louisville, Peoria, Illinois; Robert Wood Johnson Medical School, Rutgers University, New Brunswick, New Jersey; Faculty, Otolaryngology Head Neck Surgery, Michigan State University, Farmington Hills, Michigan; National Director of Head and Neck Radiology, ProScan Imaging, Carmel, Indiana

JENNY T. BENCARDINO, MD
Vice Chair of Academic Affairs, Department of Radiology, Montefiore Medical Center, Bronx, New York

EDITORS

REZA FORGHANI, MD, PhD
Professor of Radiology and Artificial Intelligence (AI) and Vice Chair of AI, Director, Radiomics and Augmented Intelligence Laboratory (RAIL), Department of Radiology, University of Florida College of Medicine, Gainesville, Florida

ASHOK SRINIVASAN, MD, FACR
Associate Chair of Operations and Quality, Professor, Department of Radiology University of Michigan, Ann Arbor, Michigan

AUTHORS

AMIT AGARWAL, MD
Associate Professor, Department of Radiology, Mayo Clinic, Jacksonville, Florida

MOHIT AGARWAL, MD
Adjunct Associate Professor, Section of Neuroradiology, Department of Radiology, Medical College of Wisconsin, Milwaukee, Wisconsin

JAYAPALLI BAPURAJ, MD
Professor Department of Radiology, University of Michigan, Ann Arbor, Michigan

ARISTIDES A. CAPIZZANO, MD, MSc
Professor Division of Neuroradiology, Department of Radiology, University of Michigan Health System, Ann Arbor, Michigan

JOHN W. CHEN, MD, PhD
Associate Professor, Institute for Innovation in Imaging, Neurovascular Research Unit, Center for Systems Biology, Division of Neuroradiology, Department of Radiology, Massachusetts General Hospital, Harvard Medical School, Boston, Massachusetts

JOHN D. COMER, MD, PhD
Clinical Assistant Professor Division of Neuroradiology, Department of Radiology, University of Michigan Health System, Ann Arbor, Michigan

AMY M. CONDOS, MD
Acting Instructor, Department of Radiology, University of Washington School of Medicine, Seattle, Washington

FRANCIS DENG, MD
Assistant Professor, Division of Neuroradiology, Russell H. Morgan Department of Radiology and Radiological Science, Johns Hopkins University School of Medicine, Baltimore, Maryland

REZA FORGHANI, MD, PhD
Professor of Radiology and Artificial Intelligence (AI) and Vice Chair of AI, Director, Radiomics and Augmented Intelligence Laboratory (RAIL), Department of Radiology, University of Florida College of Medicine, Gainesville, Florida

SONIA GILL, MD
Assistant Professor, Section of Neuroradiology, Department of Radiology, Medical College of Wisconsin, Milwaukee, Wisconsin

REBECCA L. GILLANI, MD, PhD
Instructor, Department of Neurology, Neuroimmunology and Neuro-Infectious Diseases Division, Massachusetts Institute for Neurodegenerative Disease, Massachusetts General Hospital, Harvard Medical School, Boston, Massachusetts

DAEKI KIM BS
Student, Institute for Innovation in Imaging, Neurovascular Research Unit, Center for Systems Biology, Massachusetts General Hospital, Harvard Medical School, Boston, Massachusetts

HYUNG-HWAN KIM, PhD
Associate Investigator Radiology Institute for Innovation in Imaging, Neurovascular Research Unit, Center for Systems Biology, Massachusetts General Hospital, Harvard Medical School, Boston, Massachusetts

ENRICO G. KüLLENBERG, MD
Physician Institute for Innovation in Imaging, Neurovascular Research Unit, Center for Systems Biology, Massachusetts General Hospital, Harvard Medical School, Boston, Massachusetts

DHAIRYA A. LAKHANI, MD
Fellow Division of Neuroradiology, Russell H. Morgan Department of Radiology and Radiological Science, Johns Hopkins University School of Medicine, Baltimore, Maryland

DORIS D.M. LIN, MD, PhD
Professor, Division of Neuroradiology, Russell H. Morgan Department of Radiology and Radiological Science, Johns Hopkins University School of Medicine, Baltimore, Maryland

TARA MASSINI, MD
Assistant Professor of Radiology, University of Florida, Gainesville, Florida

SHRUTI MISHRA, MD
Assistant Professor Department of Radiology, University of Michigan, Ann Arbor, Michigan

NEGIN JALALI MOTLAGH, MD
Postdoc research fellow Institute for Innovation in Imaging, Neurovascular Research Unit, Center for Systems Biology, Massachusetts General Hospital, Harvard Medical School, Boston, Massachusetts

PHUONG NGUYEN, MD
Resident Department of Radiology, University of Florida College of Medicine, Gainesville, Florida

SEPIDEH PARSI, PhD
Postdoc Institute for Innovation in Imaging, Neurovascular Research Unit, Center for Systems Biology, Massachusetts General Hospital, Harvard Medical School, Boston, Massachusetts

MAYRA MONTALVO PERERO, MD
Assistant Professor of Neurology, University of Florida at Gainesville, Gainesville, Florida

TANYA J. RATH, MD
Associate Professor, Neuroradiology Section, Department of Radiology, Mayo Clinic Arizona, Phoenix, Arizona

JOHN H. REES, MD
Associate Professor, Department of Radiology, University of Florida at Gainesville, Gainesville, Florida

TORGE REMPE, MD, PhD
Assistant Professor, William T. and Janice M. Neely Professor for Research in Multiple Sclerosis, Program Director, UF Multiple

Sclerosis, Neuroimmunology Fellowship, Department of Neurology, University of Florida College of Medicine, Gainesville, Florida

SHYAMSUNDER SABAT, MD
Associate Professor Neuroradiology, Department of Radiology, University of Florida at Gainesville, Gainesville, Florida

ASHOK SRINIVASAN, MD
Professor, Department of Radiology, University of Michigan, Ann Arbor, Michigan

IBRAHIM SACIT TUNA, MD
Associate Professor of Radiology, University of Florida at Gainesville, Gainesville, Florida

PATTANA WANGARYATTAWANICH, MD
Assistant Professor, Department of Radiology, University of Washington School of Medicine, Seattle, Washington

JOSEPH M. YETTO Jr, MD
Neuroradiology Fellow, University of Florida at Gainesville, Gainesville, Florida

CINDY ZHU
Undergraduate Intern, Institute for Innovation in Imaging, Neurovascular Research Unit, Center for Systems Biology, Massachusetts General Hospital, Harvard Medical School, Boston, Massachusetts

Contents

Foreword xiii

Suresh K. Mukherji and Jenny T. Bencardino

Preface: Demyelinating and Neuroinflammatory Diseases of the Brain and the Spine xv

Reza Forghani and Ashok Srinivasan

Multiple Sclerosis Part 1: Essentials and the McDonald Criteria 207

Sonia Gill and Mohit Agarwal

Multiple sclerosis (MS) is an inflammatory demyelinating disease of the central nervous system (CNS) characterized by relapsing-remitting or progressive neurologic symptoms and focal white matter lesions. The hallmark of the disease is the dissemination of CNS lesions in space and time, which is defined by the McDonald criteria. MRI is an essential diagnostic and prognostic biomarker for MS which can evaluate the entire CNS. MS mimics must be excluded before a diagnosis of MS is made.

Multiple Sclerosis Part 2: Advanced Imaging and Emerging Techniques 221

Shruti Mishra, Jayapalli Bapuraj, and Ashok Srinivasan

Multiple advanced imaging methods for multiple sclerosis (MS) have been in investigation to identify new imaging biomarkers for early disease detection, predicting disease prognosis, and clinical trial endpoints. Multiple techniques probing different aspects of tissue microstructure (ie, advanced diffusion imaging, magnetization transfer, myelin water imaging, magnetic resonance spectroscopy, glymphatic imaging, and perfusion) support the notion that MS is a global disease with microstructural changes evident in normal-appearing white and gray matter. These global changes are likely better predictors of disability compared with lesion load alone. Emerging techniques in glymphatic and molecular imaging may improve understanding of pathophysiology and emerging treatments.

Neuromyelitis Optica Spectrum Disorders and Myelin Oligodendrocyte Glycoprotein Antibody-Associated Disease 233

John H. Rees, Torge Rempe, Ibrahim Sacit Tuna, Mayra Montalvo Perero, Shyamsunder Sabat, Tara Massini, and Joseph M. Yetto Jr.

For over two centuries, clinicians have been aware of various conditions affecting white matter which had come to be grouped under the umbrella term multiple sclerosis. Within the last 20 years, specific scientific advances have occurred leading to more accurate diagnosis and differentiation of several of these conditions including, neuromyelitis optica spectrum disorders and myelin oligodendrocyte glycoprotein antibody disease. This new understanding has been coupled with advances in disease-modifying therapies which must be accurately applied for maximum safety and efficacy.

Toxic and Drug-Related White Matter Diseases of the Brain and Spine 253

Amit Agarwal, John H. Rees, and Shyamsunder Sabat

Toxic leukoencephalopathy and myelopathy are common neurologic complications of a wide range of chemotherapeutic and substance abuse agents. During the last decade, there has been a significant change in the profile of white matter toxins, primarily driven by the development and usage of new chemotherapeutic and immunotherapeutic agents and by the continuous increase in illicit drug abuse with contaminants. Neuroimaging in the form of MR imaging forms the cornerstone in the diagnosis of these entities, many of which are reversible and amenable to rapid correction. Chronic white matter changes are also seen with these toxins with gradually progressive clinicoradiological findings.

Uncommon and Miscellaneous Inflammatory Disorders of the Brain and Spine 277

John D. Comer and Aristides A. Capizzano

Inflammatory disorders of the brain and spine have a highly variable MRI appearance, often demonstrating significant overlap in imaging features. The resulting diagnostic dilemma is particularly challenging when considering the more uncommon neuroinflammatory entities. Diligent examination of the salient clinical presentation and signal alteration on imaging examination is necessary when considering neuroinflammation as a diagnostic possibility and may aid in raising suspicion for a particular neuroinflammatory entity. This article reviews a selection of uncommon and miscellaneous inflammatory disorders of the brain and spine to raise awareness of the clinical and imaging features that may assist in this challenging diagnostic task.

Bacterial, Viral, and Prion Infectious Diseases of the Brain 289

Amy M. Condos, Pattana Wangaryattawanich, and Tanya J. Rath

Diagnosis of brain infections is based on a combination of clinical features, laboratory markers, and imaging findings. Imaging characterizes the extent and severity of the disease, aids in guiding diagnostic and therapeutic procedures, monitors response to treatment, and demonstrates complications. This review highlights the characteristic imaging manifestations of bacterial and viral infections in the brain.

Bacterial and Viral Infectious Disease of the Spine 313

Pattana Wangaryattawanich, Amy M. Condos, and Tanya J. Rath

Spinal infections are a diverse group of diseases affecting different compartments of the spine with variable clinical and imaging presentations. Diagnosis of spinal infections is based on a combination of clinical features, laboratory markers, and imaging studies. Imaging plays a pivotal role in the diagnosis and management of spinal infections. The characteristic imaging manifestations of bacterial and viral infections in the spine are discussed with key teaching points emphasized.

Infectious Diseases of the Brain and Spine: Fungal Diseases 335

Dhairya A. Lakhani, Francis Deng, and Doris D.M. Lin

Advances in treatments of autoimmune diseases, acquired immunodeficiency syndrome, organ transplantation, and the use of long-term devices have increased the rates of atypical infections due to prolonged immune suppression. There is a significant overlap in imaging findings of various fungal infections affecting the central nervous system (CNS), often mimicking those seen in neoplastic and noninfectious inflammatory conditions. Nonetheless, there are imaging characteristics that can aid in distinguishing certain atypical infections. Hence, familiarity with a wide range of infectious agents is an important part of diagnostic neuroradiology. In this article, an in-depth review of fungal diseases of the CNS is provided.

Infectious Diseases of the Brain and Spine: Parasitic and Other Atypical Transmissible Diseases **347**

Dhairya A. Lakhani, Francis Deng, and Doris D.M. Lin

Atypical infections of the brain and spine caused by parasites occur in immunocompetent and immunosuppressed hosts, related to exposure and more prevalently in endemic regions. In the United States, the most common parasitic infections that lead to central nervous system manifestations include cysticercosis, echinococcosis, and toxoplasmosis, with toxoplasmosis being the most common opportunistic infection affecting patients with advanced HIV/AIDS. Another rare but devastating transmittable disease is prion disease, which causes rapidly progressive spongiform encephalopathies. Familiarity and understanding of various infectious agents are a crucial aspect of diagnostic neuroradiology, and recognition of unique features can aid timely diagnosis and treatment.

Multiple Sclerosis: Clinical Update and Clinically-Oriented Radiologic Reporting **363**

Phuong Nguyen, Torge Rempe, and Reza Forghani

Multiple sclerosis (MS) is a chronic inflammatory disease of the nervous system. MR imaging findings play an integral part in establishing diagnostic hallmarks of the disease during initial diagnosis and evaluating disease status. Multiple iterations of diagnostic criteria and consensus guidelines are put forth by various expert groups incorporating imaging of the brain and spine, and efforts have been made to standardize imaging protocols for MS. Emerging ancillary imaging findings have also attracted increasing interests and should be sought for on radiologic examination. In this paper, the authors review the clinical guidelines and approach to imaging of MS and related disorders, focusing on clinically impactful image interpretation and MR imaging reporting.

Basic Science of Neuroinflammation and Involvement of the Inflammatory Response in Disorders of the Nervous System **375**

Sepideh Parsi, Cindy Zhu, Negin Jalali Motlagh, Daeki Kim, Enrico G. Küllenberg, Hyung-Hwan Kim, Rebecca L. Gillani, and John W. Chen

Neuroinflammation is a key immune response observed in many neurologic diseases. Although an appropriate immune response can be beneficial, aberrant activation of this response recruits excessive proinflammatory cells to cause damage. Because the central nervous system is separated from the periphery by the blood–brain barrier (BBB) that creates an immune-privileged site, it has its own unique immune cells and immune response. Moreover, neuroinflammation can compromise the BBB causing an influx of peripheral immune cells and factors. Recent advances have brought a deeper understanding of neuroinflammation that can be leveraged to develop more potent therapies and improve patient selection.

MAGNETIC RESONANCE IMAGING CLINICS OF NORTH AMERICA

FORTHCOMING ISSUES

August 2024
Fetal MRI
Camilo Jaimes and Jungwhan J. Choi, *Editors*

November 2024
MR-Guided Focused Ultrasound
Dheeraj Gandhi and Graeme F. Woodworth, *Editors*

February 2025
MR Imaging of the Hip
Jenny T. Bencardino, *Editor*

RECENT ISSUES

February 2024
MR Perfusion
Max Wintermark and Ananth J. Madhuranthakam, *Editors*

November 2023
Clinical Value of Hybrid PET/MRI
Minerva Becker and Valentina Garibotto, *Editors*

August 2023
MR Angiography: From Head to Toe
Prashant Nagpal and Thomas M. Grist, *Editors*

PROGRAM OBJECTIVE

The goal of *Magnetic Resonance Imaging Clinics of North America* is to keep practicing physicians up to date with current clinical practice by providing timely articles reviewing the state of the art in patient care.

TARGET AUDIENCE

All practicing physicians and healthcare professionals who provide patient care utilizing findings from Magnetic Resonance Imaging.

LEARNING OBJECTIVES

Upon completion of this activity, participants will be able to:

1. Review why knowledge of the new immunotherapeutic agents and their complications is important for the radiologist.
2. Discuss the benefits of MRI as an essential component of accurate diagnosis and prognostic biomarkers for multiple sclerosis.
3. Recognize the need for increased awareness of the more uncommon neuroinflammatory entities among radiologists when evaluating MR imaging.

ACCREDITATION

The Elsevier Office of Continuing Medical Education (EOCME) is accredited by the Accreditation Council for Continuing Medical Education (ACCME) to provide continuing medical education for physicians.

The EOCME designates this journal-based CME activity enduring material for a maximum of 11 *AMA PRA Category 1 Credit*(s)™. Physicians should claim only the credit commensurate with the extent of their participation in the activity.

All other healthcare professionals requesting continuing education credit for this enduring material will be issued a certificate of participation.

DISCLOSURE OF CONFLICTS OF INTEREST

The EOCME assesses conflict of interest with its instructors, faculty, planners, and other individuals who are in a position to control the content of CME activities. All relevant conflicts of interest that are identified are thoroughly vetted by EOCME for fair balance, scientific objectivity, and patient care recommendations. EOCME is committed to providing its learners with CME activities that promote improvements or quality in healthcare and not a specific proprietary business or a commercial interest.

The planning committee, staff, authors, and editors listed below have identified no financial relationships or relationships to products or devices they or their spouse/life partner have with commercial interest related to the content of this CME activity:

Amit Agarwal, MD; Mohit Agarwal, MD; Jayapalli Bapuraj, MD; Aristides Andres Capizzano, MD; John D. Comer, MD, PhD; Amy M. Condos, MD; Francis Deng, MD; Sonia Gill, MD; Rebecca L. Gillani, MD, PhD; Daeki Kim; Hyung-Hwan Kim, PhD; Kothainayaki Kulanthaivelu, BCA, MBA; Enrico G. Küllenberg, MD; Dhairya A. Lakhani, MD; Doris D.M. Lin, MD, PhD; Michelle Littlejohn; Tara Massini, MD; Shruti Mishra, MD; Mayra Montalvo Perero, MD; Negin Jalali Motlagh, MD; Phuong Nguyen, MD; Sepideh Parsi, PhD; Tanya J. Rath, MD; John H. Rees, MD; Torge Rempe, MD, PhD; Shyamsunder Sabat, MD; Shyamsunder Sabat, MD; Ashok Srinivasan, MD; Ibrahim Tuna, MD; Pattana Wangaryattawanich, MD; Joseph M. Yetto, Jr, MD; Cindy Zhu

The planning committee, staff, authors, and editors listed below have identified financial relationships or relationships to products or devices they or their spouse/life partner have with commercial interest related to the content of this CME activity:

John W. Chen, MD, PhD: Ownership interest: Einsenca, Inc

Reza Forghani, MD, PhD: Researcher, Consultant/Speaker: Nuance Communications Inc., Canon Medical Systems Inc., GE Healthcare

UNAPPROVED/OFF-LABEL USE DISCLOSURE

The EOCME requires CME faculty to disclose to the participants:

1. When products or procedures being discussed are off-label, unlabelled, experimental, and/or investigational (not US Food and Drug Administration [FDA] approved); and
2. Any limitations on the information presented, such as data that are preliminary or that represent ongoing research, interim analyses, and/or unsupported opinions. Faculty may discuss information about pharmaceutical agents that is outside of FDA-approved labelling. This information is intended solely for CME and is not intended to promote off-label use of these medications. If you have any questions, contact the medical affairs department of the manufacturer for the most recent prescribing information.

TO ENROLL

To enroll in the *Magnetic Resonance Imaging Clinics of North America* Continuing Medical Education program, call customer service at 1-800-654-2452 or sign up online at http://www.theclinics.com/home/cme. The CME program is available to subscribers for an additional annual fee of USD 270.00.

METHOD OF PARTICIPATION

In order to claim credit, participants must complete the following:

1. Complete enrolment as indicated above.
2. Read the activity.
3. Complete the CME Test and Evaluation. Participants must achieve a score of 70% on the test. All CME Tests and Evaluations must be completed online.

CME INQUIRIES/SPECIAL NEEDS

For all CME inquiries or special needs, please contact elsevierCME@elsevier.com.

Foreword

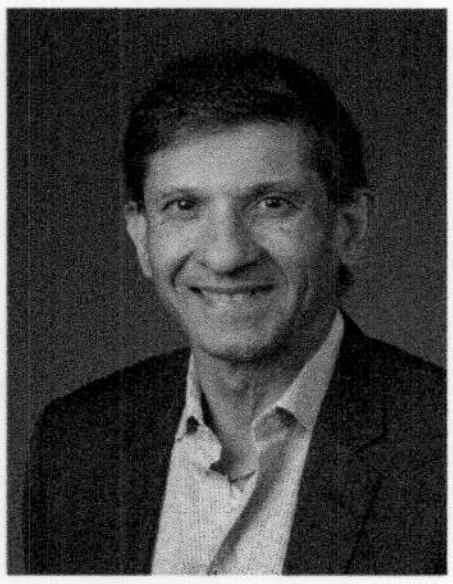
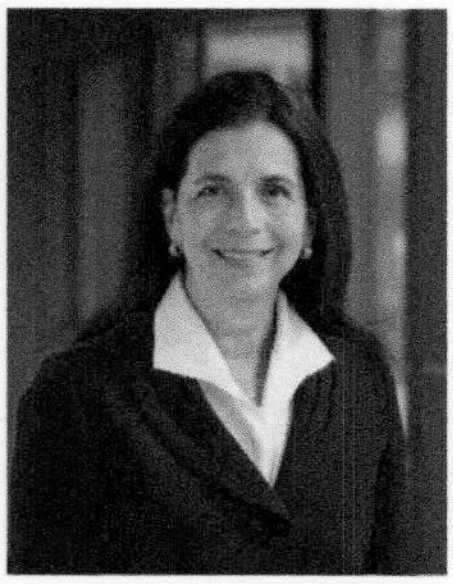

Suresh K. Mukherji, MD, MBA, FACR Jenny T. Bencardino, MD
Consulting Editors

Demyelinating and inflammatory disorders of the central nervous system (CNS) represent an important, diverse, and rather confusing (!) category of diseases. MR imaging is the optimal modality for evaluating patients with these disorders and is essential for the detection of the initial abnormality, lesion characterization, prognosis assessment, and treatment monitoring. With this in mind, we decided to devote an issue of *Magnetic Resonance Imaging Clinics of North America* to demyelinating and inflammatory diseases of the CNS and were delighted to have Drs Reza Forghani and Ashok Srinivasan accept our invitation to guest edit this important issue.

Drs Forghani and Srinivasan have masterfully created a comprehensive updated review of the imaging characteristics of a variety of inflammatory and demyelinating disorders that involve the brain and spine. Included in the issue are dedicated articles covering multiple sclerosis, neuromyelitis optica disorder, myelin oligodendrocyte gylcoprotein (MOG) antibody–associated disease, toxic and drug-related disorders, and various infections of the brain and spine (bacterial, fungal, viral, and prion). There is also an article devoted to the basic science of neuroinflammation and involvement of the inflammatory response in disorders of the nervous system.

We would like to thank all the article authors for their thorough contributions. The articles are beautifully illustrated state-of-the-art masterpieces. This issue offers our readership a comprehensive and practical overview in this important field. On a personal note, I (S.K.M.) have known both Drs Forghani and Srinivasan for many years. It has been a true pleasure seeing their careers blossom over the past 15 years, and I congratulate them both on all their accomplishments and look forward to their continuing future contributions in neuroradiology.

Suresh K. Mukherji, MD, MBA, FACR
University of Louisville
University of Illinois
ProScan Imaging
Carmel, IN 46032, USA

Jenny T. Bencardino, MD
Department of Radiology
Montefiore Medical Center
111 East 210th Street
Bronx, NY 10467-2401, USA

E-mail addresses:
sureshmukherji@hotmail.com (S.K. Mukherji)
jbencardin@montefiore.org (J.T. Bencardino)

Magn Reson Imaging Clin N Am 32 (2024) xiii
https://doi.org/10.1016/j.mric.2024.02.003
1064-9689/24/© 2024 Published by Elsevier Inc.

Preface
Demyelinating and Neuroinflammatory Diseases of the Brain and the Spine

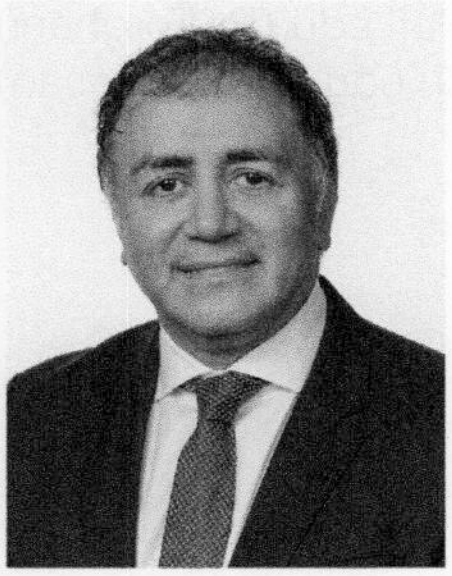
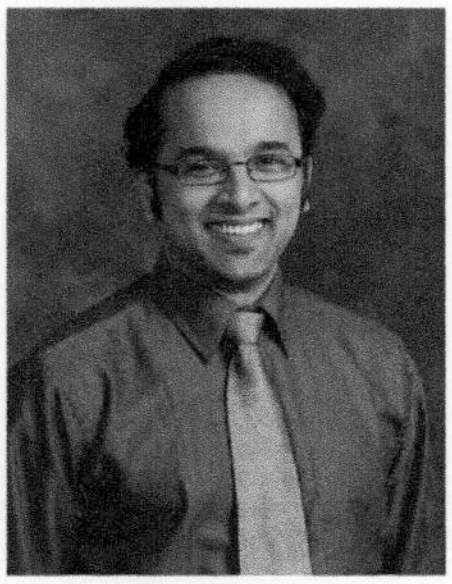

Reza Forghani, MD, PhD   Ashok Srinivasan, MD, FACR
Editors

Demyelinating and inflammatory diseases of the central nervous system (CNS) represent a diverse and important category of diseases affecting the CNS. Furthermore, inflammation has been shown to play a potentially important role in a variety of other disease states, including tumors, stroke, and neurodegenerative disorders. A fundamental understanding of the basics of demyelination and neuroinflammation, and the wide array of clinical disorders, their imaging presentation, and potential diagnostic pitfalls and their mimics is therefore essential for every practicing radiologist interpreting advanced imaging scans of the brain and spine. This issue consists of a collection of review articles written by experts across North America focused on this complex and interesting topic.

First and foremost, the articles provide a comprehensive update and review of the essential imaging characteristics of demyelinating and neuroinflammatory disorders of the brain and spine and their mimics, especially MR imaging scans, which is the most commonly used and optimal modality for noninvasive evaluation and characterization of demyelinating and complex inflammatory disorders of the brain and spine. In addition, the collection provides a concise overview of the basic science of neuroinflammation and potential advances, including novel imaging agents in development, for interested readers. It is our hope as guest editors that the collection of articles will have something to offer for radiologists from diverse backgrounds and levels of experience on this important topic, providing a comprehensive and practical overview for practicing radiologists, and in addition, a glimpse into potential future imaging agents that would enable more specific noninvasive tracking of neuroinflammation as image-based biomarkers.

We would like to conclude by expressing our gratitude to Dr Suresh K. Mukherji for the opportunity to guest edit this issue of *Magnetic Resonance Imaging Clinics of North America* and by thanking all of the authors for their excellent work and contributions. Finally, it should be emphasized that this issue would not have been possible without the support and patience of John Vassallo, Associate Publisher, and Shivank Joshi, Content Development Specialist at Elsevier, and Rajkumar Mayakrishnan, Journal Manager. We hope that

Magn Reson Imaging Clin N Am 32 (2024) xv–xvi
https://doi.org/10.1016/j.mric.2024.01.005
1064-9689/24/© 2024 Published by Elsevier Inc.

the readers will find the issue valuable and informative and useful for their clinical practice.

Reza Forghani, MD, PhD
Department of Radiology and
the Norman Fixel Institute for
Neurological Diseases
University of Florida College of Medicine
Room 221.1
3011 Southwest Williston Road
Gainesville, FL 32608, USA

Ashok Srinivasan, MD, FACR
Department of Radiology
University of Michigan
B2-A209D, Radiology
1500 East Medical Center Drive
UMHS
Ann Arbor, MI 48109, USA

E-mail addresses:
r.forghani@ufl.edu (R. Forghani)
ashoks@med.umich.edu (A. Srinivasan)

Multiple Sclerosis Part 1
Essentials and the McDonald Criteria

Sonia Gill, MD, Mohit Agarwal, MD*

KEYWORDS

• Multiple sclerosis • Demyelinating disease • McDonald criteria • Imaging recommendations • MRI
• Multiple sclerosis mimics

KEY POINTS

- The hallmark of multiple sclerosis (MS), an inflammatory demyelinating disease, is the dissemination of lesions in space and time.
- The McDonald criteria define dissemination in space and dissemination in time. The criteria combine clinical, imaging, and laboratory evidence and present a diagnostic scheme for the reliable and early diagnosis of MS.
- Imaging recommendations for MS include a contrast-enhanced MRI of the brain and spinal cord for diagnosis.
- MRI findings in MS include long time of repetition hyperintense lesions in characteristic locations in the brain including the periventricular white matter, cortical/juxtacortical region, infratentorial regions, and spinal cord. Enhancement is seen during active demyelination.
- MS mimics may be challenging to differentiate from MS but must be excluded before an MS diagnosis is made.

INTRODUCTION

Multiple sclerosis (MS) is one of the most common chronic neurologic disorders, affecting more than 2 million people worldwide and about 400,000 in the United States.[1] It is an inflammatory demyelinating disease of the central nervous system (CNS) characterized by relapsing-remitting or progressive neurologic symptoms and focal white matter lesions.[2] The McDonald criteria are the diagnostic criteria for MS that combine clinical, imaging, and laboratory evidence and present a diagnostic scheme for the reliable and early diagnosis of MS.[3] First established in 2001 by the International Panel on the Diagnosis of Multiple Sclerosis ('The Panel'), and subsequently revised several times, they have been widely accepted by practicing neurologists worldwide.

PATHOLOGY

MS lesions appear throughout the CNS as "plaque-like sclerosis" with focal areas of demyelination, inflammation, and glial reaction that evolve over time.[4] Although MS plaques are most easily recognized in the white matter, myelin is not exclusive to white matter and demyelination can also involve the gray matter. The perivascular space surrounding central veins is a favored location for inflammation and accounts for the perivenular distribution of MS plaques.

Clinical Phenotypes of Multiple Sclerosis

There are several clinical phenotypes of MS. Ranging from the least to most severe, they include clinically isolated syndrome (CIS), relapsing remitting MS (RRMS), primary progressive MS (PPMS), and secondary progressive MS.[5] These phenotypes usually exist on a continuum, with patients progressing from relapsing MS to progressive MS.[6] Patients should be assessed over time and classified and reclassified as needed according to the disease course.

Section of Neuroradiology, Medical College of Wisconsin, Milwaukee, USA
* Corresponding author. Section of Neuroradiology, Department of Radiology, Medical College of Wisconsin, Milwaukee.
E-mail address: magarwal@mcw.edu

Magn Reson Imaging Clin N Am 32 (2024) 207–220
https://doi.org/10.1016/j.mric.2023.11.002

- CIS is the first clinical presentation of a disease that has characteristics of an inflammatory/demyelinating process suggestive of MS but has yet to fulfill the criteria of dissemination in time (DIT).[5] Typical presentations include unilateral optic neuritis, focal supratentorial syndrome, focal brainstem or cerebellar syndrome or partial myelopathy.
- RRMS is characterized by alternating relapsing and remitting phases with stable neurologic disability between episodes. It is the most common initial presentation of MS, with 80% to 85% of patients falling into this category.
- PPMS is clinical progression from the onset of disease and is characterized by the absence of exacerbations prior to clinical progression. It comprises 10% to 15% of patients and has its own McDonald criteria for diagnosis.
- Secondary progressive MS is progressive worsening of neurologic function over time.

The major modifier of MS is disease activity. This can be identified by clinical relapses or MRI evidence of a gadolinium-enhancing lesion or a new/enlarging long time of repetition (TR) hyperintense lesion on a follow-up scan. Enhancing and/or enlarging lesions are accepted MRI biomarkers of new inflammation.

The distinct entity of radiologically isolated syndrome is the presence of white matter lesions suggestive of MS in a patient with no clinical signs or symptoms of demyelinating disease (**Fig. 1**).[7] It is not considered a distinct MS subtype but these patients should be followed prospectively as many of them will ultimately progress to MS. Approximately 50% experience a first clinical event within 10 years of the index MRI.[8]

Imaging Recommendations in Multiple Sclerosis

The Magnetic Resonance Imaging in Multiple Sclerosis (MAGNIMS), the Consortium of Multiple Sclerosis Centers (CMSC), and the North American Imaging in Multiple Sclerosis Cooperative (NAIMS) jointly created the 2021 MAGNIMS-CMSC-NAIMS consensus recommendations on the use of MRI in patients with MS.[9] They provide guidelines for the optimum use of MRI and outline standardized protocols for the diagnosis, prognosis, and monitoring of patients with MS. A baseline contrast MRI of the brain and spinal cord is recommended for the diagnosis of MS. If the entire cord cannot be imaged, then at least an MRI of the cervical spine should be done.

A standardized protocol for imaging the brain and spinal cord enables the accurate detection of brain and cord lesions, detects new lesions over time correlating with MS disease activity, allows for accurate comparison of the patient's MRIs between different imaging centers, and enables detection of rare complications such as progressive multifocal encephalopathy (PML). The recommended protocol is outlined in **Table 1**. 3-dimensional (3D) acquisition techniques for brain MRI are preferred to 2-dimensional acquisitions owing to their thinner slices that improve lesion detection and allow improved realignment for more accurate comparison to prior examinations. At the authors' center, the authors use 3D fluid-attenuated inversion recovery (FLAIR) images obtained in the sagittal plane with multiplanar reconstructions. These improve the visualization of corpus callosum lesions, juxta-cortical lesions, and the perivenular configuration of lesions. Before

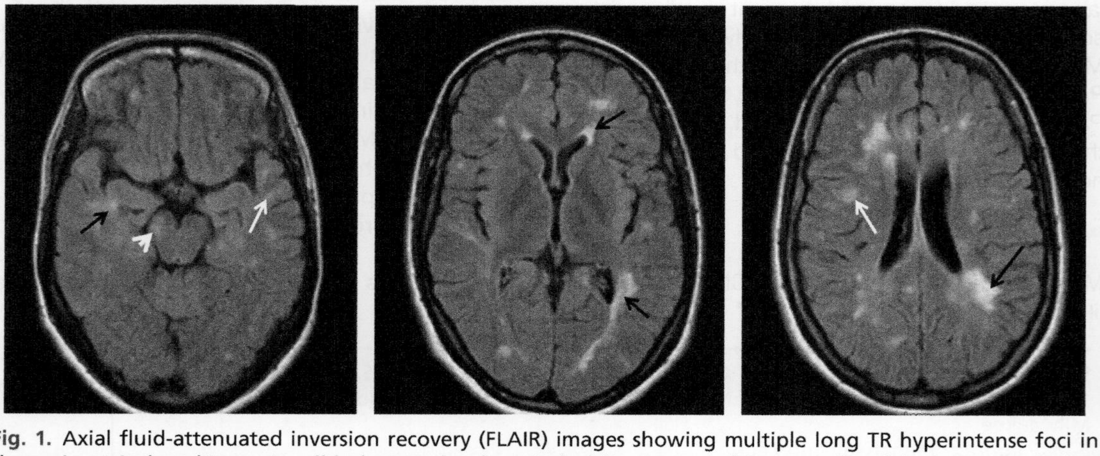

Fig. 1. Axial fluid-attenuated inversion recovery (FLAIR) images showing multiple long TR hyperintense foci in the periventricular white matter (*black arrows*), subcortical white matter (*white arrows*) and the brainstem (*white arrowhead*). The appearance and distribution of these lesions are typical of multiple sclerosis.

Table 1
Standardized brain MRI protocol for diagnosis and routine follow-up of multiple sclerosis

Parameters	Description
Field strength	>1.5 T (preferably 3T). In-plane resolution should be ≤ 1 mm × 1mm
Scan orientation	Axial images oriented along the subcallosal plane
Coverage	Whole brain and as much of the cervical cord as possible
Slice thickness & gap	For 3D imaging, 1 mm isotropic voxels. For 2D imaging, ≤3 mm with no gap.
Core sequences for diagnosis	• Sagittal 3D T2-weighted FLAIR (fat suppression optional), with multiplanar axial reconstructions • If 3D acquisition not available, then sagittal and axial T2-weighted FLAIR • Axial T2-weighted sequence: TSE or FSE • C+ axial T1-weighted sequence. Standard gadolinium dose of 0.1 mmol/kg body weight given for 30 s (5–10 min delay before obtaining postcontrast T1) • 2D axial DWI (5 mm sections, for the evaluation of acute ischemia, active demyelination)
Optional sequences	• Axial proton density • 2D axial T1 spin-echo (for chronic black holes) • SWI for identification of central vein sign and paramagnetic rims • DIR or PSIR (for detection of cortical lesions) • High resolution 3D T1 for volumetric analysis
Core sequences for follow-up	Same as for diagnosis except no contrast enhanced sequences are typically needed

Abbreviations: DIR, double inversion recovery; DWI, diffusion-weighted imaging; FLAIR, fluid-attenuated inversion recovery; FSE, fast spin echo; PSIR, phase sensitive inversion recovery; SWI, susceptibility-weighted imaging; TSE, turbo spin echo.

acquiring postcontrast sequences, a 5 to 10 minute delay is recommended after contrast injection. Axial diffusion-weighted imaging (5 mm) is recommended for the evaluation of acute ischemia and PML. Susceptibility-weighted imaging (SWI) is useful for assessing central vein sign and paramagnetic rim lesions. Optional sequences such as double inversion recovery and phase sensitive inversion recovery (PSIR) sequences improve detection of cortical lesions.

The standard spinal cord protocol (**Table 2**) should ideally include the whole cord. Sagittal long TR sequences are essential and we use short tau inversion recovery and T2-weighted sequences. Alternatives such as sagittal 3D PSIR and magnetization-prepared rapid acquisition of gradient echoes are more sensitive but remain optional. Axial gradient echo and axial T2-weighted sequences confirm and characterize lesions suspected on the sagittal images. A sagittal postcontrast T1-weighted scan is recommended for diagnosis but is optional for follow-up.

IMAGING FINDINGS

Multiple Sclerosis Lesions in the Brain

Multiple, long TR hyperintense lesions are seen in the white matter in bilateral cerebral hemispheres, often asymmetric, measuring 5 to 10 mm (**Box 1**).[10] They are typically located in the periventricular white matter in a perivenular location along the course of the medullary veins (**Fig. 2**). Ovoid lesions that radiate perpendicularly from the lateral ventricles are called "Dawson's fingers" (**Fig. 3**). Lesions at the callososeptal interface are classic of MS. The callososeptal interface is located along the inferior margin of the corpus callosum and abuts the septum pellucidum (**Fig. 4**A). They appear as thin long TR hyperintense bands along the undersurface of the corpus callosum also called subcallosal striations.[11] Lesions may be present in the brainstem, cerebellum, and cerebellar peduncles (**Fig. 5**). MS plaques may be present in the gray matter. Cortical lesions may be subpial, intracortical, or juxtacortical.[12] Standard

Table 2
Spinal cord MRI protocol

Parameter	Description
Field strength	$\geq$1.5 T with in-plane resolution $\leq$1 × 1mm
Coverage	Ideally the whole cord (cervical and thoraco-lumbar spine including conus). At least the cervical cord.
Slice thickness and gap	Sagittal: $\leq$3 mm, no gap Axial: $\leq$5 mm, no gap
Core sequences	• At least 2 of: sagittal T2-weighted, sagittal STIR, sagittal proton density–weighted sequences • Sagittal postcontrast T1-weighted sequence (5–10 min delay before obtaining postcontrast T1. Standard gadolinium dose of 0.1 mmol/kg body weight. No additional contrast needed if spinal cord MRI follows a contrast MRI of the brain)
Optional sequences	• Axial T2 or GRE to confirm and characterize lesions seen on sagittal scans • Precontrast sagittal T1-weighted sequence • Postcontrast axial T1-weighted sequence

Abbreviations: GRE, gradient echo; STIR, short tau inversion recovery.

Box 1
Imaging findings in multiple sclerosis

Brain

- Ovoid long TR hyperintense lesions in the periventricular white matter oriented perpendicular to the ventricular surface
- Dawson's fingers—radially oriented fingerlike perivenular lesions which radiate perpendicularly from the lateral ventricles
- Lesions at the callososeptal interface
- Cortical/juxtacortical lesions
- Lesions in the brainstem and brachium pontis
- Active demyelinating lesions enhance on gadolinium administration. Punctate/linear/nodular enhancement or incomplete ring with the open segment of the ring facing the cortex
- Chronic lesions may be T1 hypointense (black holes)
- Central vein sign and paramagnetic rims on SWI

Spinal cord

- Long TR hyperintense lesions along the periphery of the cord, preferentially involving the dorsolateral cord surface.
- Cervical > thoracic cord
- Lesions typically involve less than half the cross-sectional area of the cord and are less than 2 vertebral segments in length.
- Homogeneous, nodular, or ringlike enhancement in active lesions
- Mild cord edema and focal cord expansion during acute phase resolves in 6 to 8 weeks
- Cord atrophy with disease progression

Abbreviations: MS, multiple sclerosis; SWI, susceptibility-weighted imaging; TR, time of repetition.

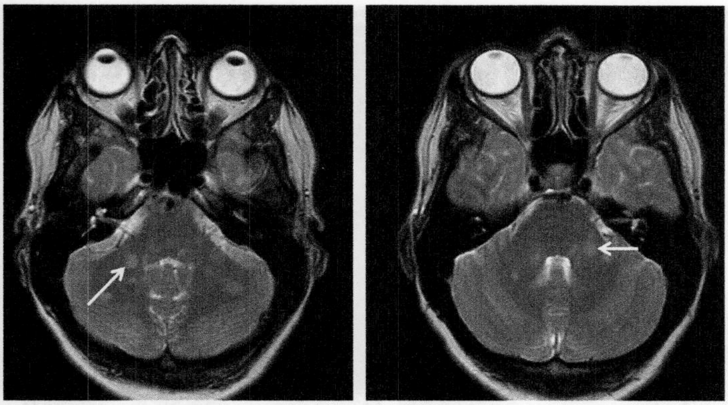

Fig. 2. Axial T2-weighted images through the posterior fossa showing infratentorial long time of repetition (TR) hyperintense lesions typical of multiple sclerosis (MS) in the cerebellar hemispheres and brachium pontis (*arrows*).

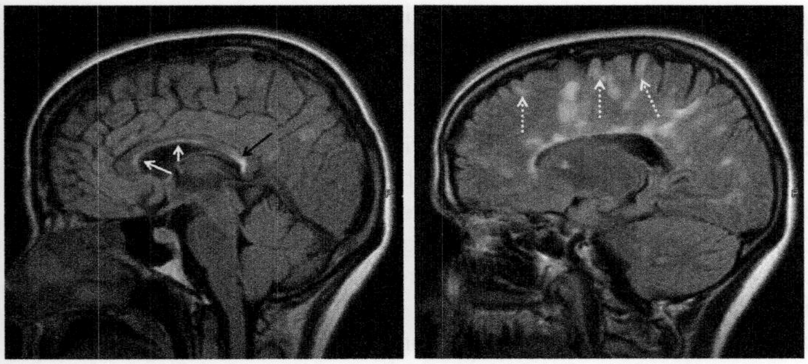

Fig. 3. Sagittal fluid-attenuated inversion recovery (FLAIR) images are particularly useful to detect lesions in the corpus callosum (*black arrow*), at the callososeptal interface (*white arrows*), and in the cortical/juxtacortical region (*dotted white arrows*).

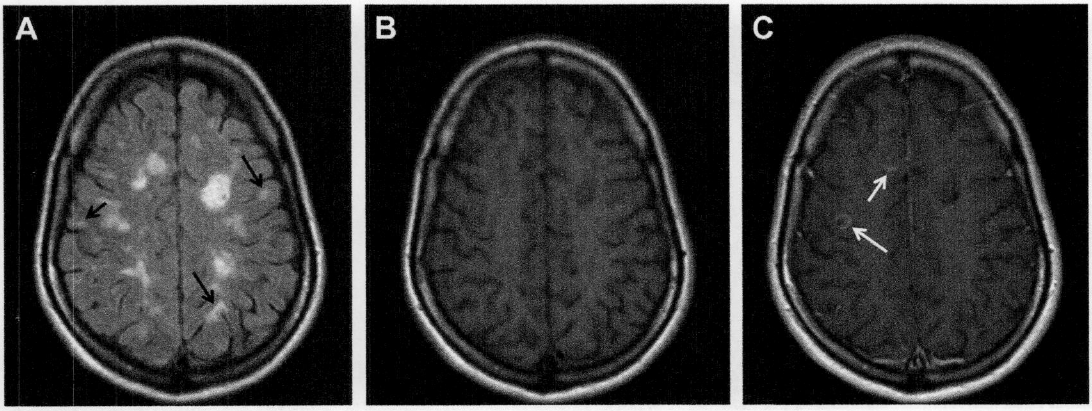

Fig. 4. Axial fluid-attenuated inversion recovery (FLAIR) image (*A*) showing cortical/juxtacortical lesions (*black arrows*). Axial T1-weighted image (*B*) and C + T1-weighted image (*C*) showing incomplete ring enhancement (*white arrows*), with the open segment of the ring facing the cortex, typical of a demyelinating lesion.

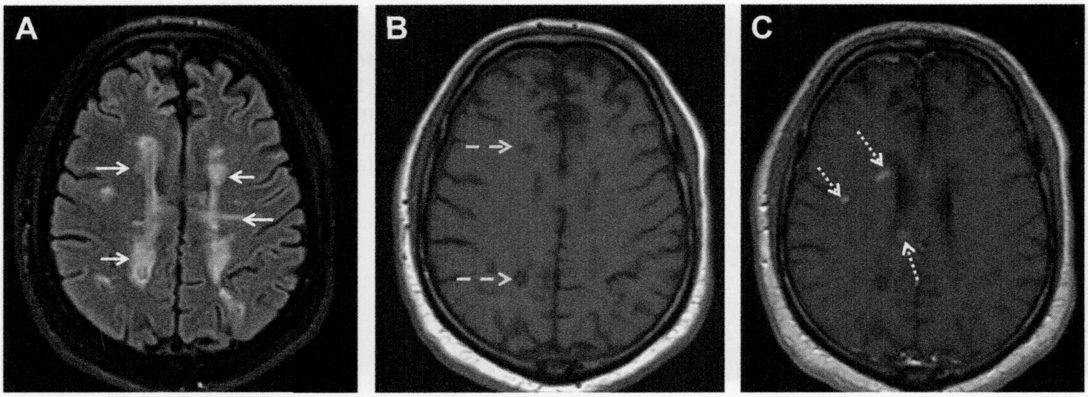

Fig. 5. (*A*) Axial fluid-attenuated inversion recovery (FLAIR) image showing extensive periventricular demyelinating lesions (*solid arrows*). (*B*) Axial T1-weighted image showing multiple "black holes" (*dashed arrows*). (*C*) Axial C + T1-weighted image showing active demyelination with linear and nodular enhancement within several lesions (*dotted arrows*).

MRI readily shows juxtacortical lesions, best seen on 3D sagittal FLAIR images (**Fig. 6**). The detection of cortical lesions requires specialized sequences. Lesions in the white matter become confluent with increasing disease severity.[13]

In the chronic phase, the lesions may become T1-hypointense with mildly hyperintense rims ("black holes") which correspond to areas of extreme demyelination and axonal destruction (**Fig.** 4B).[10] During active demyelination, the lesions enhance on contrast administration. There can be different patterns of enhancement, ranging from punctate, linear, and nodular to an incomplete ring with the open segment of the ring facing the cortex (**Fig.** 4C; see **Fig.** 6).

SWI is useful to evaluate the "central vein sign" and "paramagnetic rims." The central vein sign is the presence of central veins in MS lesions on SWI, best visualized in lesions within the periventricular and deep white matter (**Fig. 7**). A thin hypointense line or dot measuring less than 2 mm positioned centrally within a long TR hyperintense lesion on SWI images should be visualized in at least 2 perpendicular MRI planes.[14] Given the typical venocentric distribution of MS lesions, the central vein sign has been proposed as a specific imaging biomarker to distinguish MS from other MS mimics. Long TR hyperintense lesions show a paramagnetic rim on SWI, best seen on $\geq$ 3T magnets. This is an emerging marker of chronic neuroinflammation in MS, reflecting iron accumulation in microglia.[15] There is also susceptibility in the deep gray structures with advancing disease related to iron accumulation. With disease progression, there is diffuse brain atrophy and thinning of the corpus callosum.

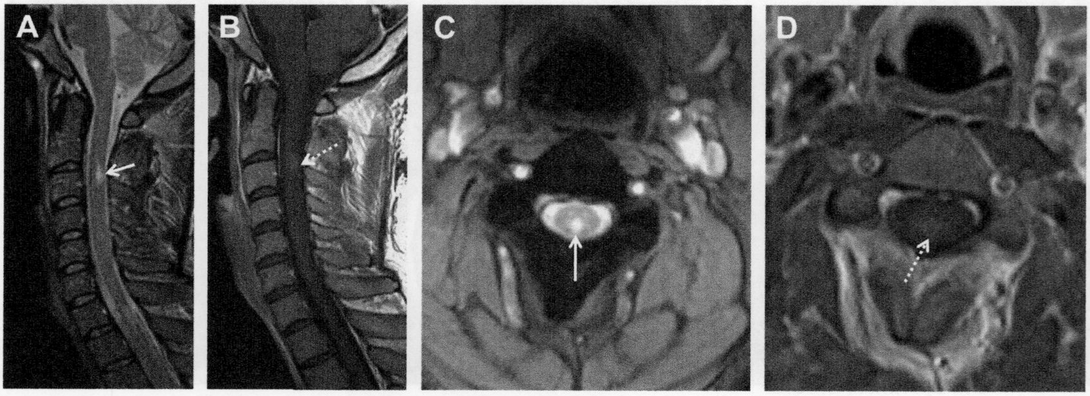

Fig. 6. Sagittal short tau inversion recovery (STIR) (*A*) & axial gradient echo (GRE) (*C*) images show an ovoid long time of repetition (TR) hyperintense lesion along the dorsal cord surface at upper C3 (*solid arrows*) with postcontrast rim enhancement on sagittal (*B*) & axial (*D*) C + T1-weighted images (*dotted arrows*).

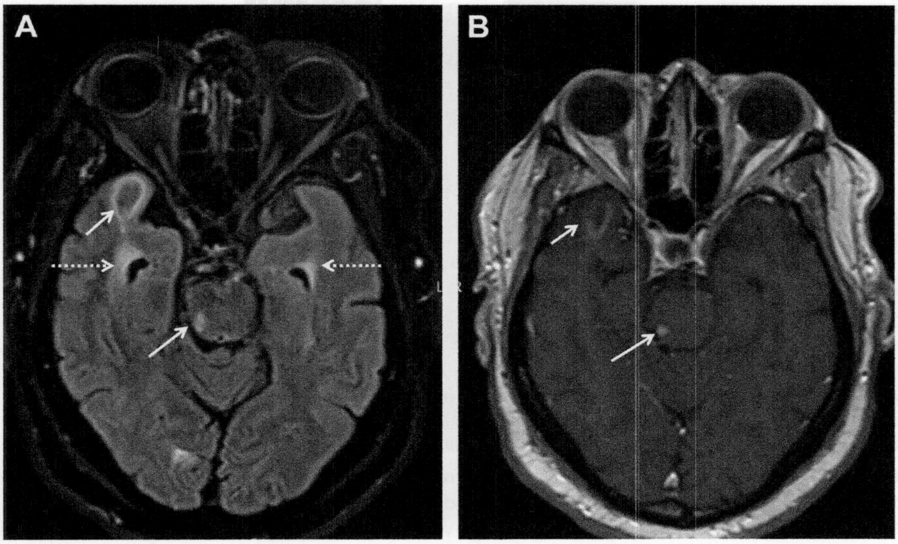

Fig. 7. (*A* and *B*) Primary progressive multiple sclerosis (MS) in a patient with progression of disease from onset a year ago. Axial fluid-attenuated inversion recovery (FLAIR) & C + T1-weighted images showing nonenhancing lesions marginating the temporal horns (*dotted arrows*) and enhancing lesions in the right anterior temporal lobe and right brainstem (*solid arrows*).

Multiple Sclerosis Lesions in the Spinal Cord

Demyelinating plaques in the cord more commonly involve the cervical cord than the thoracic cord (see **Box 1**). They appear as oval, long TR hyperintense lesions along the periphery of the cord, preferentially involving the dorsolateral cord surface (**Figs. 8** and **9**).[10] Lesions typically involve less than half the cross-sectional area of the cord and are less than 2 vertebral segments in length.[16] Enhancement of the lesions during active demyelination may be homogeneous, nodular, or ringlike (see **Figs. 8** and **9**). There may be mild cord edema and mild focal expansion

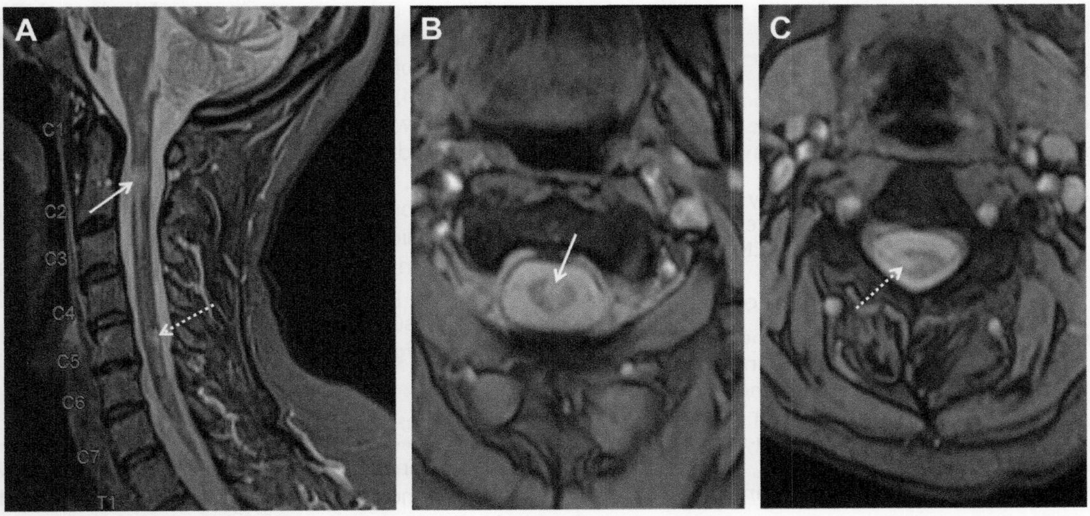

Fig. 8. (*A* and *B*) Primary progressive multiple sclerosis (MS) in a patient with progression of disease from onset a year ago. Sagittal short tau inversion recovery (STIR) (*A*) & axial gradient echo (GRE) (*B* and *C*) images showing multiple long time of repetition (TR) hyperintense lesions along the periphery of the cord, with dominant lesions at C2 (*solid arrows*) and C5 (*dotted arrows*).

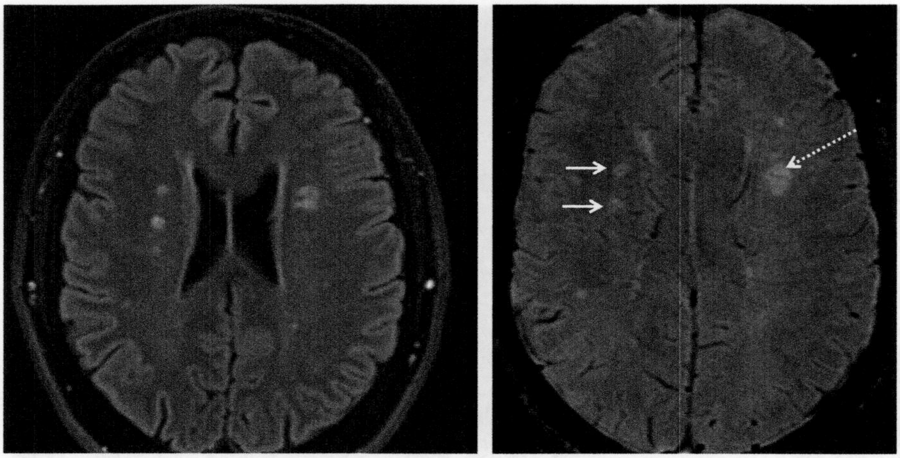

Fig. 9. Axial fluid-attenuated inversion recovery (FLAIR) image showing long time of repetition (TR) hyperintense lesions in the white matter. Axial susceptibility-weighted imaging (SWI) showing "central vein sign" of central hypointense dots (*solid arrows*) and line (*dotted arrow*) within the long time of repetition (TR) hyperintense lesions. This venocentric distribution of lesions is typical of MS.

of the cord during the acute phase that usually resolve after 6 to 8 weeks. With disease progression, there may be cord atrophy which correlates with clinical disability.

McDonald CRITERIA

The hallmark of MS is the dissemination of CNS lesions in space and time. The McDonald criteria define what is required to fulfill dissemination in space (DIS) and DIT (**Box 2**). They are applied primarily to patients presenting with a typical CIS and they stress the need to exclude alternative diagnosis.[17] DIS is defined as the development of lesions in distinct anatomic locations within the CNS. DIT is defined as the development or appearance of new CNS lesions over time.[17]

> **Box 2**
> **2017 McDonald criteria for demonstration of dissemination in space and time by MRI in a patient with clinically isolated syndrome**
>
> - DIS can be demonstrated by $\geq$ 1 long TR hyperintense lesions that are characteristic of MS in $\geq$2 of 4 areas of the CNS: periventricular, cortical/juxtacortical, infratentorial brain regions, and the spinal cord
> - DIT can be demonstrated by the simultaneous presence of gadolinium-enhancing and nonenhancing lesions, at any time or by a new long TR hyperintense or gadolinium-enhancing lesion on follow-up MRI, with reference to a baseline scan, irrespective of the timing of the baseline scan
>
> *Abbreviations:* DIS, dissemination in space; DIT, dissemination in time; MS, multiple sclerosis; TR, time of repetition.

According to the latest 2017 McDonald criteria, DIS can be demonstrated by 1 or more T2 hyperintense lesions that are characteristic of MS in 2 or more of 4 areas in the CNS: periventricular, cortical or juxtacortical, infratentorial brain regions, and the spinal cord.[18] DIT can be demonstrated by the simultaneous presence of gadolinium-enhancing and nonenhancing lesions at any time or by a new long TR hyperintense or gadolinium-enhancing lesion on follow-up MRI, with reference to a baseline scan, irrespective of the timing of the baseline MRI (case 1 & case 2—**Figs. 10–14**). Owing to the limited ability to differentiate between cortical and juxtacortical lesions on standard MRI, the Panel combined them to a single term, cortical/juxtacortical.[12]

Primary progressive MS has its own McDonald criteria outlined in **Box 3**. The criteria include lesions fulfilling DIS in the brain and spinal cord as well as the presence of cerebrospinal fluid (CSF) findings in subjects with 1 year of disease progression (see **Fig. 9**; **Fig. 15**).

Revisions of the McDonald Criteria

The McDonald criteria have been periodically reviewed and revised in 2005, 2010, and the latest in 2017, with the aim of simplifying the criteria, preserving their diagnostic sensitivity and specificity, addressing their applicability across populations, allowing earlier diagnosis, and more uniform and

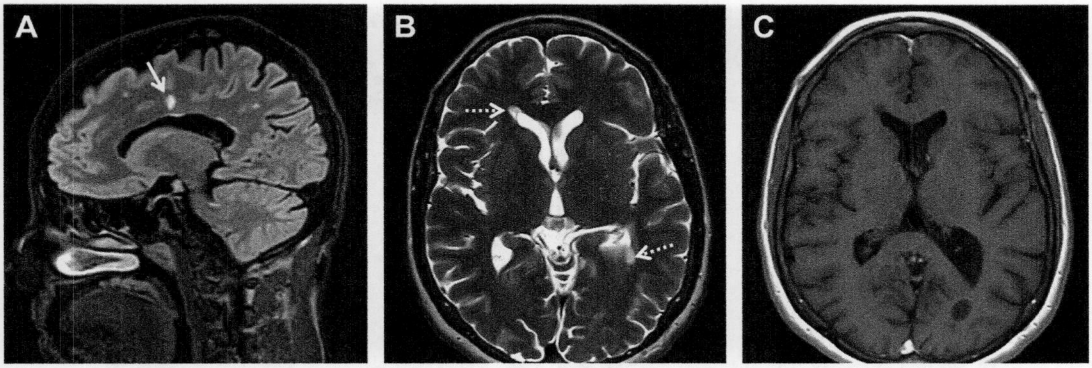

Fig. 10. Radiologically isolated syndrome. Sagittal fluid-attenuated inversion recovery (FLAIR) (*A*), axial T2 (*B*) and C+ axial T1 (*C*) weighted images showing multiple nonenhancing long time of repetition (TR) hyperintense lesions in the periventricular white matter (*dotted arrows*) and involving the corpus callosum (*solid arrow*) typical of multiple sclerosis (MS), incidentally noted in a patient imaged for trauma.

widespread use.[19] The criteria for DIS and DIT have evolved over successive revisions of the criteria, fueled by new research in MRI. Revisions to the criteria in 2017 as compared to 2010 are outlined in **Table 3**. The latest guidelines of 2017 include both symptomatic and asymptomatic lesions as well as cortical/juxtacortical lesions in the determination of DIS, with the exception of optic neuritis.[18] The Panel found insufficient evidence to include optic neuritis as a site of disease.[12] DIT can be demonstrated on a single scan by the presence of both enhancing and nonenhancing lesions (see **Figs. 10** and **11**—case 1). CSF-specific oligoclonal bands are now included in the diagnosis of MS. A provisional disease course should be specified (relapsing-remitting, primary progressive, or secondary progressive) at the time of MS diagnosis.

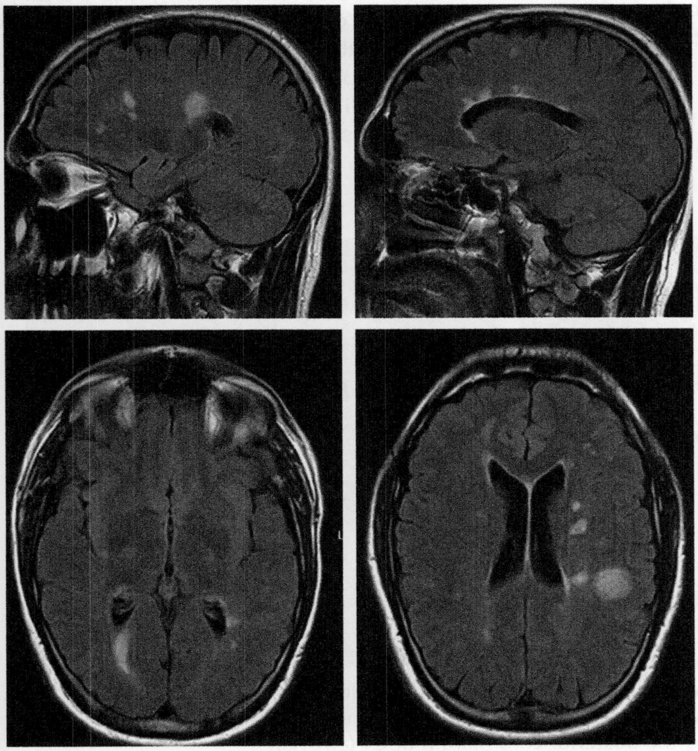

Fig. 11. Case 1. Patient with clinically isolated syndrome (CIS) presenting with bilateral upper extremity paresthesias. Sagittal and axial fluid-attenuated inversion recovery (FLAIR) images show multiple long time of repetition (TR) hyperintense lesions in the periventricular white matter, corpus callosum, and callososeptal interface fulfilling criteria for dissemination in space (DIS).

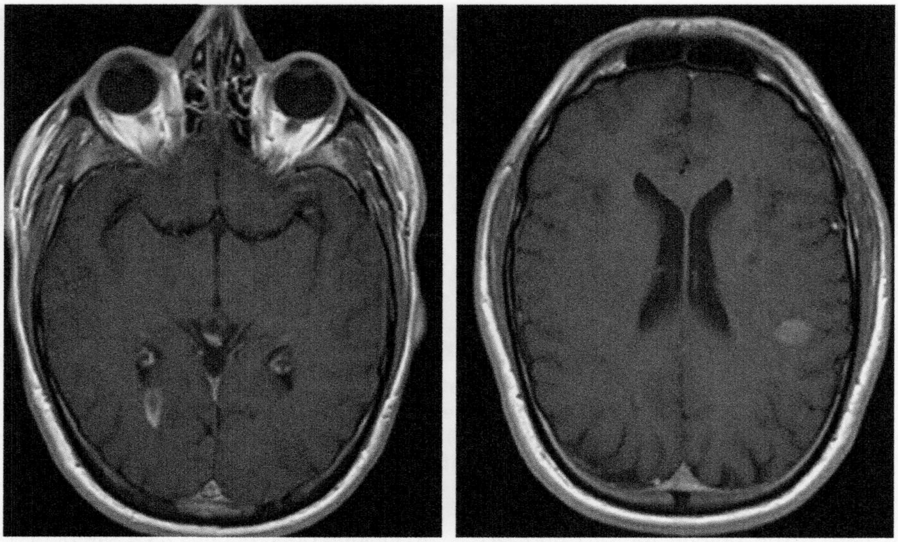

Fig. 12. Case 1. Enhancing and nonenhancing lesions on the C+ axial T1-weighted images fulfill criteria for dissemination in time (DIT). Patient was diagnosed with multiple sclerosis (MS) and started on treatment.

DIFFERENTIAL DIAGNOSIS (MULTIPLE SCLEROSIS MIMICS)

There are many clinical and radiological mimics of MS. Incidental long TR hyperintense lesions in the white matter are common and may be seen in a myriad of disease processes (Fig. 16). Differentiating these from MS can be challenging but certain imaging features may help in excluding these entities.

Small vessel disease (SVD) is usually seen with increasing age and the presence of cerebrovascular risk factors such as hypertension, diabetes and hyperlipidemia. Long TR hyperintense foci in SVD tend to spare the corpus callosum, subcortical U-fibers, and spinal cord and do not enhance.[20] Lacunar infarcts in the basal ganglia are common and brainstem involvement is often central, unlike MS.

Acute disseminated encephalomyelitis (ADEM) is typically seen in children and young adults, often triggered by a viral illness or vaccination. It classically has a monophasic course—a follow-up MRI after 6 months will show partial or complete resolution of ADEM lesions. ADEM lesions tend to be

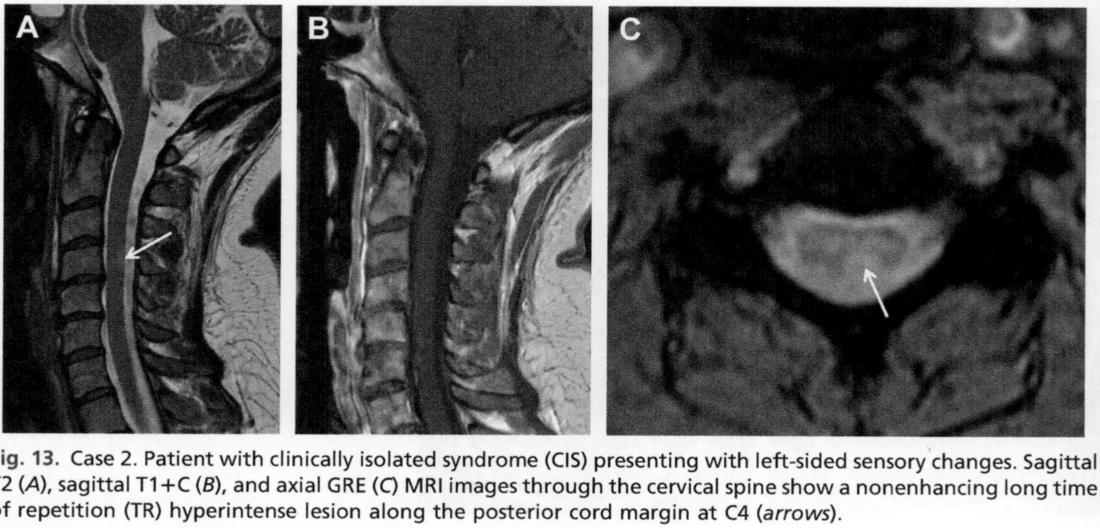

Fig. 13. Case 2. Patient with clinically isolated syndrome (CIS) presenting with left-sided sensory changes. Sagittal T2 (*A*), sagittal T1+C (*B*), and axial GRE (*C*) MRI images through the cervical spine show a nonenhancing long time of repetition (TR) hyperintense lesion along the posterior cord margin at C4 (*arrows*).

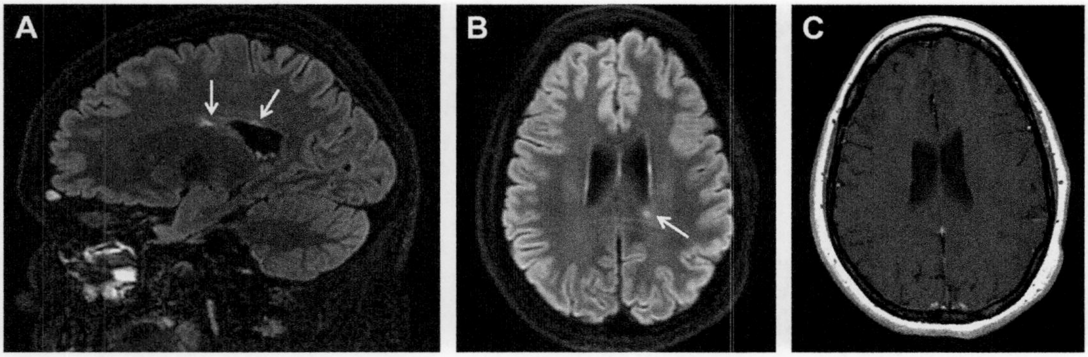

Fig. 14. Case 2. Sagittal fluid-attenuated inversion recovery (FLAIR) (*A*), axial FLAIR (*B*) and axial T1+C (*C*) MRI images of the brain show subtle long time of repetition (TR) hyperintense nonenhancing lesions (*white arrows*) in the periventricular white matter. Imaging findings fulfilled criteria for dissemination in space (DIS) but not dissemination in time (DIT).

more confluent and bilaterally symmetric than MS lesions, involve the deep white matter rather than the periventricular white matter and often enhance. They tend to involve the cortex and deep gray nuclei and rarely involve the corpus callosum.[20] Spinal cord lesions in ADEM are longitudinally extensive, centrally located, and favor the thoracic cord.

Susac syndrome or retinocochleocerebral vasculopathy is a rare autoimmune endotheliopathy affecting small blood vessels in the brain, retina, and inner ear. Multiple small long TR hyperintensities are seen in the periventricular white matter with the majority showing restricted diffusion, unlike MS lesions. Lesions in Susac involve the central fibers in the corpus callosum and spare the peripheral fibers.

CADASIL (Cerebral autosomal dominant arteriopathy with subcortical infarcts and leukoencephalopathy) is an inherited microangiopathy that presents in early adulthood with transient ischemic attacks and strokes. Long TR hyperintensities classically involve the subinsular white matter and external capsule with symmetric lesions in the frontal and anterior temporal white matter. The corpus callosum and infratentorial brain are usually spared. There are lacunar infarcts in the basal ganglia and microbleeds scattered in the infratentorial and supratentorial brain.[20]

Lyme disease is a tick-borne systemic inflammatory disorder that is characterized by meningitis, cranial nerve involvement, and radiculoneuritis. Nonspecific long TR hyperintensities in the white matter are indistinguishable from MS. The presence of nerve root enhancement and the absence of myelitis may help in narrowing the differential.

Vasculitis is characterized by inflammation of vessel walls. Imaging usually shows infarctions and hemorrhage, but nonspecific long TR hyperintensities often with enhancement in the white matter and cortex can be confused with MS. The enhancement in vasculitis is often linear or radial, unlike the ringlike enhancement seen in MS.[20] The diagnosis rests on the clinical presentation, laboratory results, and arterial abnormalities on catheter angiography.

The main problematic differential diagnosis for MS is neuromyelitis optica spectrum disorder (NMOSD). In the 2010 revision of the McDonald criteria, the Panel separated NMOSD from typical

Box 3
McDonald criteria for diagnosis of multiple sclerosis in patients with a disease course characterized by progression from onset (primary progressive multiple sclerosis)

PPMS can be diagnosed in patients with

- 1 year of disability progression (retrospectively or prospectively determined) independent of clinical relapse

Plus 2 of the following criteria

- ≥1 T2 hyperintense lesions characteristic of multiple sclerosis in ≥1 of the following brain regions: periventricular, cortical/juxtacortical, or infratentorial
- ≥2 T2 hyperintense lesions in the spinal cord
- Presence of CSF-specific oligoclonal bands

Abbreviations: CSF, cerebrospinal fluid; PPMS, primary progressive multiple sclerosis.

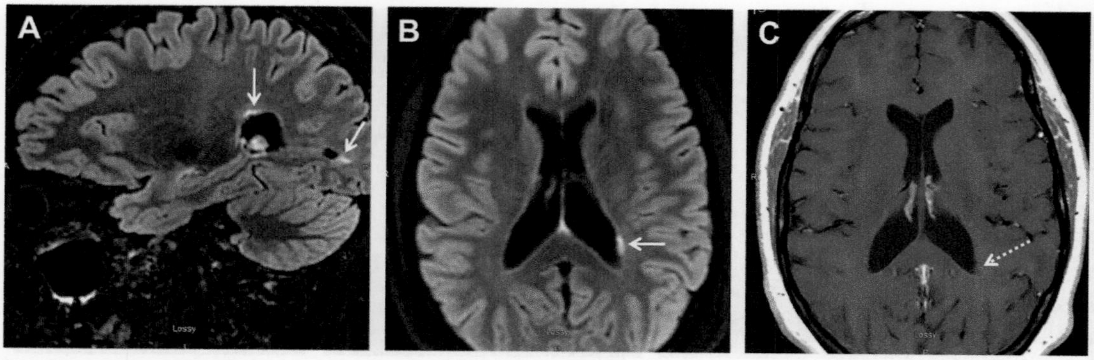

Fig. 15. Case 2. MRI of the brain done 6 months later showed new long time of repetition (TR) hyperintense lesions scattered in the periventricular white matter on sagittal & axial fluid-attenuated inversion recovery (FLAIR) (*solid arrows* in *A* and *B*) with subtle rim enhancement on axial C + T1-weighted images (*dotted arrow* in *C*). Imaging findings fulfilled criteria for dissemination in space (DIS) & dissemination in time (DIT). The patient was started on disease-modifying therapy.

MS as the 2 entities have a very different clinical course, prognosis, and underlying pathophysiology,[12] with NMOSD also having a poor response to some available disease-modifying MS drugs.[21] These patients have severe, often bilateral, optic neuritis and severe myelopathy. They characteristically have longitudinally extensive MRI cord lesions that span greater than 3 segments and are located centrally within the cord, unlike MS. Brain MRI is often normal. A majority of these patients test positive for serum aquaporin-4 antibody (AQP4)[22] with some testing positive for anti-myelin oligodendrocyte antibodies.[12] The panel recommended that NMOSD should be considered in the differential diagnosis of all potential MS patients presenting with a longitudinally extensive cord lesion, bilateral and severe optic neuritis, and MRI evidence of a periaqueductal medullary lesion and should be tested for AQP4 autoantibodies.[17]

Table 3
McDonald 2010 versus McDonald 2017

McDonald 2010	McDonald 2017
Lesions in *asymptomatic* regions considered in DIS and DIT. Lesions in symptomatic regions were excluded.	All *symptomatic and asymptomatic* lesions can be considered in the determination of DIS and DIT. Exception: optic neuritis
Juxtacortical lesions can be used in fulfilling criteria for DIS. Cortical lesions cannot be used.	Both *cortical and juxtacortical* lesions can be used in fulfilling the criteria for DIS.
DIT can be demonstrated on a single scan by the presence of enhancing and nonenhancing *asymptomatic* lesions.	DIT can be demonstrated on a single scan by the presence of enhancing and nonenhancing lesions, both *symptomatic and asymptomatic*.
CSF-specific oligoclonal bands *not* used for fulfilling the criteria	In a patient with CIS who has clinical or MRI demonstration of DIS, the presence of *CSF-specific oligoclonal bands* allows a diagnosis of multiple sclerosis.
	Additional recommendation: At the time of diagnosis, a provisional disease course should be specified, and whether active or not, and progressive or not. This *phenotype* should be periodically reevaluated.

Abbreviations: CIS, clinically isolated syndrome; CSF, cerebrospinal fluid; DIS, dissemination in space; DIT, dissemination in time.

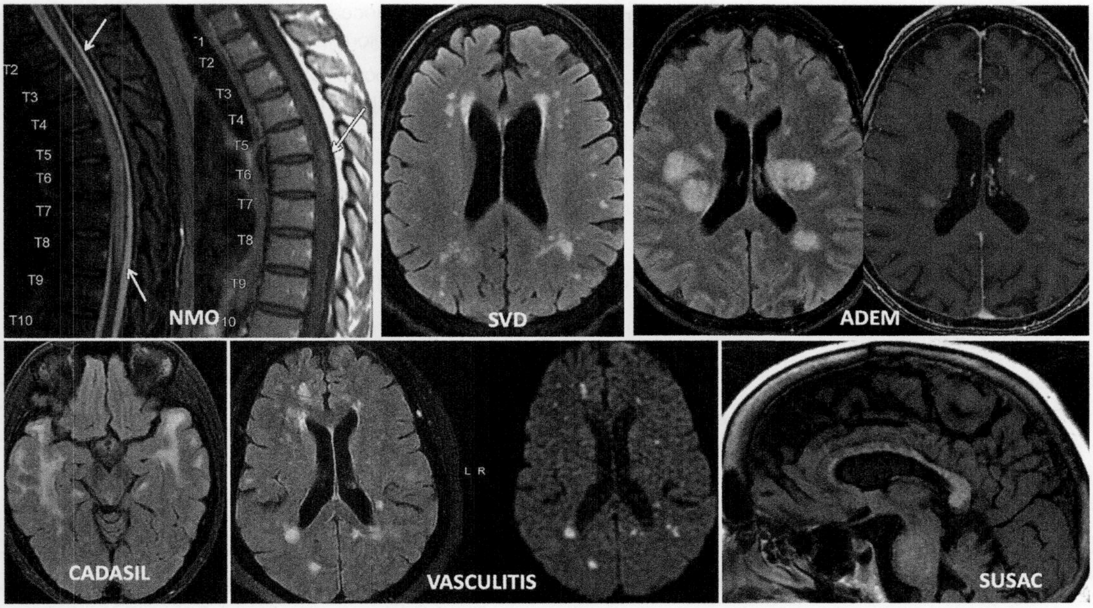

Fig. 16. Montage of multiple sclerosis (MS) mimics. Longitudinally extensive cord lesion with patchy post contrast enhancement (*white arrows first image*) typical of NMO.

SUMMARY

MS is an inflammatory demyelinating disease of the CNS characterized by relapsing or progressive neurologic symptoms and focal white matter lesions. The hallmark of the disease is the dissemination of CNS lesions in space and time. The McDonald criteria define what is required to fulfill DIS and DIT. MRI is the most important diagnostic and prognostic biomarker for MS which can interrogate the entire CNS. MS mimics must be excluded before a diagnosis of MS is made.

CLINICS CARE POINTS

The hallmark of MS is the dissemination of CNS lesions in space and time.

- The *McDonald criteria* define DIS and DIT

DIS is demonstrated by

- $\geq$1 long TR hyperintense lesions that are characteristic of MS in $\geq$2 of 4 areas of the CNS: periventricular, cortical/juxtacortical, infratentorial brain regions, and the spinal cord

DIT is demonstrated by

- The simultaneous presence of gadolinium-enhancing and nonenhancing lesions, at any time or by a new long TR hyperintense or gadolinium-enhancing lesion on follow-up MRI, with reference to a baseline scan, irrespective of the timing of the baseline scan.

Primary progressive MS can be diagnosed in patients with

- 1 year of disability progression (retrospectively or prospectively determined) independent of clinical relapse.
- Plus 2 of the following criteria:
  1. $\geq$1 long TR hyperintense lesions characteristic of multiple sclerosis in $\geq$1 of the following brain regions: periventricular, cortical/juxtacortical, or infratentorial
  2. $\geq$2 long TR hyperintense lesions in the spinal cord
  3. Presence of CSF-specific oligoclonal bands

MS plaques are present in both white matter and gray matter.

- The 2017 McDonald criteria recommended that cortical lesions could be included along with juxtacortical lesions to fulfill criteria for DIS and combined them to a single term, cortical/juxtacortical.

The "central vein sign" has been proposed as a specific imaging biomarker to distinguish MS from other MS mimics.

- The perivascular space surrounding central veins is a favored location for inflammation and accounts for the perivenular distribution of MS plaques.

"Paramagnetic rims" is an emerging marker of chronic neuroinflammation in MS, best seen on ≥3T magnets.

- They reflect iron accumulation in microglia.

Accepted MRI biomarkers of new inflammation include

- Enhancing lesions and/or
- Changes in long TR hyperintense lesions

MRI is the most important diagnostic and prognostic biomarker for MS. It is used to

- Diagnose MS.
- Assess treatment response.
- Guide new disease modifying therapies.

REFERENCES

1. Group GBDNDC. Global, regional, and national burden of neurological disorders during 1990-2015: a systematic analysis for the Global Burden of Disease Study 2015. Lancet Neurol 2017;16(11):877–97.
2. Thompson AJ, Baranzini SE, Geurts J, et al. Multiple sclerosis. Lancet 2018;391(10130):1622–36.
3. Polman CH, Reingold SC, Edan G, et al. Diagnostic criteria for multiple sclerosis: 2005 revisions to the "McDonald Criteria". Ann Neurol 2005;58(6):840–6.
4. Reich DS, Lucchinetti CF, Calabresi PA. Multiple Sclerosis. N Engl J Med 2018;378(2):169–80.
5. Lublin FD, Reingold SC, Cohen JA, et al. Defining the clinical course of multiple sclerosis: the 2013 revisions. Neurology 2014;83(3):278–86.
6. Vollmer TL, Nair KV, Williams IM, et al. Multiple sclerosis phenotypes as a continuum: the role of neurologic reserve. Neurol Clin Pract 2021;11(4):342–51.
7. Okuda DT, Mowry EM, Beheshtian A, et al. Incidental MRI anomalies suggestive of multiple sclerosis: the radiologically isolated syndrome. Neurology 2009;72(9):800–5.
8. Lebrun-Frenay C, Kantarci O, Siva A, et al, 10-year RISC study group on behalf of SFSEP, OFSEP. Radiologically Isolated Syndrome: 10-Year Risk Estimate of a Clinical Event. Ann Neurol 2020;88(2):407–17.
9. Wattjes MP, Ciccarelli O, Reich DS, et al. MAGNIMS-CMSC-NAIMS consensus recommendations on the use of MRI in patients with multiple sclerosis. Lancet Neurol 2021;20(8):653–70.
10. Filippi M, Rocca MA. MR imaging of multiple sclerosis. Radiology 2011;259(3):659–81.
11. Ho ML, Moonis G, Ginat DT, et al. Lesions of the corpus callosum. AJR Am J Roentgenol 2013;200(1):W1–16.
12. McNicholas N, Hutchinson M, McGuigan C, et al. 2017 McDonald diagnostic criteria: A review of the evidence. Mult Scler Relat Disord 2018;24:48–54.
13. Ge Y. Multiple sclerosis: the role of MR imaging. AJNR Am J Neuroradiol 2006;27(6):1165–76.
14. Sati P, Oh J, Constable RT, et al. The central vein sign and its clinical evaluation for the diagnosis of multiple sclerosis: a consensus statement from the North American Imaging in Multiple Sclerosis Cooperative. Nat Rev Neurol 2016;12(12):714–22.
15. Hemond CC, Reich DS, Dundamadappa SK. Paramagnetic Rim Lesions in Multiple Sclerosis: Comparison of Visualization at 1.5-T and 3-T MRI. AJR Am J Roentgenol 2022;219(1):120–31.
16. Ciccarelli O, Cohen JA, Reingold SC, et al, International Conference on Spinal Cord Involvement and Imaging in Multiple Sclerosis and Neuromyelitis Optica Spectrum Disorders. International Conference on Spinal Cord I, Imaging in Multiple S, et al. Spinal cord involvement in multiple sclerosis and neuromyelitis optica spectrum disorders. Lancet Neurol 2019;18(2):185–97.
17. Polman CH, Reingold SC, Banwell B, et al. Diagnostic criteria for multiple sclerosis: 2010 revisions to the McDonald criteria. Ann Neurol 2011;69(2):292–302.
18. Thompson AJ, Banwell BL, Barkhof F, et al. Diagnosis of multiple sclerosis: 2017 revisions of the McDonald criteria. Lancet Neurol 2018 Feb;17(2):162–73.
19. Hawkes CH, Giovannoni G. The McDonald Criteria for Multiple Sclerosis: time for clarification. Mult Scler 2010;16(5):566–75.
20. Chen JJ, Carletti F, Young V, et al. MRI differential diagnosis of suspected multiple sclerosis. Clin Radiol 2016 Sep;71(9):815–27.
21. Shimizu J, Hatanaka Y, Hasegawa M, et al. IFNβ-1b may severely exacerbate Japanese optic-spinal MS in neuromyelitis optica spectrum. Neurology 2010 Oct 19;75(16):1423–7.
22. Lennon VA, Wingerchuk DM, Kryzer TJ, et al. A serum autoantibody marker of neuromyelitis optica: distinction from multiple sclerosis. Lancet 2004;364(9451):2106–12.

Multiple Sclerosis Part 2
Advanced Imaging and Emerging Techniques

Check for updates

Shruti Mishra, MD*, Jayapalli Bapuraj, MD, Ashok Srinivasan, MD

KEYWORDS

• Multiple sclerosis • Susceptibility-weighted imaging • Diffusion tensor imaging
• Glymphatic imaging • Magnetization transfer imaging • Myelin water imaging • Molecular imaging

KEY POINTS

- Multiple advanced imaging techniques have been in investigation including advanced diffusion-weighted techniques, myelin quantification methods, proton magnetic resonance spectroscopy and molecular imaging, and glymphatic and perfusion imaging. Imaging techniques are focused on early disease detection, prediction of disease prognosis, and imagingspecific tissue components of the central nervous system.
- Alterations in metrics derived from diffusion tensor imaging (DTI), myelin quantification techniques including magnetization transfer and myelin water imaging, proton MR spectroscopy, and MR perfusion within normal-appearing white matter on T2-weighted imaging supports the notion that multiple sclerosis (MS) is a global disease with microstructural alterations distinct from MS plaques. Microstructural alteration may prove a better predictor of disability compared with lesion load alone.
- Glymphatic system impairment in MS has been suggested based on DTI along the perivascular space. Further investigation with gold-standard contrast-enhanced techniques is required.
- Although MS is considered a white matter demyelinating disorder, metabolic derangements in gray matter structures as demonstrated by proton MR spectroscopy suggest that gray matter abnormalities contribute significantly to the pathophysiology of the disease.
- Molecular imaging techniques with both advanced MR spectroscopy and PET are in development as novel imaging methods for the assessment of treatment efficacy in clinical trials.

INTRODUCTION

Conventional MR imaging methods of multiple sclerosis (MS), such as T1-weighted, T2-weighted, fluid-attenuated inversion recovery [FLAIR], and T1 postcontrast, provide valuable information for diagnosis[1] and monitoring of disease activity[2] while on therapy. Conventional sequences are used to identify the number, location, and enhancement of lesions as well as detection of new lesions. Although conventional MR imaging sequences have been used as a surrogate outcome measure in clinical trials, the association between clinical disability and MR imaging findings is poor, resulting in the "clinico-radiological paradox."[3] Multiple contributing reasons have been proposed, including underestimation of disease involvement in normal-appearing brain tissue on T2-weighted imaging as well as insensitivity to specific contributors of pathophysiology (ie, myelination and axonal loss).[3,4] Multiple advanced MR imaging techniques have been in development with a focus on early disease detection, improved correlation with clinical disability, prediction of disease prognosis, and

Department of Radiology, University of Michigan, 1500 East Medical Center Drive, UH B2A209, Ann Arbor, MI 48109-5030, USA
* Corresponding author. Department of Radiology, Medical Science, Unit 1, Room #3125, 1301 Catherine Street, Ann Arbor, MI 48109.
E-mail address: mishruti@med.umich.edu

Magn Reson Imaging Clin N Am 32 (2024) 221–231
https://doi.org/10.1016/j.mric.2024.01.002
1064-9689/24/

greater specificity to different tissue components of the central nervous system (CNS). In this review, focus will be on iron-sensitive techniques (susceptibility weighted imaging and quantitative susceptibility mapping [QSM]), advanced diffusion-weighted techniques including diffusion tensor imaging (DTI), myelin quantification methods, glymphatic imaging, and perfusion imaging.

IRON-SENSITIVE TECHNIQUES

Susceptibility-Weighted Imaging

Susceptibility-weighted imaging (SWI) is a combination of a particular sequence and postprocessing techniques to enhance the contrast in T2*-weighted images. The premise of SWI postprocessing is using high-pass filtering of the phase data to create a mask that either highlights paramagnetic (eg, hemosiderin) or diamagnetic (eg, white matter [WM] tracts, and calcium) substances based on their positive or negative phase shifts. The creation of SWI data then involves multiplying the phase mask several times with the magnitude image to obtain the desired contrast. To enhance the visibility of veins, SWI is often postprocessed by using a minimum-intensity projection over multiple sections.[5]

SWI in MS can be used to distinguish demyelinating lesions from T2/FLAIR hyperintense lesions that are vascular/ischemic in etiology. The central vein sign is characteristically found in MS lesions and characterized by a central hypointensity on SWI scans at the center of the lesion, and is best depicted at 3T.[6] Although characteristic, the central vein sign is not specific for MS and has been reported to be present in 27.2% of vascular lesions related to small vessel ischemic disease. For this reason, a threshold of 45% or more of lesions demonstrating central vein sign has been suggested to discriminate MS from nonspecific WM lesions.[6]

Another diagnostic and prognostic sign that has been described with SWI in MS is the paramagnetic rim sign (**Fig. 1**). The basis of the paramagnetic rim surrounding a WM lesion is iron deposition within macrophages and has been postulated to reflect chronically active MS lesions that are linked with a worse prognosis.[7,8]

Quantitative Susceptibility Mapping

QSM is an extension of SWI, which allows for quantification of concentration of iron, calcium, and myelin based on changes in local susceptibility. Histopathologic studies with QSM in MS have demonstrated that both demyelination and iron contribute to QSM signal alteration.[7] In vivo evaluation of QSM has found that susceptibility values as determined by QSM is substantially different between enhancing and nonenhancing lesions, and has been suggested as an alternative method for imaging blood–brain barrier breakdown.[9] Although brain QSM measurements have been found to be highly reproducible across MR imaging scanners, required offline reconstructions and lack of consensus on the optimal algorithm present barriers for clinical translation.[4]

DIFFUSION-BASED TECHNIQUES

Diffusion Tensor Imaging

DTI is an advanced application of diffusion-weighted imaging (DWI), which measures the diffusion of water molecules in tissue.[10] DWI makes use of gradient pulses to introduce a phase difference to detect water motion. DTI uses the principles of DWI with additional gradient pulses to estimate diffusion along different gradient directions. Measurements on 3 orthogonal planes are fitted to a 3D ellipsoid using a 3×3 symmetric matrix called a tensor, which yields the length and orientation of diffusion (eigenvalues and eigenvectors, respectively) at each voxel.[10] In white matter, diffusion is hindered by presence of highly organized myelinated axonal fiber tracts resulting in greater water diffusion along the direction of the fiber tracts.[11] Multiple quantitative scalar indices can be extracted from DTI with the 2 most common representing mean diffusivity (MD) and fractional anisotropy (FA). MD is a mean of eigenvalues with higher MD corresponding to diminished local anisotropy.[10,12] FA provides a measure of anisotropy and is highest in voxels containing highly ordered fiber tracts.

DTI has been extensively studied in MS to assess its utility for early disease diagnosis, assessment of disease severity, and prediction of prognosis. DTI has been used in the evaluation of different MS lesion types.[11] MS lesions are associated with elevated MD and low FA compared with normal-appearing white matter[11] (**Fig. 2**). FA and MD values can distinguish between enhancing and nonenhancing lesions and nonenhancing T1-hypointense lesions compared with T1 isointense lesions.[13] Others have attempted to use DTI metrics for differentiating lesion types in different phenotypes of MS. For example, greater change has been identified in MD and FA compared with unaffected white matter in patients with secondary-progressive MS compared with relapsing-remitting MS[14] (RRMS).

DTI may detect subtle changes in white matter that is undetectable on routine FLAIR or T2-weighted imaging.[13,15] Normal-appearing white matter (NAWM) on conventional T1-and T2-weighted imaging demonstrates altered tissue

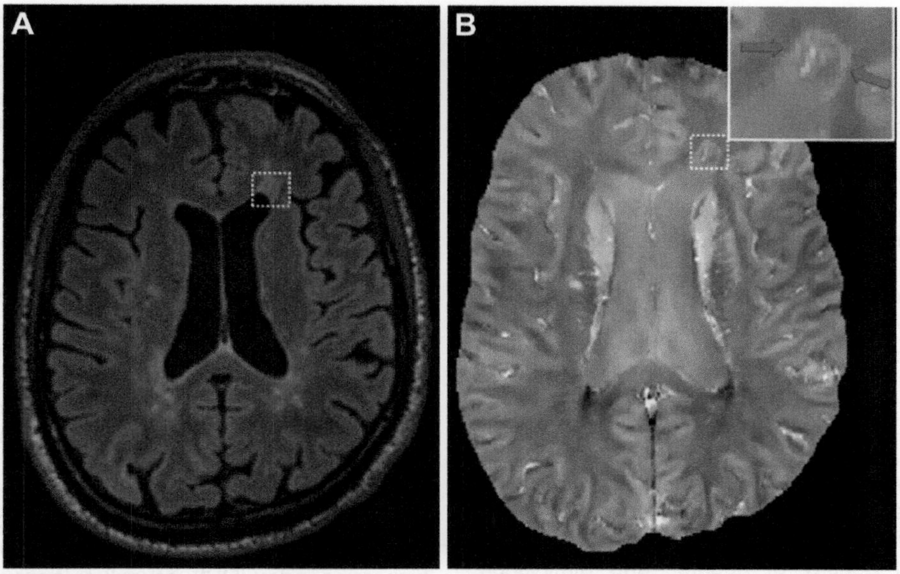

Fig. 1. Example of Paramagnetic-Rim Lesion in MS. (*A*) FLAIR axial image with demonstrating multiple periventricular and deep white matter MS lesions. (*B*) Susceptibility-weighted image of left periventricular lesion demonstrating paramagnetic rim, associated with chronically active lesion (*red arrow*). (Rahmanzadeh, R. et al., (2022), A New Advanced MRI Biomarker for Remyelinated Lesions in Multiple Sclerosis. Ann Neurol, 92: 486-502. https://doi.org/10.1002/ana.26441.)

microstructure as evidenced by diminished FA, elevated MD when compared with healthy controls.[16,17] Although the mechanism and pathologic correlation of these DTI changes is not fully understood, myelin and axonal loss are thought to contribute.[11] DTI metrics have been evaluated in normal-appearing corpus callosum (NACC), given the propensity of demyelinating lesions in MS to occur at the callosomarginal or callososeptal interface. NACC demonstrates abnormalities in DTI not demonstrated in other NAWM regions and has been proposed as a marker of disease burden because it has been found to correlate with cerebral WM lesion load.[18] Microstructural alterations in NACC may predict conversion to MS in patients presenting with clinically isolated syndrome.[19] DTI may provide an alternative, more specific imaging metric for disease burden

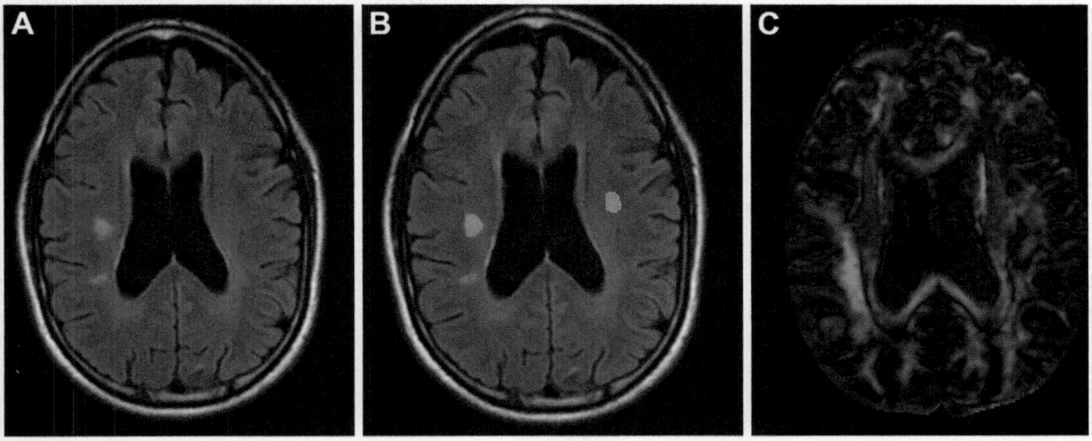

Fig. 2. DTI in MS. (*A*) FLAIR image of a patient with RRMS demonstrating multiple FLAIR-hyperintense MS plaques. (*B*) Locations of regions of interest of MS plaque (*green*) and NAWM (*yellow*). (*C*) Color FA map derived from DTI. Mean FA in the MS plaque is lower (0.33) compared with NAWM (0.46). MD in the lesion is higher (0.0013) compared with NAWM (0.0009).

corresponding to clinical disability compared with WM lesion load.[11,20]

Despite the extensive investigation of DTI as an advanced method for early detection and disease burden monitoring, its use has remained investigational and is not used in routine clinical imaging to date. However, the quantitative nature of DTI may play a role in assessing the outcome of clinical trials particularly its advantages in assessing microstructural damage, in monitoring of therapeutic response of future and ongoing therapies.

Advanced Diffusion MR Imaging Analytical Methods

Although DTI has been the most extensively studied in MS, DTI has several disadvantages. First, the DTI metrics (FA and MD) are nonspecific, and the decreased FA in the white matter of MS patients may be sequela of multiple factors including decreased density of neurites and diminished myelin.[12] Therefore, advanced diffusion MR imaging techniques have been in development to capture more specific white matter changes.[21]

Q-space imaging

The DTI model assumes that the displacement probability of water molecules is Gaussian, whereas experimental evidence points to the presence of non-Gaussian diffusion in white matter.[10] Q-space imaging (QSI) an analytical method of DWI, which resolves this limitation. The technique uses high b-values and does not introduce the assumption of Gaussian diffusion in calculation of quantitative metrics.[22] QSI has been found to be very sensitive to MS lesions compared with conventional MR imaging as well as demonstrating abnormalities in the NAWM of brains of MS. QSI's potential advantage is its greater sensitivity in comparison to DTI and potential to differentiate plaques of different pathologic states such as degree of myelination.[22] However, the larger number of high magnitude b-values (ie, b-values in 6000s compared with 1000–1500 in DTI and 2500–3000 in diffusion kurtosis imaging [DKI]) and subsequently long imaging time are disadvantages.[22]

Diffusion kurtosis imaging

DKI is related to QSI and is a mathematical extension of the DTI also allowing for the quantification of non-Gaussian diffusion.[21,22] It is advantageous compared with QSI in that it does not require as high b-values making it more feasible for clinical translation. Similar to QSI, DKI is more sensitive than DTI for the detection of microstructural abnormalities in NAWM. DKI metrics are also less susceptible to crossing fibers compared with DTI.[22]

Neurite orientation dispersion and density imaging

Neurite orientation dispersion and density imaging (NODDI) is a new technique that incorporates a biophysical model[21,22] for mapping of neurite morphology. Neurites refer to projections from the cell body of a neuron and include axons in the white matter and both axons and dendrites in the gray matter (GM). In NODDI, the diffusion signal is modeled as a sum of the contribution of 3 compartments: intraneurite, extraneurite, and cerebrospinal fluid (CSF). The intraneurite space is modeled using zero-radius cylinders and the extraneurite space is modeled as a symmetric diffusion tensor (ie, similar to DTI if eigenvalues in 2 directions were the same). The CSF compartment is modeled as an isotropic diffusion tensor with a predefined diffusivity. Fitting the NODDI model voxel-by-voxel provides maps quantifying degree of orientation coherence of neurites, that is, orientation dispersion index (ODI), as well as density, that is, neurite density index (NDI) or intraneurite volume fraction (INVF).[21]

In MS, studies have found diminished INVF / NDI in both MS plaques (eg, **Fig. 3**) compared with NAWM and diminished INVF in NAWM compared with age-matched controls. Changes in INVF demonstrate more widespread variability compared with DTI metrics and, therefore, is postulated as a superior method for evaluating microstructural changes. Histopathologic correlation studies in the postmortem spinal cord of patients with MS found correlation between ODI with histologic neurite orientation dispersion.[23] Additionally they found decreased NDI and ODI within lesions compared with nonlesional areas while FA values from DTI showed mixed changes, suggesting dispersion indices from NODDI may be more sensitive to microstructural change.[23] However, further studies in vivo are required to assess its utility in monitoring disease progression or predicting prognosis.

MYELIN QUANTIFICATION WITH MR IMAGING

Standard T1-weighted and T2-weighted imaging provides qualitative information on myelin content but are nonspecific. The previously described diffusion approaches, the most studied being DTI, yield measures that are sensitive to but nonspecific for myelination because additional factors such as axonal density and fiber orientation affect DTI metrics.[24] Various myelin quantification methods using MR imaging have been in development to improve characterization of MS lesions in vivo, motivated by the development of novel therapeutic

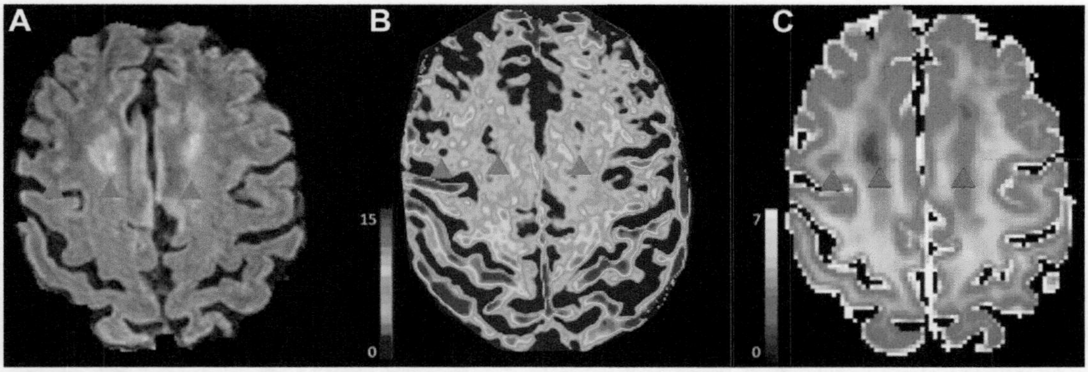

Fig. 3. MWI and NODDI in MS. (*A*) Axial FLAIR image with multiple confluent deep white matter MS lesions (*red arrowheads*). (*B*) MWF map derived from MWI. (*C*) NDI map derived from NODDI (*blue arrowheads* correspond to MS lesions). (Reza Rahmanzadeh et al., Myelin and axon pathology in multiple sclerosis assessed by myelin water and multi-shell diffusion imaging, Brain, Volume 144, Issue 6, June 2021, Pages 1684–1696, https://doi.org/10.1093/brain/awab088.)

interventions targeting promotion of repair through remyelination.

Magnetization Transfer Imaging

Magnetization transfer (MT) imaging exploits magnetization exchange between mobile water and immobile macromolecules. An off-resonance radiofrequency (RF) pulse is used to preferentially saturate the immobile protons. MT subsequently occurs between the immobile protons to the mobile protons resulting in a loss of signal. MT ratio (MTR) is calculated by computing the difference in signal intensity before and after the application of the RF pulse, and it reflects the efficiency of the magnetization exchange.[25] A low MTR is associated with a reduced proportion of bound immobile protons and is correlated with demyelination and axonal loss in MS.[26] MTR has been found to correlate with degree of myelination in histopathologic correlation studies.[27] In vivo studies have found that MTR is reduced in enhancing lesions and increases subsequently, suggesting that demyelination and remyelination may be the predominant feature underlying these changes. MTR has been evaluated both within lesions as well as NAWM. Lowlesional MTR has been found to correlate with the degree of clinical disability as well as with the severity of the clinical phenotype, with lower MTR seen in the progressive forms of MS.[13,28] An example of an MTR map is depicted in **Fig. 4**.

In NAWM, MTR reduction has been predictive of subsequent plaque development.[29] MTR reduction is more pronounced with more severe primary and secondary progressive phenotypes.[30] MTR alterations have been shown to be associated with the degree of clinical disability, particular locomotor disability.[31] Extent of MTR change in NAWM in patients with clinically isolated syndrome has been suggested to predict subsequent evolution to definite MS.[28]

MTR has some intrinsic limitations. The nature of the measured signal makes it an indirect measure of myelin. It is not capable of differentiating healthy myelin from myelin debris, and is influenced by edema and inflammation.[4] More advanced approaches of MT include quantitative MT and inhomogeneous MT, which may provide greater specificity for myelin. However, such approaches are more time-consuming and require more complex postprocessing resulting in barriers to clinical translation. Compared with other advanced MR imaging methods, MTR is limited by low reproducibility across different centers.[32] More studies are therefore required to establish feasibility and reproducibility before larger scale clinical implementation.

Myelin Water Imaging

Myelin water imaging (MWI) can be T2-weighted, T2*-weighted, or T1-weighted, and it exploits signal decay curves to estimate the contribution of water trapped within myelin sheaths, characterized by short relaxation times, compared with water trapped in other tissue compartments. The fraction of water signal originating from myelin sheaths is defined as the myelin water fraction (MWF).[33,34] Various implementation techniques have been in development for MWI with suggestion of greater specificity to myelin, good correlation with histopathology, and greater reproducibility when compared with other myelin quantification techniques.[32]

MWI has been found to be sensitive to different MS lesion types, for example, periventricular lesions demonstrate lower MWF compared with juxtacortical lesions. Lesions with paramagnetic rims

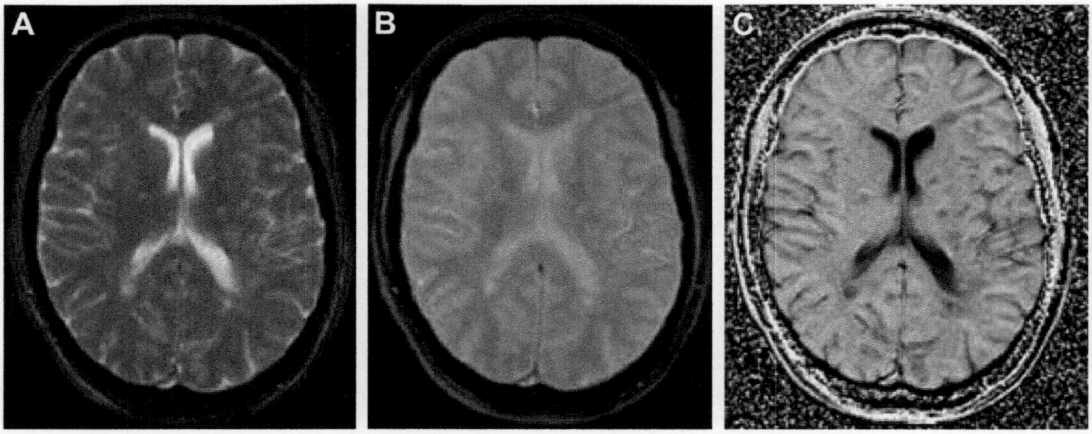

Fig. 4. MT in MS. (*A*) Axial gradient echo image without RF saturation pulse. (*B*) Axial gradient echo image with RF saturation pulse. (*C*) MT ratio map in a patient with MS. (Filippi, M. and Agosta, F. (2007), Magnetization Transfer MRI in Multiple Sclerosis. Journal of Neuroimaging, 17: 22S-26S. https://doi.org/10.1111/j.1552-6569.2007.00132.x.)

show lower MWF compared with lesions without paramagnetic rims.[35] MWI has also shown diminished MWF in NAWM compared with healthy controls.[35] MWF may be more sensitive in differentiating T2/FLAIR lesions compared with NAWM compared with MTR and metrics derived from DTI (FA and radial diffusivity).[36] An example of an MWF map in an patient with MS is depicted in **Fig. 3**. Systematic reviews comparing different myelin quantification methods suggest MWF may be superior method based on in vivo studies[32]; however, head-to-head comparison studies of MWF with other myelin quantification techniques are required in humans. A limitation of MWI is its sensitivity to iron content and therefore further studies are required to evaluate utility in correction for iron content.[32]

G-Ratio

G-ratio is a marker of myelination, which attempts to combine myelin-sensitive measures with axonal-sensitive measures to disentangle ambiguities of myelin measurements, which may be secondary to a decrease in the number of axons.[37] G-ratio refers to the ratio between the inner axon radius and the outer radius of the axon surrounding the myelin sheath to estimate degree of myelination and is derived by combining myelin volume fraction from myelin-sensitive measures with axonal density derived from diffusion-based techniques, such as NODDI.[22] Various methods for calculating g-ratio have demonstrated good correlation with histology. However, g-ratios computed from different techniques have shown significant differences across techniques and in some cases divergent results in MS lesions and NAWM (ie, higher g-ratio values in some parameter maps and lower values in others).[37] Therefore, more studies are required to compare different g-ratio modalities.

MOLECULAR IMAGING

Proton MR spectroscopy

Proton MR spectroscopy (1H-MRS) allows in vivo quantification of certain cerebral metabolites with the most common clinically relevant being N-acetyl-aspartate (NAA), choline (Ch), creatinine (Cr), and inositol (In). NAA is considered a marker of neuronal integrity and Ch and In are affected by damage and repair of nonneuronal cells. 1H-MRS is used to evaluate metabolites in MS lesions as well as NAWM. Specifically, 1H-MRS has been used to distinguish different stages of MS lesions. Acute demyelinating lesions demonstrate elevated lactate, Ch, myo-inositol peaks and diminished NAA peaks.[38] The changes in lactate may reflect metabolism from active inflammatory cells.[38,39] Elevated Ch peak may be secondary to elevated levels of membrane phospholipids released from myelin breakdown. The decrease in NAA signal has been postulated to be secondary to axonal injury. Reported changes in Cr in acute lesions are more variable with report of Cr increase in the acute phase[40,41] and other reports of Cr decreasing.[38] Cr is present in both neuronal and glial cells, and as such, divergent reports of Cr changes may reflect heterogeneity in the evolution of plaques. During evolution of a lesion from acute to chronic phase, there is a progressive decrease and/or normalization of the lactate, Ch, and lipid peaks.[38] Cr peaks have been shown to increase between 3 and 12 months, which may reflect developing gliosis.[41]

In NAWM, there is a decrease in NAA or NAA/Cr ratio compared with controls, which are more pronounced in progressive phenotypes[42] but can also be seen in the earliest stage of the disease.[43] The degree of decrease of the NAA peak correlates with disability scores and lesion load.[44] Evaluation of metabolites in segmented NACC found diminished NAA/Cho ratio and increased Cho/Cr ratio in the splenium and central portions of the corpus callosum compared with healthy controls while controlling for CC volume,[19] suggesting the presence of microstructural change in the corpus callosum at the earliest stages of the disease.

Some studies focused on metabolic changes in the GM support that GM pathology has a substantial contribution to the pathophysiology of MS. Decrease in NAA peaks within deep GM structures, particularly the thalamus, has been demonstrated.[45,46] Decreased NAA peaks have also been demonstrated in global cortical GM with the NAA peak correlating with the degree of disability.[47] These results support the notion that while MS is a demyelinating condition of the white matter, it is associated with GM damage not visualized on conventional MR sequences and may play a role in disease pathophysiology.[48]

1H-MRS changes have been used as a secondary endpoint in clinical trials. For example, interferon-beta therapy has shown an increase in Cr and Ch levels and glatiramer acetate has resulted in higher NAA:Cr ratio.[49] Longitudinal monitoring of NAA:Cr ratio found it to be a better predictor of disability compared with lesion load for patients on glatiramer acetate therapy.[50]

1H-MRS has important technical limitations. The minimum volume of the region of interest is typically 1 cm^3 to obtain a useful spectrum and have a reasonable acquisition time. However, most MS lesions are smaller than this. Therefore, metabolite profiles of MS lesions are likely affected by partial volume effects.[39,51]

Emerging molecular imaging techniques

Although 1H-MRS is widely used clinically and as a surrogate imaging marker in clinical trials, its lack of specificity results in limited assessment of specific treatment mechanisms and efficacy. Multiple MR imaging and PET molecular imaging biomarkers have been in development in mouse models with early human studies to assess their utility in evaluating treatment response to both existing and developing therapies.[49] Hyperpolarization is an emerging MR imaging technique, which allows for the detection of nonproton nuclei probes in MRS imaging. The most studied in humans and murine models is hyperpolarized 13C-pyruvate, which has shown promise in the detection of neuroinflammatory lesions in a mouse model for MS.[52] Studies in human patients with MS are still required for validation. Additionally, this imaging technique requires specialized equipment only available in a few clinical centers, which will be a hurdle for clinical translation.

Multiple imaging targets have been in development, which attempt to target the markers of inflammation for both elucidating pathophysiology and identifying potential therapeutic targets. The enzyme myeloperoxidase (MPO) is a proinflammatory enzyme expressed by monocytes, macrophages, microglia, and neutrophils and has been explored as a possible novel therapeutic target.[53,54] MPO inhibition is associated with diminished inflammatory response and decreased demyelination, as well as reduced severity of clinical symptoms and improved survival in murine models of MS.[54] Multiple imaging modalities have been investigated for targeting MPO in vivo including fluorescence, PET, and MR imaging, with the MR imaging agent bis-5-HT-Gd-DTPA (MPO-Gd) demonstrating promise as an imaging biomarker of MS in murine models.[54] Novel MR imaging agents are in development, which are not linear gadolinium-based contrast agents, a potential limitation of MPO-Gd given safety concerns of nephrogenic systemic fibrosis with existing linear agents, although further in vivo studies are required for validation.[55]

Multiple PET tracers have been developed with a wide range of molecular targets ranging from physiologic metabolites to small molecules, designed to monitor different aspects of pathophysiology, for example, demyelination or glial activity or to assess efficacy of drug therapies. For example, dalfampridine is a potassium-channel blocker approved for use in MS and has been radiolabeled with 18F for PET imaging and used in a mouse model to show probe uptake in demyelinated brain regions.[56] Development of novel molecular imaging targets is an active area of research and will provide novel imaging biomarkers for clinical trials. Of the PET molecular imaging targets, probes targeting translocator protein (TSPO) has been the most widely studied with currently more than 10 TSPO-targeting probes with 18F and 11C, which have been evaluated in humans. TSPO is a mitochondrial protein involved in steroid metabolism and is upregulated in the brain with microglia activation and reactive astrocyte upregulation. TSPO PET has been used as a secondary biomarker in multiple ongoing clinical trials of in vivo neuroinflammation. However, there is little consensus on which TSPO radioligand is optimal and to date there are no MS therapies that share molecular targets with TSPO.[49]

GLYMPHATIC IMAGING

Recent evidence has suggested the presence of a waste clearance system in the CNS, referred to as the glymphatic system. In the proposed glymphatic exchange pathway, CSF penetrates brain parenchyma via perivascular spaces surrounding arteries and communicates with interstitial space via an astrocytic aquaporin 4-dependent process. Interstitial fluid drains along perivenous spaces to meningeal lymphatic vessels located in proximity to major venous sinuses.

Multiple imaging techniques have been used to assess glymphatic function in vivo, including dynamic PET imaging with 11C-PiB PET[57] and intravenous gadolinium-enhanced MR imaging as well as less-invasive noncontrast MR techniques including arterial spin labeling and DTI.[58] Preliminary evidence of glymphatic system impairment in MS has been suggested with 11C-PiB PET[57] as well as DTI.[59] The basic principles of DTI are discussed elsewhere in this article. DTI has been proposed as a noninvasive method to measure of glymphatic function by quantifying diffusivity along the perivascular space. This technique exploits the fact that diffusion along the perivascular space surrounding the medullary veins in the periventricular white matter subjacent to the lateral ventricles course perpendicular to the traversing white matter fibers. Dividing the diffusivity along the perivascular axis from the perpendicular y-axis projecting fibers and the z-axis associative fibers yields the diffusion along the perivascular space (DTI-APLS) index.[59]

Assessment of in vivo glymphatic system function with DTI in MS overall demonstrated impaired glymphatic function with diminished APLS index in patients with relapsing remitting and primary progressive MS compared with healthy controls, with greater decrease in the primary progressive subgroup. Lower DTI-APLS correlated with higher disability scores, longer disease duration, and higher white matter and cortical lesion volumes.[59]

These results suggest that glymphatic function as measured by the surrogate marker of DTI-APLS may provide insight into pathophysiology of the disease as well as provide a novel imaging biomarker for disease monitoring and treatment response. However further research is required to better understand the differences in the noninvasive approach with that of intrathecal contrast enhanced technique, which is considered the gold standard.[60] Future studies will be required to assess its potential role in predicting disease progression.

PERFUSION IMAGING

Blood perfusion to the brain can be assessed with MR imaging, both with noncontrast techniques (arterial spin labeling) and contrast-enhanced techniques (T1-weighted dynamic contrast-enhanced sequence or T2*-weighted dynamic susceptibility contrast [DSC] sequence). In MS, various studies have evaluated the utility of perfusion imaging for the prediction of plaque development, evaluation of normal-appearing brain tissue, and correlation with clinical disability.[4] Perfusion studies in MS have shown that MS lesion hyperperfusion precedes the development of an enhancing lesion or lesion appearance on T2-weighted images.[61,62] Chronic lesions demonstrate hypoperfusion

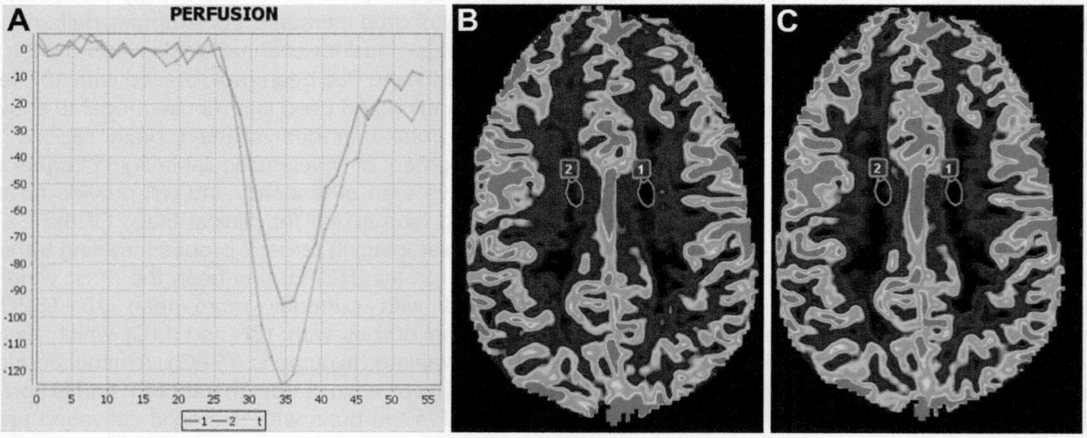

Fig. 5. DSC perfusion imaging in RRMS. (*A*) Signal intensity vs time after injection of the MS plaque (*red*, region 1) compared with NAWM (*blue*, region 2). (*B*) Color map of relative cerebral blood volume (rCBV). (*C*) Color map of relative cerebral blood flow (rCBF). Both rCBV and rCBF are diminished in MS plaques compared with NAWM, 0.39 and 6.86 compared with 0.57 and 9.91, respectively.

compared with NAWM (**Fig. 5**).[62] Evaluation of NAWM with DSC perfusion has demonstrated diminished perfusion metrics in NAWM in primary-progressive and RRMS compared with normal controls, with greater degree of hypoperfusion in the primary-progressive MS cohort,[63] supporting MR perfusion sensitivity to white matter microstructural damage. Multiple studies have demonstrated correlation between degree of hypoperfusion and degree of disability,[4,63] with changes more pronounced at 3T.[64] The cause of these perfusion changes has been hypothesized to be secondary to axonal degeneration and vascular degeneration.[62] However, further studies are required for clarification of the pathogenesis.

SUMMARY

In summary, multiple advanced imaging methods have been in investigation to identify new imaging biomarkers for early disease detection, predicting disease prognosis, and for clinical trial endpoints. The discussed advanced imaging techniques including advanced diffusion-weighted techniques, myelin quantification methods, proton magnetic resonance spectroscopy and molecular imaging, and glymphatic and perfusion imaging are investigational in nature. Multiple imaging techniques probing different aspects of tissue microstructure (ie, DTI, MT, MWI, MRS, glymphatic imaging, and perfusion) support the notion that MS is a global disease with microstructural alterations distinct from MS plaques seen in both white matter and GM, which seems unaffected on conventional T1-and T2-weighted sequences. These global changes are likely better predictors of disability compared with lesion load seen on conventional imaging alone. However, many of these techniques provide complimentary information and more multimodality studies are required to determine which technique(s) have potential to provide unique, reproducible, quantitative information that can be readily translated to the clinic. Currently, heterogeneity in imaging protocols and postprocessing techniques are barriers to widespread adoption. Emerging techniques, particularly glymphatic imaging, may improve understanding of disease pathophysiology. Novel molecular imaging techniques have potential to assess efficacy of specific treatments in clinical trials.

CLINICS CARE POINTS

- Advanced MR imaging techniques in MS are focused on early disease detection, predicting disease prognosis, increasing understanding of pathophysiology, and novel imaging biomarkers for clinical trials.
- Advanced diffusion methods, myelin quantification methods, and 1H-MRS demonstrate microstructural alterations in normal-appearing brain tissue suggesting MS is a global disease.
- Microstructural changes in NAWM may be a better predictor of clinical disability than white matter lesion load alone.
- Recent evidence suggests glymphatic system impairment, as measured by DTI in the perivascular space, contributes to the pathophysiology of MS.
- Novel molecular imaging techniques include hyperpolarized 13C-pyruvate and novel PET tracers may represent more specific targets for clinical trial endpoints.

DISCLOSURE

The authors have no relevant financial disclosures.

REFERENCES

1. Rovira Á, Wattjes MP, Tintoré M, et al. Evidence-based guidelines: MAGNIMS consensus guidelines on the use of MRI in multiple sclerosis - Clinical implementation in the diagnostic process. Nat Rev Neurol 2015;11(8):471–82.
2. Wattjes MP, Rovira À, Miller D, et al. Evidence-based guidelines: MAGNIMS consensus guidelines on the use of MRI in multiple sclerosis - Establishing disease prognosis and monitoring patients. Nat Rev Neurol 2015;11(10):597–606.
3. Barkhof F. The clinico-radiological paradox in multiple sclerosis revisited. Curr Opin Neurol 2002;15(3):239–45.
4. Granziera C, Wuerfel J, Barkhof F, et al. Quantitative magnetic resonance imaging towards clinical application in multiple sclerosis. Brain 2021;144(5):1296–311.
5. Haller S, Haacke EM, Thurnher MM, et al. Susceptibility-weighted imaging: technical essentials and clinical neurologic applications. Radiology 2021;299(1):3–26.
6. Sparacia G, Agnello F, Gambino A, et al. Multiple sclerosis: high prevalence of the 'central vein' sign in white matter lesions on susceptibility-weighted images. NeuroRadiol J 2018;31(4):356–61.
7. Wisnieff C, Ramanan S, Olesik J, et al. Quantitative susceptibility mapping (QSM) of white matter multiple sclerosis lesions: Interpreting positive susceptibility and the presence of iron. Magn Reson Med 2015;74(2):564–70.

8. Rahmanzadeh R, Galbusera R, Lu PJ, et al. A new advanced MRI biomarker for remyelinated lesions in multiple sclerosis. Ann Neurol 2022;92(3):486–502.
9. Zhang Y, Gauthier SA, Gupta A, et al. Magnetic susceptibility from quantitative susceptibility mapping can differentiate new enhancing from nonenhancing multiple sclerosis lesions without gadolinium injection. Am J Neuroradiol 2016;37(10):1794–9.
10. Mori S, Zhang J. Principles of diffusion tensor imaging and its applications to basic neuroscience research. Neuron 2006;51(5):527–39.
11. Ge Y, Law M, Grossman RI. Applications of diffusion tensor MR imaging in multiple sclerosis. Ann N Y Acad Sci 2005;1064:202–19.
12. Assaf Y, Pasternak O. Diffusion tensor imaging (DTI)-based white matter mapping in brain research: A review. J Mol Neurosci 2008;34(1):51–61.
13. Filippi M, Iannucci G, Cercignani M, et al. A quantitative study of water diffusion in multiple sclerosis lesions and normal-appearing white matter using echo- planar imaging. Arch Neurol 2000; 57(7):1017–21.
14. Scanderbeg AC, Tomaiuolo F, Sabatini U, et al. Demyelinating plaques in relapsing-remitting and secondary-progressive multiple sclerosis: Assessment with diffusion MR imaging. Am J Neuroradiol 2000;21(5):862–8.
15. Cercignani M, Iannucci G, Rocca MA, et al. Pathologic damage in MS assessed by diffusion-weighted and magnetization transfer MRI. Neurology 2000; 54(5):1139–44.
16. Rocca MA, Cercignani M, Iannucci G, et al. Weekly diffusion- white matter in MS. J Magn Reson Imag 1998;6–8.
17. Guo AC, MacFall JR, Provenzale JM. Multiple sclerosis: diffusion tensor MR imaging for evaluation of normal-appearing white matter. Radiology 2002; 222(3):729–36.
18. Ge Y, Law M, Johnson G, et al. Preferential occult injury of corpus callosum in multiple sclerosis measured by diffusion tensor imaging. J Magn Reson Imag 2004;20(1):1–7.
19. Ranjeva JP, Pelletier J, Ibarrola D, et al. MRI/MRS of corpus callosum in patients with clinically isolated syndrome suggestive of multiple sclerosis. Mult Scler 2003;9:554–65.
20. Cercignani M, Bozzali M, Iannucci G, et al. Magnetisation transfer ratio and mean diffusivity of normal appearing white and grey matter from patients with multiple sclerosis. J Neurol Neurosurg Psychiatry 2001;70(3):311–7.
21. Martinez-Heras E, Grussu F, Prados F, et al. Diffusion-weighted imaging: recent advances and applications. Semin Ultrasound CT MRI 2021;42(5): 490–506.
22. Hori M, Maekawa T, Kamiya K, et al. Advanced Diffusion MR Imaging for Multiple Sclerosis in the Brain and Spinal Cord. Magn Reson Med Sci 2022;21(1): 58–70.
23. Grussu F, Schneider T, Tur C, et al. Neurite dispersion: a new marker of multiple sclerosis spinal cord pathology? Ann Clin Transl Neurol 2017;4(9): 663–79.
24. De Santis S, Drakesmith M, Bells S, et al. Why diffusion tensor MRI does well only some of the time: Variance and covariance of white matter tissue microstructure attributes in the living human brain. Neuroimage 2014;89:35–44.
25. Wolff SD, Balaban RS. Magnetization transfer imaging: Practical aspects and clinical applications. Radiology 1994;192(3):593–9.
26. Filippi M, Agosta F. Magnetization transfer MRI in multiple sclerosis. J Neuroimaging 2007;17(22S-26S). https://doi.org/10.1111/j.1552-6569.2007.00132.x.
27. Schmierer K, Scaravilli F, Altmann DR, et al. Magnetization transfer ratio and myelin in postmortem multiple sclerosis brain. Ann Neurol 2004;56(3):407–15.
28. Iannucci G, Tortorella C, Rovaris M, et al. Prognostic value of MR and magnetization transfer imaging findings in patients with clinically isolated syndromes suggestive of multiple sclerosis at presentation. Am J Neuroradiol 2000;21(6):1034–8.
29. Filippi M, Rocca MA, Martino G, et al. Magnetization transfer changes in the normal appearing white matter precede the appearance of enhancing lesions in patients with multiple sclerosis. Ann Neurol 1998; 43(6):809–14.
30. Filippi M, Iannucci G, Tortorella C, et al. Comparison of MS clinical phenotypes using conventional and magnetization transfer MRI. Neurology 1999;52(3): 588–94.
31. Rocca MA, Falini A, Colombo B, et al. Adaptive functional changes in the cerebral cortex of patients with nondisabling multiple sclerosis correlate with the extent of brain structural damage. Ann Neurol 2002;51(3):330–9.
32. van der Weijden CWJ, García DV, Borra RJH, et al. Myelin quantification with MRI: A systematic review of accuracy and reproducibility. Neuroimage 2021; 226:117561.
33. Mackay A, Whittall K, Adler J, et al. In vivo visualization of myelin water in brain by magnetic resonance. Magn Reson Med 1994;31(6):673–7.
34. Balaji S, Johnson P, Dvorak AV, et al. Update on myelin imaging in neurological syndromes. Curr Opin Neurol 2022;35(4):467–74.
35. Rahmanzadeh R, Lu PJ, Barakovic M, et al. Myelin and axon pathology in multiple sclerosis assessed by myelin water and multi-shell diffusion imaging. Brain 2021;144(6):1684–96.
36. Lipp I, Jones DK, Bells S, et al. Comparing MRI metrics to quantify white matter microstructural damage in multiple sclerosis. Hum Brain Mapp 2019;40(10): 2917–32.

37. Berg RC, Menegaux A, Amthor T, et al. Comparing myelin-sensitive magnetic resonance imaging measures and resulting g-ratios in healthy and multiple sclerosis brains. Neuroimage 2022;264. https://doi.org/10.1016/j.neuroimage.2022.119750.
38. De Stefano N, Matthews PM, Antel JP, et al. Chemical pathology of acute demyelinating lesions and its correlation with disability. Ann Neurol 1995;38(6):901–9.
39. De Stefano N, Filippi M. MR spectroscopy in multiple sclerosis. J Neuroimaging 2007;17(2):31–5.
40. Srinivasan R, Sailasuta N, Hurd R, et al. Evidence of elevated glutamate in multiple sclerosis using magnetic resonance spectroscopy at 3 T. Brain 2005;128(5):1016–25.
41. Mader I, Roser W, Kappos L, et al. Serial proton MR spectroscopy of contrast-enhancing multiple sclerosis plaques: Absolute metabolic values over 2 years during a clinical pharmacological study. Am J Neuroradiol 2000;21(7):1220–7.
42. Fu L, Matthews PM, De Stefano N, et al. Imaging axonal damage of normal-appearing white matter in multiple sclerosis. Brain 1998;121(1):103–13.
43. De Stefano N, Narayanan S, Francis GS, et al. Evidence of axonal damage in the early stages of multiple sclerosis and its relevance to disability. Arch Neurol 2001;58(1):65–70.
44. Sarchielli P, Presciutti O, Pelliccioli GP, et al. Absolute quantification of brain metabolites by proton magnetic resonance spectroscopy in normal-appearing white matter of multiple sclerosis patients. Brain 1999;122(Pt 3):513–21.
45. Wylezinska M, Cifelli A, Jezzard P, et al. Thalamic neurodegeneration in relapsing-remitting multiple sclerosis. Neurology 2003;60(12):1949–54.
46. Inglese M, Liu S, Babb JS, et al. Three-dimensional proton spectroscopy of deep gray matter nuclei in relapsing-remaining MS. Neurology 2004;63(1):170–2.
47. Sastre-Garriga J, Ingle GT, Chard DT, et al. Metabolite changes in normal-appearing gray and white matter are linked with disability in early primary progressive multiple sclerosis. Arch Neurol 2005;62(4):569–73.
48. Filippi M. Multiple sclerosis: a white matter disease with associated gray matter damage. J Neurol Sci 2001;185(1):3–4.
49. Thomas AM, Barkhof F, Bulte JWM. Opportunities for molecular imaging in multiple sclerosis management: linking probe to treatment. Radiology 2022;303(3):486–97.
50. Khan O, Seraji-Bozorgzad N, Bao F, et al. The relationship between brain MR spectroscopy and disability in multiple sclerosis: 20-year data from the U.S. glatiramer acetate extension study. J Neuroimaging 2017;27(1):97–106.
51. Rovira À, Alonso J. 1H magnetic resonance spectroscopy in multiple sclerosis and related disorders. Neuroimaging Clin 2013;23(3):459–74.
52. Guglielmetti C, Najac C, Didonna A, et al. Hyperpolarized 13C MR metabolic imaging can detect neuroinflammation in vivo in a multiple sclerosis murine model. Proc Natl Acad Sci U S A 2017;114(33):E6982–91.
53. Rodríguez E, Nilges M, Weissleder R, et al. Activatable magnetic resonance imaging agents for myeloperoxidase sensing: Mechanism of activation, stability, and toxicity. J Am Chem Soc 2010;132(1):168–77.
54. Forghani R, Wojtkiewicz GR, Zhang Y, et al. Demyelinating diseases: Myeloperoxidase as an imaging biomarker and therapeutic target. Radiology 2012;263(2):451–60.
55. Wang C, Cheng D, Jalali Motlagh N, et al. Highly efficient activatable mri probe to sense myeloperoxidase activity. J Med Chem 2021;64(9):5874–85.
56. Brugarolas P, Sánchez-Rodríguez JE, Tsai HM, et al. Development of a PET radioligand for potassium channels to image CNS demyelination. Sci Rep 2018;8(1):1–16.
57. Schubert JJ, Veronese M, Marchitelli L, et al. Dynamic 11C-PIB PET shows cerebrospinal fluid flow alterations in Alzheimer disease and multiple sclerosis. J Nucl Med 2019;60(10):1452–60.
58. Naganawa S, Taoka T. The Glymphatic system: a review of the challenges in visualizing its structure and function with mr imaging. Magn Reson Med Sci 2022;21(1):182–94.
59. Carotenuto A, Cacciaguerra L, Pagani E, et al. Glymphatic system impairment in multiple sclerosis: relation with brain damage and disability. Brain 2022;145(8):2785–95.
60. Rocca MA, Margoni M, Battaglini M, et al. Emerging perspectives on MRI application in multiple sclerosis: moving from pathophysiology to clinical practice. Radiology 2023;307(5):e221512.
61. Wuerfel J, Bellmann-Strobl J, Brunecker P, et al. Changes in cerebral perfusion precede plaque formation in multiple sclerosis: a longitudinal perfusion MRI study. Brain 2004;127(1):111–9.
62. Lapointe E, Li DKB, Traboulsee AL, et al. What have we learned from perfusion MRI in multiple sclerosis? Am J Neuroradiol 2018;39(6):994–1000.
63. Adhya S, Johnson G, Herbert J, et al. Pattern of hemodynamic impairment in multiple sclerosis: dynamic susceptibility contrast perfusion MR imaging at 3.0 T. Neuroimage 2006;33(4):1029–35.
64. Lagana M, Pelizzari L, Baglio F. Relationship between MRI perfusion and clinical severity in multiple sclerosis. Neural Regen Res 2020;15(4):646–52.

Neuromyelitis Optica Spectrum Disorders and Myelin Oligodendrocyte Glycoprotein Antibody-Associated Disease

John H. Rees, MD[a,*], Torge Rempe, MD, PhD[b], Ibrahim Sacit Tuna, MD[c], Mayra Montalvo Perero, MD[c], Shyamsunder Sabat, MD[c], Tara Massini, MD[d], Joseph M. Yetto Jr, MD[c]

KEYWORDS

- Aquaporin-4 • Myelin oligodendrocyte glycoprotein
- Neuromyelitis optica spectrum disorders (NMOSD)
- Myelin oligodendrocyte glycoprotein antibody disease (MOGAD) • Optic neuritis

KEY POINTS

- Our understanding of white matter disease targeting the visual apparatus and the spinal cord has undergone substantial advances over the last 20 years.
- Antibodies against specific proteins: aquaporin-4 and myelin oligodendrocyte glycoprotein have been identified as pathologic, and serum assays are currently an important diagnostic tool for clinicians, in association with MR imaging.
- The pathogenesis of these processes, as well as related conditions including multiple sclerosis, acute disseminated encephalomyelitis (ADEM), seems to be a combined cellular and humoral autoimmune process which breaches the central nervous system immune barrier to attack white matter; however, research and clinical investigations are active and ongoing.
- Therapeutic regimens have shown substantial growth and development which is ongoing.

INTRODUCTION

Neuromyelitis optica and the more general term neuromyelitis optica spectrum disorders (NMOSD) refers to a group of auto immune neuroinflammatory diseases which target the optic nerves, the spinal cord, the brainstem, as well as the brain, in the order of decreasing frequency. The nomenclature, diagnostic criteria, clinical features, and treatment modalities for these conditions have undergone many iterations and modulations over the last two centuries since their initial clinical descriptions in the early 1800s.

The development of MR imaging in the 1980s greatly enhanced our ability to identify and characterize these conditions in living patients, and more recently we have achieved a higher degree of clarification and specificity due to the identification of specific antibody populations such as aquaporin-4 (AQP4) immunoglobulin (IgG) and myelin oligodendrocyte glycoprotein (MOG) antibodies found to be present in many patients.

Despite powerful and ongoing scientific advances, however, this group of conditions remains in the words of Jarius “etiopathogenetically heterogeneous,” and by this, we mean that there may be

[a] Neuroradiology, Department of Radiology, University of Florida College of Medicine; [b] UF Multiple Sclerosis / Neuroimmunology Fellowship, Department of Neurology, University of Florida, College of Medicine; [c] University of Florida at Gainesville, Gainesville, FL, USA; [d] University of Florida, Gainesville, FL, USA
* Corresponding author. UF Shands, Department of Radiology, Box 100374, Gainesville, FL 32614-0374.
E-mail address: jree0002@radiology.ufl.edu

Magn Reson Imaging Clin N Am 32 (2024) 233–251
https://doi.org/10.1016/j.mric.2023.12.001
1064-9689/24/

more than one etiology with varying degrees of penetrance and virulence within these conditions.[1,2] The science is incomplete and new data continues to be integrated into the conceptual frameworks used to diagnose, categorize, and treat these individuals with these conditions. Because the science is incomplete, the nomenclature remains imperfect and continues to evolve. Most of the cases we will discuss will be antibody-positive AQP4 or MOG-ab positive; however, there are a substantial number of similar cases which are seronegative to either marker. Based on what we do know, it is likely that we will discover other specific antibody targets in the future, such as glial fibrillary acidic protein (GFAP).[3]

The purpose of this work is to summarize and present the current state of our knowledge about these conditions and specifically to detail the variety and characteristics of the imaging findings seen in these patients and the implications for therapy and prognosis. In order to understand the present, we must at least glance at the past so we will begin with a brief recounting of the development of the nomenclatures which have been used up to the present.[4,5]

HISTORY

Beginning in the early 1800s diagnostic medicine and specifically diagnosis of neurologic conditions underwent substantial development in Europe. Cruveilhier, Carswell, Charcot, and other clinicians were aware of many patients who suffered from debilitating, variably progressive, neurologic injury and decline, and when these patients were studied postmortem, they were found to have multiple areas of focal injury in the white matter of the brain which had the tactile characteristic of hardening or scarring and this class of diseases became known as "multiple sclerosis" (MS), which literally means "multiple hardenings."[6]

Contemporaneous with the growth in understanding and diagnostic labeling of MS, a somewhat smaller cohort of patients was identified by a number of clinicians in a number of scattered reports who had somewhat similar pattern of intermittent progression of different symptoms primarily involving the visual apparatus and the spinal cord. These patients' symptoms had significant overlap with, and were sometimes grouped with, MS patients. The earliest distinct diagnostic label for these patients was "spinal amaurosis" in the 1837 by Sichel,[7] which signified that these patients suffered visual loss and spinal cord injury resulting in paraparesis sometimes progressing to paraplegia.

The first reported clinical description of this spinal amaurosis category of patients may have been by Antoine Portal who notably described a patient with visual loss, and spinal cord symptoms specifically without brain involvement for the first time in 1804.[8] Spinal amaurosis was mentioned again by John Abercrombie in his 1829 2nd edition text, with later reports including in 1844 by Giovanni Pescetto, in 1850 by Christopher Durant, and in1862 by Jacob Clarke.[9]

In 1894, Eugene Devic, in conjunction with his graduate student Fernand Gault, published a description of a patient with visual loss and spinal cord symptoms and for the first time used the term neuro myelitis Optica ("neuro-myelite optique aigue" in the original French), and in 1907 Peppo Achiotte, a Turkish neurologist published a similar case and made the suggestion that these conditions be eponymously described as Devic's disease.[9]

For more than a century "Devic's disease" was considered by most to be a subtype or variant of MS, although ironically Devic himself considered them to be separate and distinct in 1894.

In 2005, the discovery of AQP4 antibodies (ab) in patients with NMO symptoms[10] and subsequent studies showing distinct pathologic differences led to the final separation of NMOSD from MS.[11] This separation was made complex however by the undeniable presence of patients who were AQP4-ab negative, some of whom were simply MS patients with optic neuritis (ON), some who may have suffered from acute disseminated encephalomyelitis (ADEM), and some of whom would fall into other diagnostic categories.

In 2011, it was found that specific subtypes of MOG antibodies were elevated in patients with ON and cord lesions,[12] and this led to MOGs initial inclusion as a subtype of NMO; however, further work demonstrated that MOG, although exhibiting significant overlap with AQP4 disease, had other distinct imaging and clinical manifestations. This led to the term MOG antibody-associated disease (MOGAD), distinct from NMOSD. MOG had previously been found in patients with MS, and potentially implicated with classic MS as well as with ADEM,[13] but was initially determined not to be pathogenic. In 2011, this was clarified when it was found that only antibodies to a certain conformational state of MOG were pathogenic.[12] This emphasizes the important of correct and specific forms of antibody testing in these conditions.

The question of categorization of other non-AQP4 non-MOG-ab positive "seronegative NMO patients" remains to be fully understood. AQP4-ab-positive patients may have antibodies also to GFAP which is a ubiquitous component of glial cells; however, at the present time, this does not seem to contribute to active autoimmune reaction.

In summary, the current state of the science and of the terminology has advanced greatly but is still in flux. NMOSD is a broad category which means either NMOSD (disorder or disorders) and includes primarily AQP4-ab-positive patients as well as some seronegative patients. Some have suggested the term AQP4 channelopathy as a distinct entity but this has not been widely adopted. MOGAD is now recognized to be a separate condition with some clinical overlap with NMOSD. Both of these groups must be differentiated from MS patients with ON, and from ADEM, although MOG AD may overlap substantially with ADEM. In subsequent sections, we focus on AQP4 and MOGAD separately from a clinical standpoint and then evaluate and demonstrate their shared or overlapping imaging findings. It is reasonable to expect that these diagnostic categories will gain further specificity and change over time as our knowledge grows.

Aquaporin-4

Basic science

In 1992, Agre and colleagues discovered a cellular membrane protein which confers a high water permeability in central nervous system (CNS) tissues,[14] later designated AQP1 which was found to be one of a large family of proteins which facilitate bidirectional water movement across the

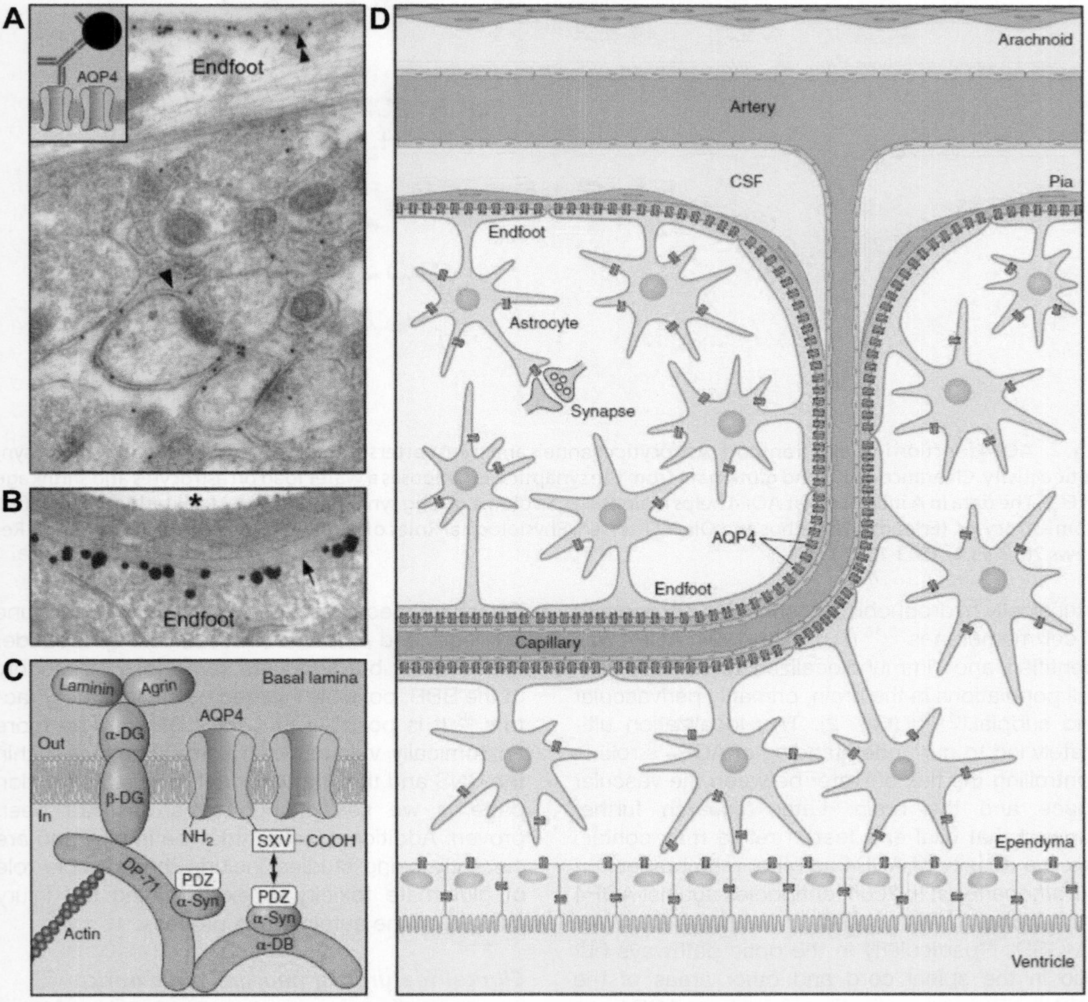

Fig. 1. AQP4 location on cell surfaces. (Søren Nielsen et al. Specialized Membrane Domains for Water Transport in Glial Cells: High-Resolution Immunogold Cytochemistry of Aquaporin-4 in Rat Brain. Journal of Neuroscience 1 January 1997, 17 (1) 171-180; DOI: 10.1523/JNEUROSCI.17-01-00171.1997. Copyright 1997 Society for Neuroscience.) (*A, B*) Electron micrograph showing AQP-4, (*C*) Diagram of AQP-4 in water channel, (*D*) Larger view of distribution of AQP-4 along water channels. (C, D) (Erlend A. Nagelhus and Ole P. Ottersen, Physiological Roles of Aquaporin-4 in Brain. Physiological Reviews 2013 93:4, 1543-1562.)[19,80]

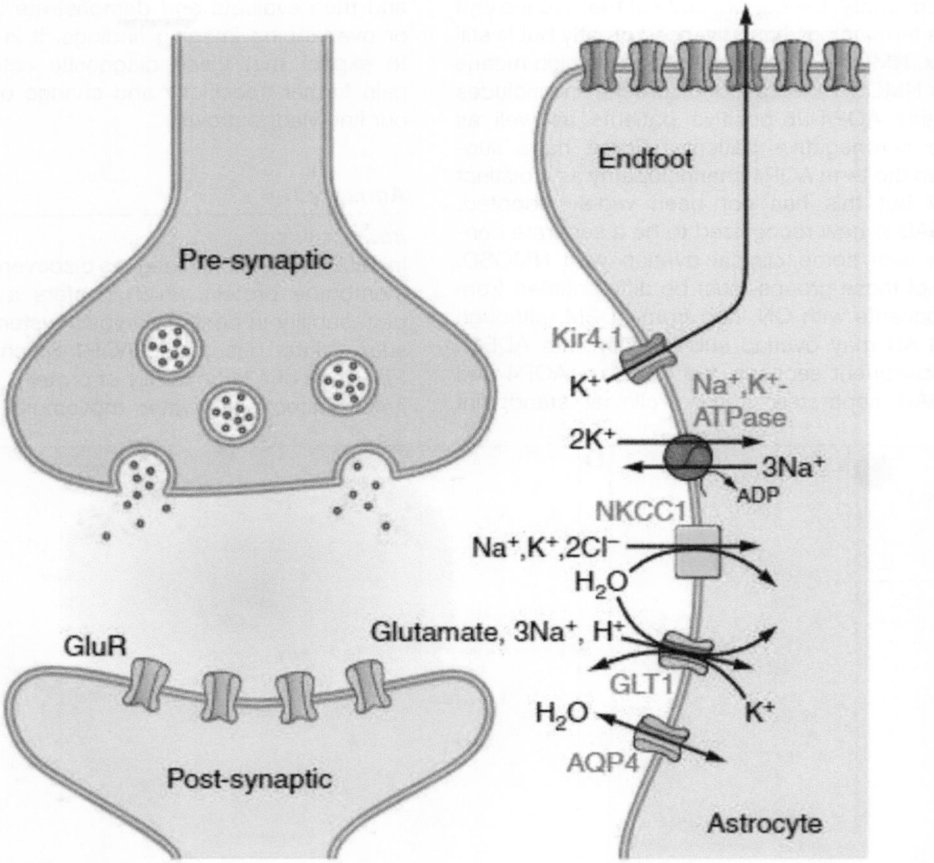

Fig. 2. AQP4 function in water transport. Astrocytic channels and transporters relevent for water transport during synaptic activity. Clearance ok K^+ and glutamate from the synaptic cleft imposes a water load on astrocytes and shrinkage of ECS. The data in A indicate that AQP4 helps maintain ECS volume during synaptic activity by facilitating water efflux from astrocytes. (Erlend A. Nagelhus and Ole P. Ottersen, Physiological Roles of Aquaporin-4 in Brain. Physiological Reviews 2013 93:4, 1543-1562.) [19,80]

intrinsically hydrophobic phospholipid component of cell membranes[15,16] (**Fig. 1**). In 1994, AQP4 was identified and "immunolocalized to specific glial cell populations in the brain, primarily perivascular and subpial."[17,18] (**Fig. 2**). This localization ultimately led to our understanding of AQP4's role in controlling the flux of water between the vascular space and the brain. Later research further showed that glial end feet in retina may contain 10x the density of AQP4 as other membranes.

Pathogenesis: In 2004, antibodies against AQP4 were found in high concentrations in patients with NMOSD,[20] particularly in the optic pathways but also in the spinal cord and other areas of the CNS.[10] The demyelination found in AQP4-ab-positive NMOSD occurs through a combined autoimmune response involving both activated T cells and IgG antibodies produced by B cells in the periphery which cross the blood brain barrier (BBB) in a primarily perivenous pattern[21] (**Fig. 3**). The exact mechanism of this loss of CNS immune privilege and immune cell trafficking is under active study but suggests some loss of integrity of the BBB, possibly initiated by inflammatory factors.[22] It is possible that the BBB may be more anatomically vulnerable in some locations within the CNS and this may account for the distribution patterns we see although this has not been proven. Additional factors may be in play and are currently being studied include the possible role of glutamate toxicity in exacerbating the injury caused by the autoimmune process.

Clinical features of neuromyelitis optica spectrum disorders

Epidemiology The age range for disease onset in NMOSD is wide (3–80 years) with an average age of onset at 40 years. There is a strong female predominance after adolescence with women constituting 70% to 90% of patients and a 9:1 female to

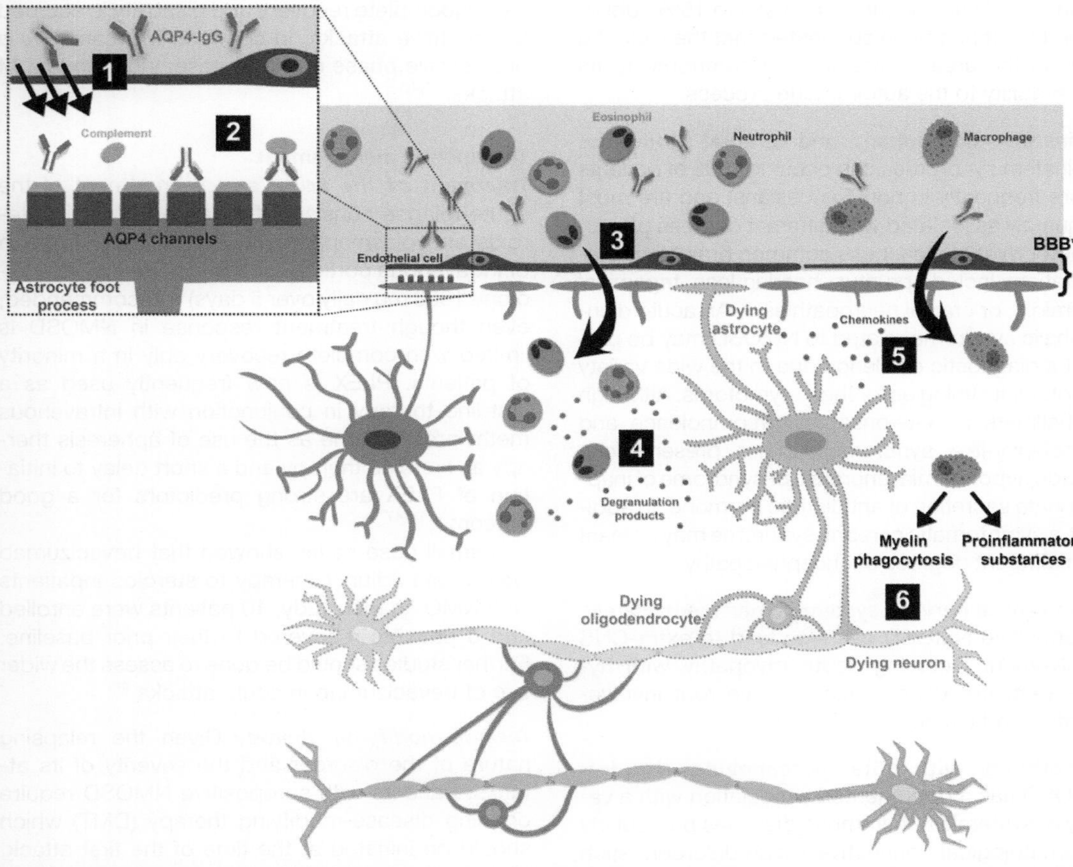

Fig. 3. Pathophysiology of AQP4 antibody disease (NMOSD).[23] (*From* Dutra BG, da Rocha AJ, Nunes RH, Maia ACM. Neuromyelitis optica spectrum disorders: spectrum of MR imaging findings and their differential diagnosis. Radiographics. 2018;38(1):169–93.)

male ratio. The prevalence ranges from 0.5/100.000 to 4/100.000 with significantly higher risk in patients of African-Caribbean background.[3,24,25]

Clinical presentation The six core clinical syndromes of NMOSD are (1) acute myelitis, (2) ON, (3) area postrema syndrome, (4) brainstem syndrome, (5) diencephalic syndrome, and (6) symptomatic cerebral syndrome.[26] An acute onset is characteristic for an NMOSD exacerbation, whereas hyperacute or prolonged (<4 hours and >4 weeks from onset to nadir, respectively) disease course is highly atypical and considered a red flag.[3,26]

Acute myelitis Acute myelitis is the most common presentation of NMOSD. Patients generally develop a severe acute myelopathy and present with a complete spinal cord syndrome with involvement of motor, sensory, and autonomic pathways with resulting sensorimotor para- or tetraparesis and bowel and bladder dysfunction.[3,27] The classic description of transverse myelitis in NMOSD is longitudinally extensive (extending more than three vertebral segments on MR imaging); however, short lesions and asymptomatic myelitis have been described in patients with positive AQP4 IgG.[28]

Optic neuritis ON is the second most common presentation of NMOSD. Commonly, it leads to severe vision loss in the bilateral eyes. As it primarily affects the posterior optic pathway, vision loss is often painless and disc edema is frequently absent in fundoscopic examination. Recovery is poor with a high rate (historically 41%) of NMOSD patients becoming legally blind.[3,27] However, the spectrum of the disease continues to grow and there is evidence of asymptomatic ON in approximately 17% of patients.[29]

Area postrema syndrome Area postrema syndrome characteristically presents with intractable nausea, vomiting, and/or hiccupping, and a gastrointestinal etiology may erroneously be presumed, leading to a delay in diagnosis.[25] Isolated area postrema syndrome can be seen in 7% to 10% of patients at initial diagnosis and 9% to 15% subsequently.[30] It has been suggested that the lack of a BBB in the area postrema may contribute to its vulnerability to the autoimmune process.[31]

Brainstem, diencephalic, and cerebral syndromes Brainstem syndromes can occur in 30% of patients (more frequently in non-Caucasians) and are most frequently associated with different degrees of oculomotor dysfunction. Less common brainstem presentations include pruritus, hearing loss, trigeminal neuralgia, or cranial neuropathies.[32] An acute diencephalic syndrome related to NMOSD may be present a diagnostic challenge due to the wide variety of potential etiologies for these symptoms. Although its hallmark is new-onset hypersomnolence and narcolepsy-like syndromes, other presentations include hypothermia, anorexia, or syndrome of inappropriate secretion of antidiuretic hormone. In addition, a symptomatic cerebral syndrome may present with different degrees of encephalopathy.[33]

Extra-central nervous system involvement Rarely, seropositive NMOSD can also lead to extra-CNS involvement including acute myopathy with hyper-creatinine-kinase-emia,[34] nerve root involvement,[35] and uveitis.[36]

Comorbidity with other autoimmune disorders NMOSD has a documented association with a variety of systemic autoimmune diseases particularly rheumatological connective tissue disorders such as systemic lupus erythematosus, Sjögren syndrome,[27] and myasthenia gravis.[37]

Racial and ethnic disparities African American patients are disproportionally likely to develop NMOSD. Furthermore, there are data that patients of African ancestry have a higher mortality rate.[38] A recent cohort showed that patients of black race were more likely to require ventilatory support.[39] Brain abnormalities in NMOSD are also more frequently observed in patients of African and Asian backgrounds.[40,41]

Laboratory data Cerebrospinal fluid (CSF) is significant for variable pleocytosis and increased total protein. In contrast to MS, cell counts greater than 50 cell/uL are commonly seen in up to 35% of patients. CSF-restricted oligoclonal bands are only present in approximately less than 20% of patients.[25,27] AQP4 antibodies have 83% sensitivity and 100% specificity; therefore, it is a great tool for diagnosis.[42]

Disease course Up to 96% of patients develop a relapsing disease course with the majority of patients experiencing the second attack within the first year of disease onset.[43] The attacks can often have incomplete recovery and disability is accrued by repetitive attacks. In contrast, MS can have a progressive phase of the disease, independent of attacks.[44,45]

Therapeutic management

Treatment of the acute attack Treatment of the acute relapse consists of intravenous corticosteroids and plasmapheresis (PLEX). Early initiation of intravenous corticosteroids (eg, methylprednisolone 1000 mg daily over 5 days) is recommended, even though treatment response in NMOSD is limited with complete recovery only in a minority of patients. PLEX is now frequently used as a first-line therapy in conjunction with intravenous methylprednisolone as the use of apheresis therapy as first-line therapy and a short delay to initiation of PLEX are strong predictors for a good outcome.[46,47]

A small case series showed that bevacizumab was a safe adjunct therapy to steroids inpatients with NMO. In this study, 10 patients were enrolled and 3 patients recovered to their prior baseline. Further studies should be done to assess the wider use of bevacizumab in acute attacks.[48]

Disease-modifying therapy Given the relapsing nature of the disorder and the severity of its attacks, patients with seropositive NMOSD require ongoing disease-modifying therapy (DMT) which should be initiated at the time of the first attack. Historically, azathioprine, mycophenolate mofetil (MMF), and prednisolone have been used,[3] but their use is nowadays discouraged given the availability of highly efficacious monoclonal antibodies. There are three main mechanisms of action that have been proven effective: (1) B-cell depletion, (2) interleukin-6 inhibition, and (3) complement inhibition.

B-cell depletion The chimeric anti-CD20 monoclonal antibody rituximab is not approved for the treatment of NMOSD by the Food and Drug Administration or the European Medicines Agency. However, its efficacy is overall well-documented in multiple randomized controlled trials[49,50] and meta-analyses.[51,52] The anti-CD19 monoclonal antibody inebilizumab is approved by the regulatory agencies of the United States and Europe after it has been shown superior to placebo in the pivotal N-Momentum trial.[53]

Interleukin-6 inhibition The subcutaneous anti-interleukin-6 monoclonal antibody satralizumab has also been shown to be effective in NMOSD in its two pivotal trials.[54,55] Limited data from a Phase 2 trial also exist for the anti-interleukin-6 monoclonal antibody tocilizumab.[56]

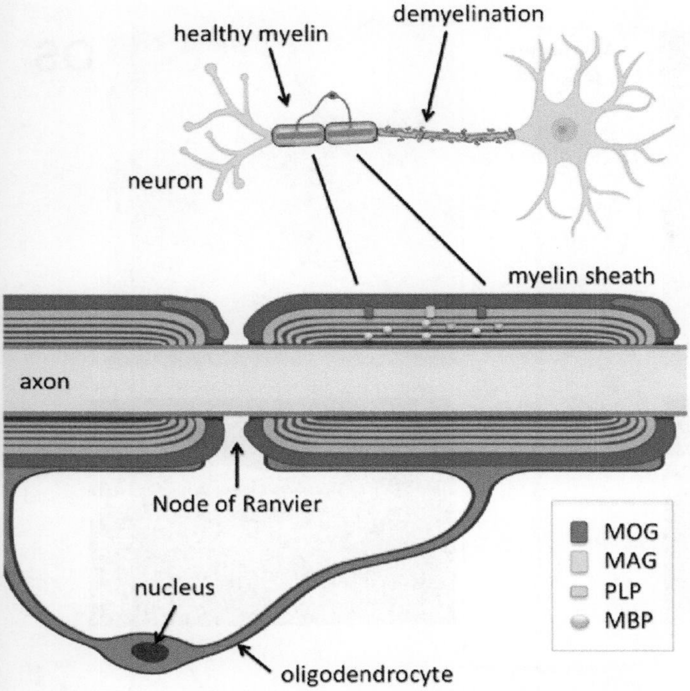

Fig. 4. Location of MOG on cell surface.[62]

Complement inhibition Complement inhibition has been proven to be a viable instrument for NMOSD disease modification. By binding C5 and inhibiting cleavage, the monoclonal antibodies eculizumab (PREVENT trial[57]) and ravulizumab (CHAMPION-NMOSD[58]) have been shown to be highly effective in NMOSD.

Multiple sclerosis disease-modifying therapies Of note, several MS DMT have been shown to potentially exacerbate NMO including interferon beta, natalizumab, and fingolimod.[59] This emphasizes the importance to evaluate for presence of the AQP4 antibody in demyelinating diseases with characteristics of NMOSD.

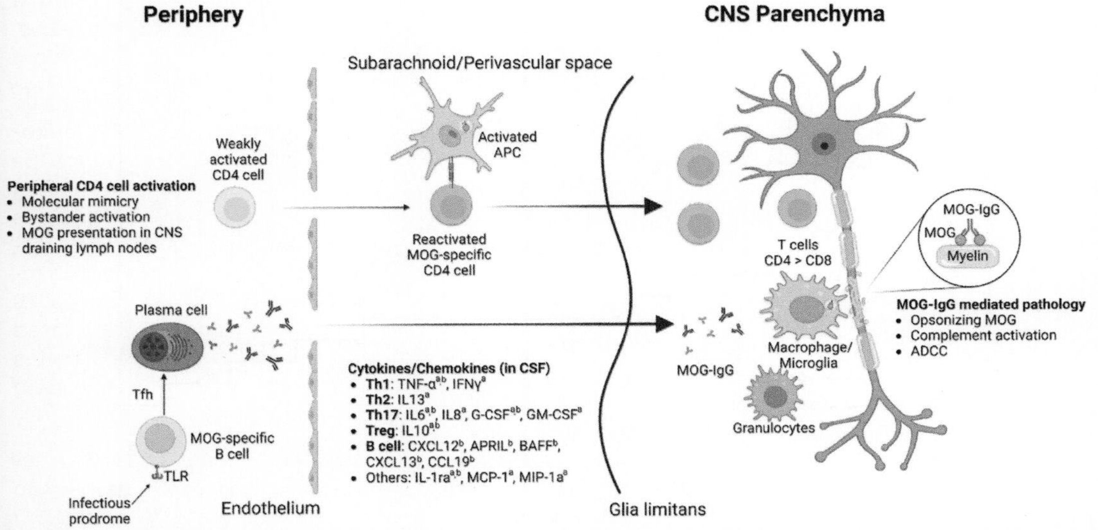

Fig. 5. Pathophysiology of MOGAD.[63] [a]Increased compared to MS. [b]Increased compared to MOG-ab negative demyelination. (*From* Corbali O, Chitnis T. Pathophysiology of myelin oligodendrocyte glycoprotein antibody disease. Front Neurol. 2023 Feb 28;14:1137998.)

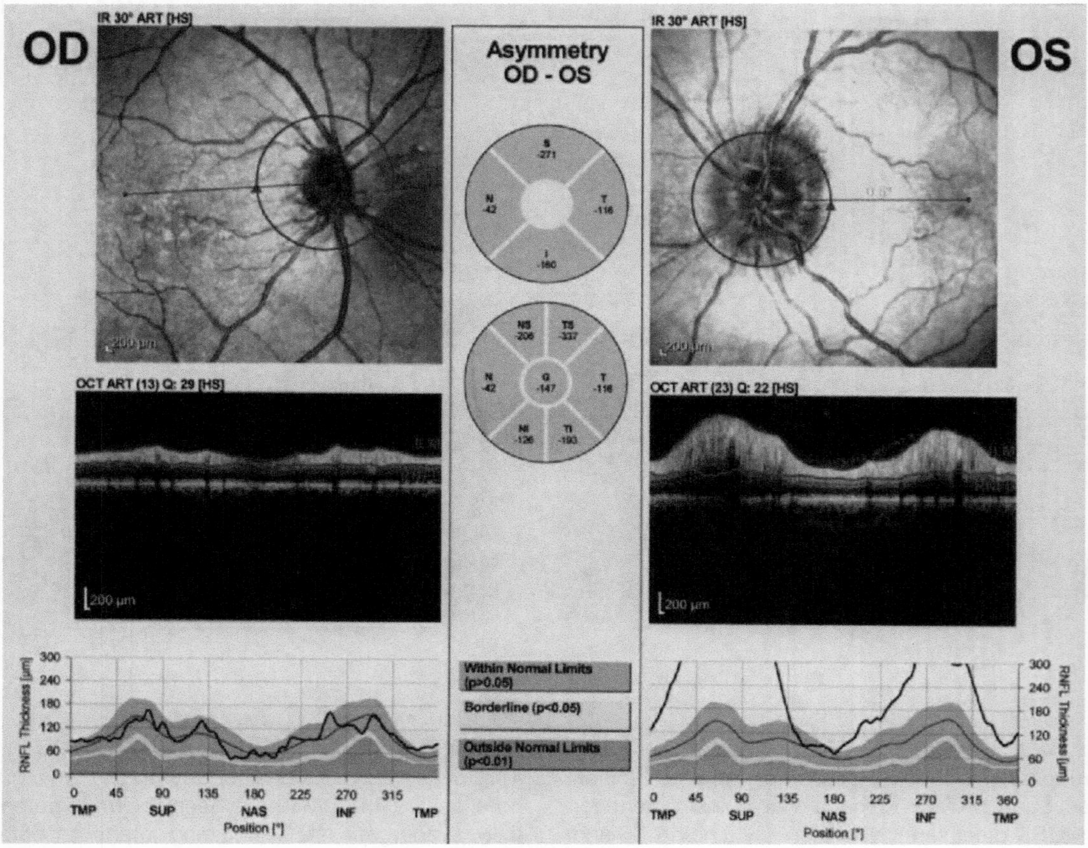

Fig. 6. Optical coherence tomography (OCT) shows left optic disc edema in MOGAD.

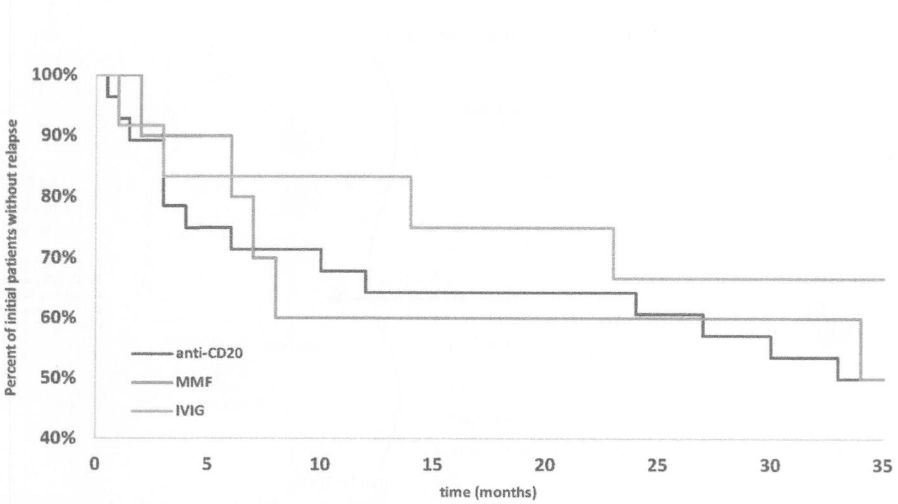

Fig. 7. Treatment failure for different immunotherapies in MOGAD over 3 years.[76] (*From* Elfasi A, Alkabie S, Rodriguez E, Kinkel R, Graves J, Rempe T. Treatment Response to Different Immunotherapies in Relapsing Myelin-Oligodendrocyte Glycoprotein Antibody - Associated Disease (MOGAD). ACTRIMS Forum 2023; 2023 Feb 24.)

	MOGAD	NMOSD	MS
Clinical findings			
Presentation at onset	Optic neuritis	Optic neuritis	Optic neuritis
	Transverse myelitis	Transverse myelitis	Transverse myelitis
	Brainstem demyelination	Brainstem demyelination	Brainstem demyelination
	ADEM	Area postrema syndrome	Internuclear ophthalmoplegia
	Cerebral cortical encephalitis		
Infectious Prodrome (6–14)	37.5–70% (at least once)	15–35% (at least once)	27–48% (of all relapses)
Course (6, 15–17)	Monophasic (40–50%)	Monophasic (10%)	Relapsing Remitting (90%)
	Relapsing (50–55%)	Relapsing (90%)	Secondary Progressive (half of relapsing remitting patients develop secondary progressive disease)
			Primary Progressive/Relapsing Progressive (10%)
Annualized Relapse Rate (excluding the first attack) (5, 18, 19) [Overall: treated and untreated]	0.23 (pediatric, overall) 0.35 (adult, overall)	0.91 (adult, untreated) 0.18 (adult, treated)	1.13 (pediatric, overall) 0.40 (adult, overall)
Progression independent of relapse activity (PIRA) (20, 21)	No	No	Yes

Fig. 8. Comparison of clinical findings in MOGAD, NMOSD, and MS, respectively.[63] (*From* Corbali O, Chitnis T. Pathophysiology of myelin oligodendrocyte glycoprotein antibody disease. Front Neurol. 2023 Feb 28;14:1137998.)

	MOGAD	NMOSD	MS
Radiology			
Optic nerve (22, 23)	Bilateral	Bilateral	Unilateral
	Lengthier	Lengthier	Shorter
	Anterior optic pathway involvement	Posterior optic pathway involvement	
	ON head swelling		
	Perineural sheath enhancement		
Spinal cord (22, 24, 25)	LETM	LETM	Shorter lesions
	Multiple lesions	Central cord	Multiple lesions
	H-sign (gray matter restricted lesion)		Dorsal/lateral lesions
	Central cord		Conus medullaris
	Conus medullaris		
Brain (22, 26, 27)	Less supratentorial lesions	Less supratentorial lesions	More supratentorial lesions
	ADEM-like lesions	Diencephalon (i.e., hypothalamus and thalamus)	Cortical/juxtacortical lesions
		Dorsal midbrain (i.e., area postrema)	
Contrast Enhancement rate within 4 weeks of the attack (Indication of BBB damage) (23, 24, 28)	ON (94%) Myelitis (26–70%)	ON (100%) Myelitis (78%)	ON (75%) Myelitis (75%)
Leptomeningeal enhancement (29–31)	33% (Pediatric)	6%	21% (1.5 or 3 T field)
	6% (Adult)		79% (7 T field)
Central Vein sign (average CVS+ rate) (22)	≈10%	<10%	>40%
Slowly expanding lesions (25, 32)	No	Not studied	Yes
Paramagnetic rim lesions (32–34)	Not studied	Rare	Yes (due to iron laden microglia/macrophage)

Fig. 9. Comparison of imaging findings between MOGAD, NMOSD, and MS, respectively.[63] (*From* Corbali O, Chitnis T. Pathophysiology of myelin oligodendrocyte glycoprotein antibody disease. Front Neurol. 2023 Feb 28;14:1137998.)

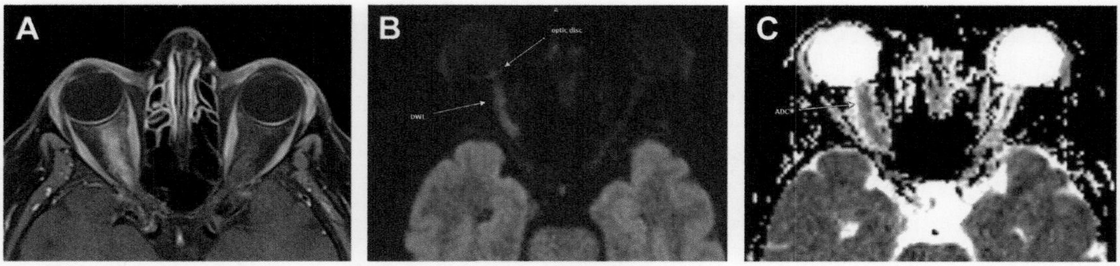

Fig. 10. Optic neuritis in MOGAD. (*A–C*) Axial post-gadolinium, DWI, and ADC images showing enhancement and restricted diffusion in the R optic nerve and sheath. ADC, automated diffusion coefficient; DWI, diffusion weighted imaging.

Myelin Oligodendrocyte Glycoprotein Antibody-Associated Disease

Basic science

"Myelin oligodendrocyte glycoprotein (MOG) is a quantitatively minor component of CNS myelin whose function remains relatively unknown."[60] The exact function of MOG is uncertain with primary hypothesis some aspect of myelin "sheath completion and/or maintenance"[61] with more detailed considerations such as (1) a cellular adhesive molecule, (2) a regulator of oligodendrocyte microtubule stability, and (3) a mediator of interactions between myelin and the immune system, in particular, the complement cascade."[60] Key features include peripheral location on the myelin sheath and relatively late addition to the developing myelin which may play a role in antigenicity (**Fig. 4**).

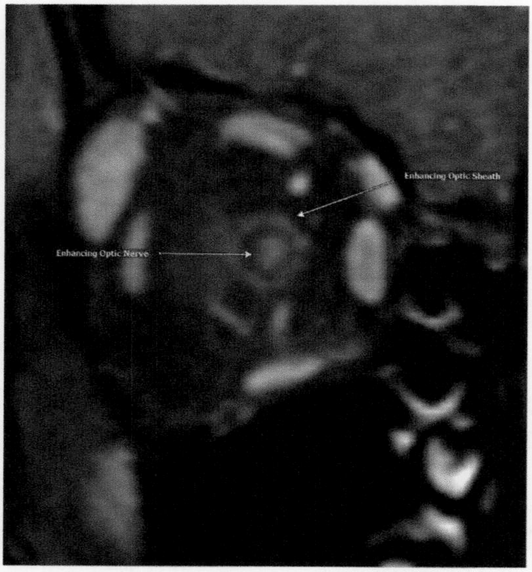

Fig. 11. Optic perineuritis in MOGAD: Coronal T1 post-gadolinium fat-saturated image shows shaggy corona of enhancement in the optic nerve sheath.

Pathogenesis:MOGAD proceeds by a complex interplay of cellular and humoral immunity. In the peripheral blood, activation of T cells and production of IgG antibodies by B cells occurs. These both enter the CNS and initiate an inflammatory complement cascade attacking the myelin sheath. The pattern of injury is typically perivenous but surrounding small veins, lacking the central vein location which produces the "central vein sign" and the appearance of Dawson's finger in MS (**Fig. 5**).

Clinical features of myelin oligodendrocyte glycoprotein antibody-associated disease

Epidemiology MOGAD patients are overall younger than NMOSD patients at disease onset and the first manifestation of the disorder will frequently occur in childhood as early as in infancy.[25] The female-to-male ratio is approximately 1:1 and there does not seem to be a predominance related to different ethnic or racial backgrounds.[64]

Clinical presentation The core clinical demyelinating events of MOGAD are defined as ON, transverse myelitis, ADEM, cerebral monofocal or polyfocal deficits, brainstem or cerebellar deficits, and cerebral cortical encephalitis (CCE).[65]

Optic neuritis ON is by far the most common clinical syndrome of adult MOGAD patients and the disease has a remarkable predilection for the visual pathway. It is frequently bilateral with either bilateral simultaneous or bilateral sequential occurrence. It predominantly affects the anterior optic pathway, and optic disc edema is frequently present[25,64] and may be detected on direct ophthalmoscopy and confirmed on optical coherence tomography (OCT) (**Fig. 6**). In contrast to MS, disc edema can be accompanied by peripapillary hemorrhages and macular star.[66] ON in MOGAD will usually lead to significant clinical deficit with reduction to finger counting in most cases and patients frequently develop pain with extraocular movements.[64] Of note, new-onset, often severe periorbital and

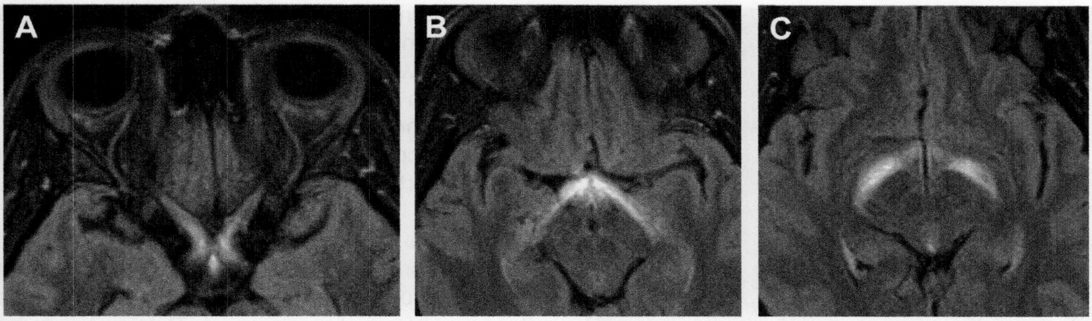

Fig. 12. Retrochiasmatic involvement in MOGAD. (*A–C*) Axial FLAIR images show hyperintensity in the chiasm, immediately posterior to the chiasm, and following visual pathways into the basal forebrain and thalami, respectively.

frontotemporal headache is often described a few days before the visual deficit. MOGAD can present as a chronic relapsing inflammatory optic neuropathy-like phenotype.[64] Of note, relapsing ON can present in 30% to 50% of patient with MOGAD and can be seen in pediatric patients with ON presenting concomitantly with ADEM and adult or pediatric patients that present with ON and transverse myelitis.[65]

Myelitis Acute myelitis in MOGAD is the second most common presentation in adults and frequently leads to severe acute myelopathy with sensorimotor para- or tetraparesis with associated bowel and bladder dysfunction. Longitudinally extensive (involving three or more spinal segments) myelitis occurs in approximately 60% of patients, but short lesions can occur. Short lesions are more common in MOGAD than AQP4 disease.[65,67] Rarely, myelitis may also lead to associated nerve root involvement in the context of combined central and peripheral demyelination.[25,68]

Brainstem and cerebellar syndrome MOGAD can lead to a brainstem syndrome that most frequently presents with ophthalmoplegia as well as a cerebellar syndrome with varying degrees of truncal and appendicular ataxia.[25] One case series showed that brainstem or cerebellar involvement was present in 34% of MOGAD patients and approximately 40% were asymptomatic and it usually does not present in isolation but rather as a multifocal demyelination.[69]

Acute disseminated encephalomyelitis ADEM leading to varying degrees of encephalopathy and associated multifocal neurologic deficits is the most common pediatric presentation in more than 50% of cases[64] and occurs less common in adults. MOGAD seems to be the most common cause of ADEM and MOG-IgG1 seropositivity has been reported in up to 50% of ADEM cases.[70]

Meningoencephalitis MOGAD can rarely (<10%) present with the clinical syndrome of meningoencephalitis including a variety of meningo-cortical (unilateral CCE, fluid attenuated inversion recovery [FLAIR]-hyperintense Lesions in Anti-MOG-associated Encephalitis with Seizures [FLAMES]) and predominantly meningeal (FLAIR-variable Unilateral Enhancement of the Leptomeninges, MOG antibody-associated aseptic meningitis) presentations. Patients will present with headaches,

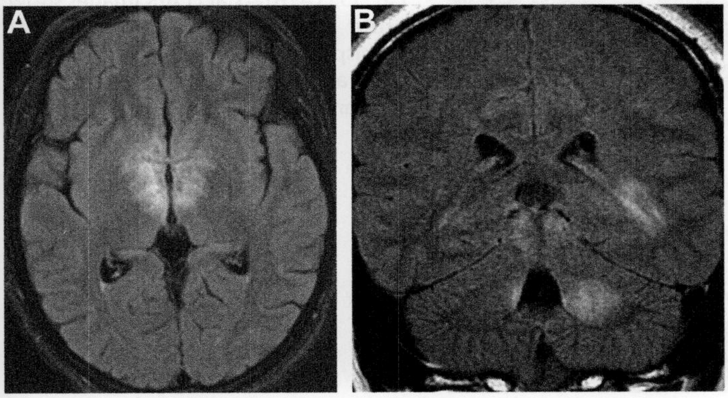

Fig. 13. (*A, B*) Axial and coronal FLAIR images in AQP4 positive patient showing involvement of the bilateral thalami and deep cerebellar nuclei.

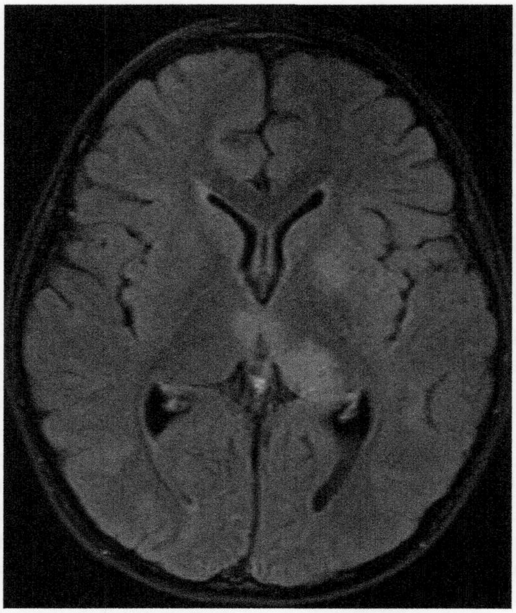

Fig. 14. Axial FLAIR image showing left thalamic and basal ganglia involvement in MOGAD.

encephalopathy, meningismus, nausea, and vomiting as well as seizures. CSF is usually significant for a marked (>100 cells/mm^3) neutrophilic (>25% neutrophils) pleocytosis.[71]

One study showed that 10% of patients with MOGAD present with acute symptomatic seizures and all of those patients had encephalitis features either CCE or ADEM on MR imaging. Eighty-three percentage of patients had pediatric disease onset, and focal motor seizures were the most common semiology with the majority (91%) of patients being seizure free at last follow-up.[72]

Laboratory data Similarly to NMOSD, pleocytosis can be pronounced (>50 cells/mm^3) in approximately 35% of MOGAD cases. There has also been described a rare co-seropositivity of MOG and N-methyl-D-aspartate receptor antibodies.[64,71] Of note, low titers such as 1:20–1:40 can be associated with false positives, especially in patients with MS; therefore, careful interpretation of the results and correlation with the clinical picture is of great importance.[73,74]

Disease course A relapsing disease course occurs in approximately two-thirds of patients. The first relapse usually occurs within the first 6 months to a year from disease onset. Relapses can be seen after steroid taper.[75] However, some patients may experience their first relapse multiple years after their initial presentation.[72,76] There is some evidence that associates persistent seropositivity with disease relapses but further studies are needed to assess the implications of persistent seropositivity with response to treatment and prognosis.[70]

Therapeutic management

Treatment of the acute attack The mainstay of treatment of the acute attack is intravenous methylprednisolone 1000 mg daily for 5 days, and most of the MOGAD patients experience an excellent response to corticosteroids.[25] The use of oral prednisolone may also be effective.[64] There are limited data that PLEX and intravenous immunoglobulins can be helpful as treatment of acute exacerbations if the response to intravenous methylprednisolone is insufficient. Usually, a taper of oral prednisolone is initiated over 3 months to prevent the risk of an early relapse.[77,78]

Disease-modifying therapy Generally, initiation of immunotherapy should be considered once a relapsing course of the disorder has been established. However, data for DMT in MOGAD are limited as there are mainly data from retrospective case series available to date. Although efficacy of B-cell depletion in an antibody-mediated demyelinating

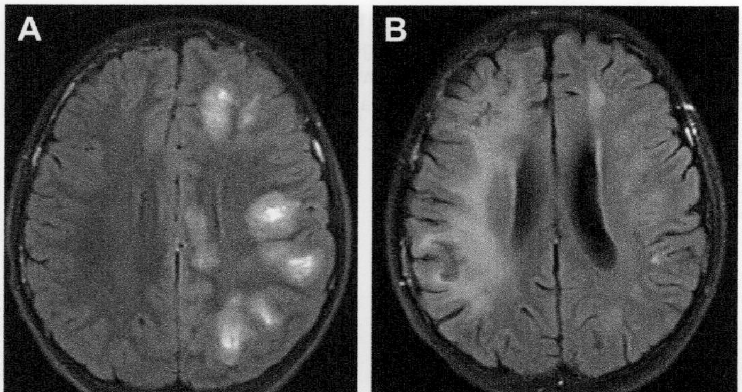

Fig. 15. (*A, B*) Axial FLAIR images show acute white matter lesions in left hemisphere and chronic encephalomalacia and gliosis right hemisphere in the same MOGAD patient.

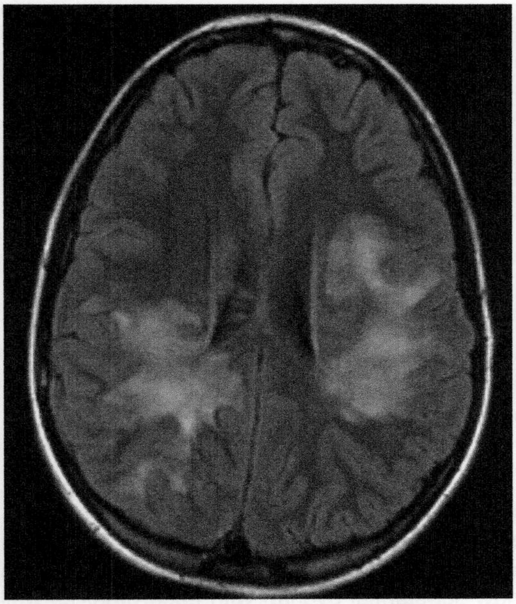

Fig. 16. Patchy bilateral areas of white matter hyperintensity in AQP4 NMOSD.

disorder could be expected, data of anti-CD20 therapy has not been convincing in MOGAD with treatment failure in ≥50% of cases. Similarly, MMF also showed high relapse rates ≥50%. Intravenous immunoglobulins seem to have the best data so far with the majority of patients remaining relapse-free on treatment.[76,79]

Clinical trials There are two ongoing Phase 3 trials to evaluate satralizumab (METEOROID: A Study to Evaluate the Efficacy, Safety, Pharmacokinetics, and Pharmacodynamics of Satralizumab in Patients With Myelin Oligodendrocyte Glycoprotein Antibody-Associated Disease) and rozanolixizumab (cosMOG: A Study to Evaluate the Efficacy and Safety of Rozanolixizumab in Adult Participants With Myelin Oligodendrocyte Glycoprotein [MOG] Antibody-associated Disease) in MOGAD (**Fig. 7**).

Comparison and Differences Between Neuromyelitis Optica Spectrum Disorders, Myelin Oligodendrocyte Glycoprotein Antibody-Associated Disease, and Multiple Sclerosis: Clinical and Imaging

Separating and distinguishing between these entities on a clinical basis is by no means simple, but as the table points out (**Fig. 8**), there are a few criteria which, if present, may help. MOGAD is more commonly associated with an ADEM like episode and in younger patients. NMOSD is more likely to produce the area postrema syndrome. Patients with typical MS not infrequently exhibit internuclear ophthalmoplegia. In addition, both NMOSD and MOGAD typically are more likely to exhibit a monophasic time course, whereas MS is more commonly relapsing and remitting.

Also, on imaging, there is more similarity than there are distinctive differences, but some features may be helpful as shown in **Fig. 9**. MS typically shows a preponderance of supratentorial lesions including "Dawsons Fingers." MOGAD and NMOSD both favor longer and bilateral areas of ON, although not necessarily simultaneous, and optic perineuritis (OPN) is more typical for MOGAD. MOGAD tends to involve anterior optic nerve

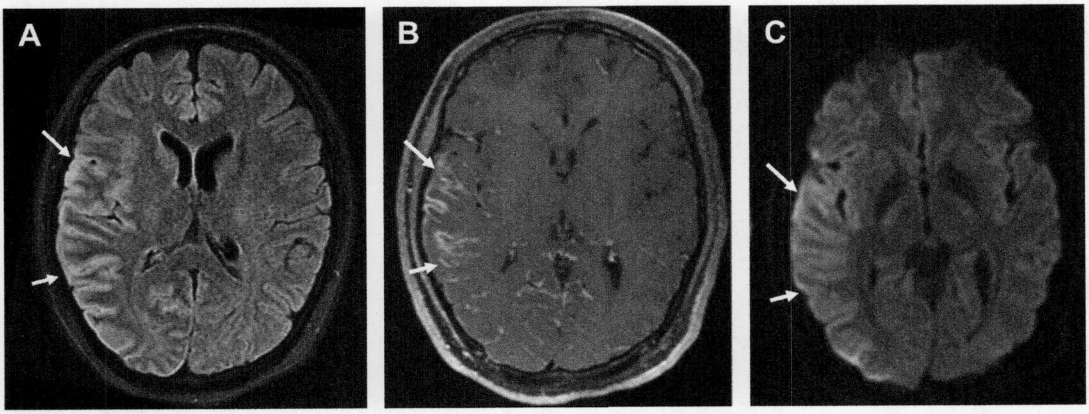

Fig. 17. Axial FLAIR (*A*), post-contrast T1 (*B*), and DWI (*C*) demonstrate asymmetric right temporal cortical swelling with FLAIR hyperintensity, cortical/leptomeningeal enhancement, and diffusion restriction in a patient with MOGAD and seizures. These combined imaging and clinical findings represent "FLAIR Hyperintensity in MOGAD Encephalitis with Seizures" (FLAMES). *Arrows* indicate (*A*) cortical FLAIR hyperintensity; (*B*) Cortical enhancement; (*C*) cortical diffusion restriction.

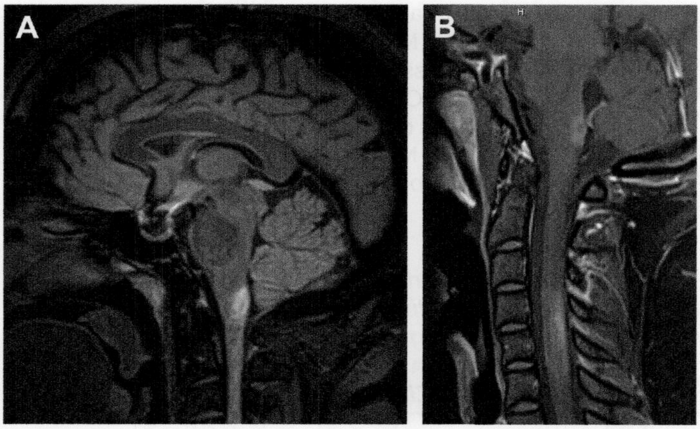

Fig. 18. Area postrema involvement in AQP4 positive NMOSD patients. (*A*) Sagittal FLAIR image shows hyperintensity in lower medulla in the expected location of the area postrema. (*B*) Sagittal and axial post-gad images in a different patient showing enhancement in area postrema and also in cervical cord.

segments and AQP4 tends to be more posterior and even retrochiasmatic. MOGAD and NMOSD also both tend to produce more and longer areas of transverse myelitis than MS, referred to as longitudinally extensive transverse myelitis (LETM), and MOGAD in particular is associated with lower cord lesions including the conus medullaris. NMOSD is suggested by the presence of abnormality in the lower medulla in the expected location of the area postrema.

Imaging examples

As we have detailed above, the imaging findings in patients with NMOSD/AQP4 and MOGAD patients show substantial overlap with each other as well as with other neuroinflammatory conditions such as typical MS and ADEM. MOG specifically may also be implicated in the etiology of ADEM as discussed above.

One primary common imaging and clinical feature of these conditions is ON which can be

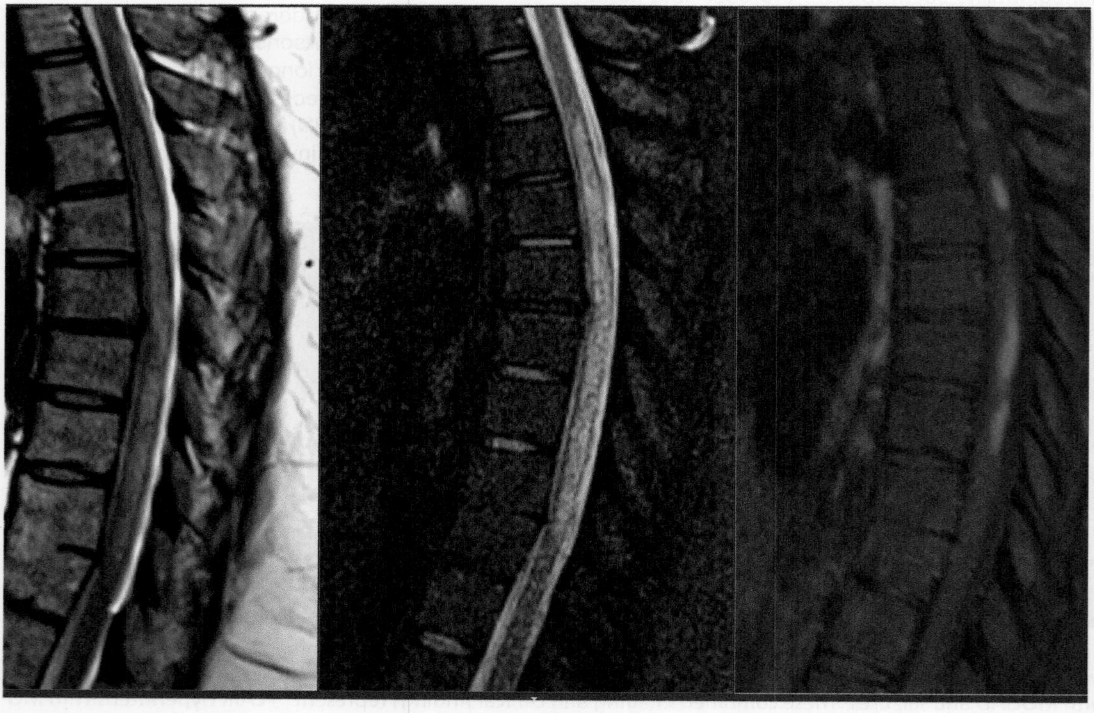

Fig. 19. Sagittal T2, FLAIR, and post-gad T1 images in AQP4 patient with LETM showing diffuse patchy T2 and FLAIR hyperintensity with patchy enhancement over at least seven vertebral levels in the thoracic cord.

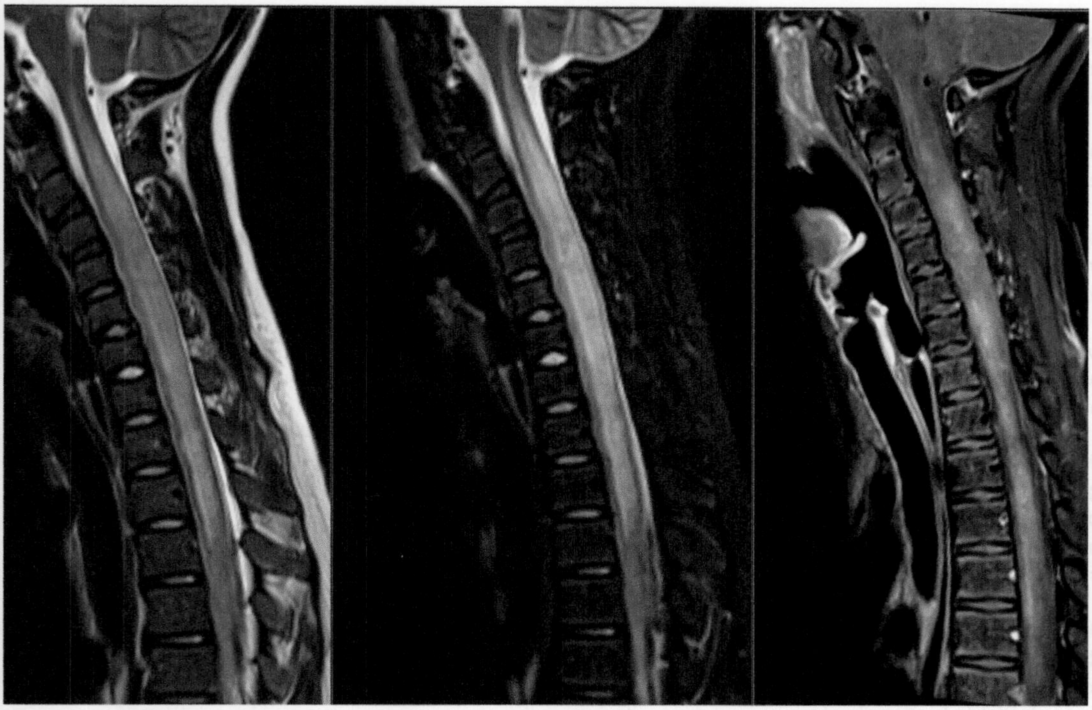

Fig. 20. Sagittal T2, FLAIR, and post-gad T1 images in MOGAD patient with LETM showing extensive T2 and FLAIR hyperintensity with cord swelling and diffuse heterogeneous enhancement extending from the craniocervical junction into the upper thoracic cord.

unilateral or bilateral, diffuse or focal, and may be asynchronous. MR imaging findings of ON are diffuse or focal T2 hyperintensity, and enhancement of the optic nerve, usually imaged on post-gad fat-sat axial and coronal images as well as diffusion restriction (**Fig. 10**).

Often, we see not only enhancement of the optic nerve itself but also a corona like enhancement and short tau inversion recovery (STIR) signal in the optic nerve sheath which is referred to as OPN. The exact etiology of OPN is uncertain; however, it may represent a sympathetic inflammation

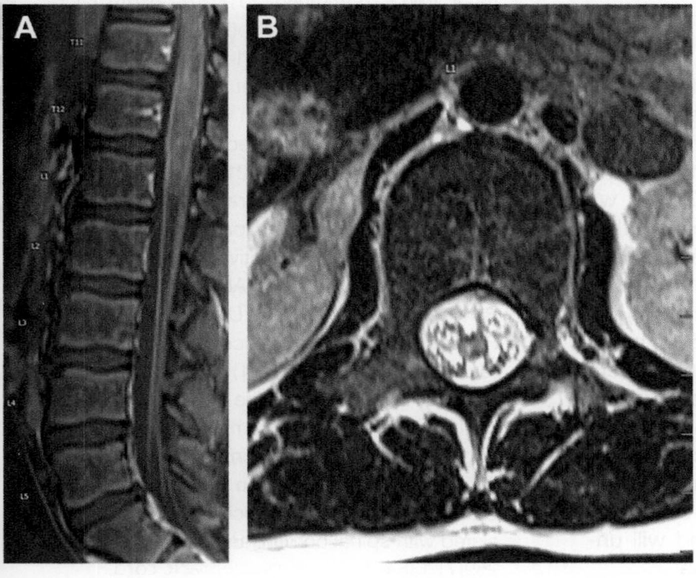

Fig. 21. (*A*) Sagittal T1 post-gad fat-saturated image shows enhancing conus medullaris and cauda equina, and (*B*) axial T2 image at the conus shows T2 hyperintensity with the distal most cord typical for MOGAD.

of the sheath due to adjacent optic nerve inflammation similar to leptomeningeal enhancement which may be seen in the brain (**Fig. 11**).

The inflammatory changes in the optic nerves may extend to the chiasm and further to the retrochiasmatic optic pathways as well (**Fig. 12**).

Within brain parenchyma, both AQP4 and MOGAD may involve basal ganglia, bilateral, thalami, and other gray matter structures including the deep cerebellar nuclei (**Figs. 13** and **14**).

Both NMOSD and MOGAD may acutely involve patchy areas of supratentorial white matter (WM) and may also cause permanent visible damage as evidence of chronic injury (**Figs. 15** and **16**).

In a small number of patients, estimated at less than 10%, MOGAD can cause a superficial meningoencephalitis resulting in seizures, and this has been given the acronym FLAMES for "FLAIR-hyperintense Lesions in Anti-MOG-associated Encephalitis with Seizures" (**Fig. 17**).

In the brainstem, involvement may focally involve the area postrema or chemoreceptor trigger zone in the lower medulla adjacent to the obex, and this may result in a clinical presentation of vomiting or uncontrollable hiccupping known as area postrema syndrome (**Fig. 18**).

Spinal involvement is relatively typical in both AQP4 and MOGAD and may be focal or commonly present as longitudinally extensive transverse myelitis (LETM) with typical imaging features of hyperintensity on T2 and inversion recobery (IR) and diffuse or patchy enhancement (**Figs. 19** and **20**).

More characteristically in MOGAD, involvement of the conus medullaris and cauda equina may be seen (**Fig. 21**).

SUMMARY

Our understanding of the spectrum of CNS inflammatory autoimmune demyelinating disease has broadened greatly over the last 10 to 20 years. As we explore the clinical, laboratory, and imaging manifestations of both NMOSD and MOGAD, we broaden our understanding of the complex pathophysiology of these conditions and their clinical and imaging manifestations. As we learn more, new questions arise which include our growing understanding of the breakdown of CNS immune integrity, which allows peripheral immune system components to enter and cause damage within the CNS and the interplay of different components of the immune response in different clinical entities. The attempt to clarify the category of seronegative syndromes and to identify additional specific antibody targets is ongoing and will undoubtedly bear fruit in the years to come.

CLINICS CARE POINTS

- MR imaging is the preferred imaging modality in patients with optic neuritis, transverse myelitis, and associated brain syndromes with specific targeted protocols including the use of gadolinium providing higher degrees of diagnostic specificity.
- Serum antibody testing in association with careful clinical evaluation can provide highly specific information, which can guide various therapeutic algorithms.
- There is substantial overlap both in imaging and in clinical features between these various entities.
- Neuroimaging may also display certain more specific patterns which can be useful in combination with clinical data to provide accurate and specific diagnoses.

DISCLOSURE

No commercial or financial conflicts of interest for any authors.

REFERENCES

1. Jarius S, Wildemann B. Aquaporin-4 antibodies (NMO-IgG) as a serological marker of neuromyelitis optica: a critical review of the literature. Brain Pathol 2013;23(6):661–83.
2. Jarius S, Wildemann B, Paul F. Neuromyelitis optica: clinical features, immunopathogenesis and treatment. Clin Exp Immunol 2014;176(2):149–64.
3. Costello F. Neuromyelitis optica spectrum disorders. Continuum 2022;28(4):1131–70.
4. Kaseka ML, Ly M, Yea C, et al. Impact of COVID-19 public health measures on myelin oligodendrocyte glycoprotein IgG-associated disorders in children. Mult Scler Relat Disord 2021;56:103286.
5. Messina S, Mariano R, Geraldes R, et al. The influence of smoking on the pattern of disability and relapse risk in AQP4-positive Neuromyelitis Optica Spectrum Disorder, MOG-Ab Disease and Multiple Sclerosis. Mult Scler Relat Disord 2021;49:102773.
6. Pearce JMS. Historical descriptions of multiple sclerosis. Eur Neurol 2005;54(1):49–53.
7. Jarius S, Wildemann B. The history of neuromyelitis optica. Part 2: "Spinal amaurosis". or how it all began. J Neuroinflammation 2019;16(1):280.
8. Jarius S, Wildemann B. The case of the Marquis de Causan (1804): an early account of visual loss associated with spinal cord inflammation. J Neurol 2012;259(7):1354–7.

9. Jarius S, Wildemann B. The history of neuromyelitis optica. J Neuroinflammation 2013;10:8.
10. Lennon VA, Kryzer TJ, Pittock SJ, et al. IgG marker of optic-spinal multiple sclerosis binds to the aquaporin-4 water channel. J Exp Med 2005; 202(4):473–7.
11. Lopez JA, Denkova M, Ramanathan S, et al. Pathogenesis of autoimmune demyelination: from multiple sclerosis to neuromyelitis optica spectrum disorders and myelin oligodendrocyte glycoprotein antibody-associated disease. Clin Transl Immunology 2021; 10(7):e1316.
12. Mader S, Gredler V, Schanda K, et al. Complement activating antibodies to myelin oligodendrocyte glycoprotein in neuromyelitis optica and related disorders. J Neuroinflammation 2011;8:184.
13. Egg R, Reindl M, Deisenhammer F, et al. Anti-MOG and anti-MBP antibody subclasses in multiple sclerosis. Mult Scler 2001;7(5):285–9.
14. Preston GM, Carroll TP, Guggino WB, et al. Appearance of water channels in Xenopus oocytes expressing red cell CHIP28 protein. Science 1992; 256(5055):385–7.
15. King LS, Kozono D, Agre P. From structure to disease: the evolving tale of aquaporin biology. Nat Rev Mol Cell Biol 2004;5(9):687–98.
16. Solenov E, Watanabe H, Manley GT, et al. Sevenfold-reduced osmotic water permeability in primary astrocyte cultures from AQP-4-deficient mice, measured by a fluorescence quenching method. Am J Physiol Cell Physiol 2004;286(2):C426–32.
17. Nielsen S, Nagelhus EA, Amiry-Moghaddam M, et al. Specialized membrane domains for water transport in glial cells: high-resolution immunogold cytochemistry of aquaporin-4 in rat brain. J Neurosci 1997;17(1):171–80.
18. Nagelhus EA, Veruki ML, Torp R, et al. Aquaporin-4 water channel protein in the rat retina and optic nerve: polarized expression in Müller cells and fibrous astrocytes. J Neurosci 1998;18(7):2506–19.
19. Wolburg H, Wolburg-Buchholz K, Fallier-Becker P, et al. Structure and functions of aquaporin-4-based orthogonal arrays of particles. Int Rev Cell Mol Biol 2011;287:1–41.
20. Lennon VA, Wingerchuk DM, Kryzer TJ, et al. A serum autoantibody marker of neuromyelitis optica: distinction from multiple sclerosis. Lancet 2004;364(9451):2106–12.
21. Louveau A, Harris TH, Kipnis J. Revisiting the mechanisms of CNS immune privilege. Trends Immunol 2015;36(10):569–77.
22. Marchetti L, Engelhardt B. Immune cell trafficking across the blood-brain barrier in the absence and presence of neuroinflammation. Vasc Biol 2020; 2(1). H1–18.
23. Dutra BG, da Rocha AJ, Nunes RH, et al. Neuromyelitis optica spectrum disorders: spectrum of MR imaging findings and their differential diagnosis. Radiographics 2018;38(1):169–93.
24. Pandit L, Asgari N, Apiwattanakul M, et al. Demographic and clinical features of neuromyelitis optica: A review. Mult Scler 2015;21(7):845–53.
25. Rempe T, Tarhan B, Rodriguez E, et al. Anti-MOG associated disorder-Clinical and radiological characteristics compared to AQP4-IgG+ NMOSD-A single-center experience. Mult Scler Relat Disord 2021; 48:102718.
26. Wingerchuk DM, Banwell B, Bennett JL, et al. International consensus diagnostic criteria for neuromyelitis optica spectrum disorders. Neurology 2015; 85(2):177–89.
27. Chen H, Liu S-M, Zhang X-X, et al. Clinical Features of Patients with Multiple Sclerosis and Neuromyelitis Optica Spectrum Disorders. Chin Med J 2016; 129(17):2079–84.
28. Flanagan EP, Weinshenker BG, Krecke KN, et al. Asymptomatic myelitis in neuromyelitis optica and autoimmune aquaporin-4 channelopathy. Neurol Clin Pract 2015;5(2):175–7.
29. Shah SS, Morris P, Buciuc M, et al. Frequency of Asymptomatic Optic Nerve Enhancement in a Large Retrospective Cohort of Patients With Aquaporin-4+ NMOSD. Neurology 2022;99(8):e851–7.
30. Shosha E, Dubey D, Palace J, et al. Area postrema syndrome: Frequency, criteria, and severity in AQP4-IgG-positive NMOSD. Neurology 2018; 91(17):e1642–51.
31. Popescu BFG, Lennon VA, Parisi JE, et al. Neuromyelitis optica unique area postrema lesions: nausea, vomiting, and pathogenic implications. Neurology 2011;76(14):1229–37.
32. Zekeridou A, Lennon VA. Aquaporin-4 autoimmunity. Neurol Neuroimmunol Neuroinflamm 2015;2(4): e110.
33. Tarhan B, Rempe T, Rahman S, et al. A Comparison of Pediatric- and Adult-Onset Aquaporin-4 Immunoglobulin G-Positive Neuromyelitis Optica Spectrum Disorder: A Review of Clinical and Radiographic Characteristics. J Child Neurol 2022;37(8–9):727–37.
34. Guo Y, Lennon VA, Popescu BFG, et al. Autoimmune aquaporin-4 myopathy in neuromyelitis optica spectrum. JAMA Neurol 2014;71(8):1025–9.
35. Takai Y, Misu T, Nakashima I, et al. Two cases of lumbosacral myeloradiculitis with anti-aquaporin-4 antibody. Neurology 2012;79(17):1826–8.
36. Carey AR, Arevalo JF. Neuromyelitis optica spectrum disorder and uveitis. Ocul Immunol Inflamm 2022;30(7–8):1747–50.
37. McKeon A, Lennon VA, Jacob A, et al. Coexistence of myasthenia gravis and serological markers of neurological autoimmunity in neuromyelitis optica. Muscle Nerve 2009;39(1):87–90.
38. Mealy MA, Kessler RA, Rimler Z, et al. Mortality in neuromyelitis optica is strongly associated with

African ancestry. Neurol Neuroimmunol Neuroinflamm 2018;5(4):e468.
39. Zhao-Fleming HH, Valencia Sanchez C, Sechi E, et al. CNS Demyelinating Attacks Requiring Ventilatory Support With Myelin Oligodendrocyte Glycoprotein or Aquaporin-4 Antibodies. Neurology 2021; 97(13):e1351–8.
40. Kim S-H, Mealy MA, Levy M, et al. Racial differences in neuromyelitis optica spectrum disorder. Neurology 2018;91(22):e2089–99.
41. Flanagan EP, Cabre P, Weinshenker BG, et al. Epidemiology of aquaporin-4 autoimmunity and neuromyelitis optica spectrum. Ann Neurol 2016;79(5): 775–83.
42. Redenbaugh V, Montalvo M, Sechi E, et al. Diagnostic value of aquaporin-4-IgG live cell based assay in neuromyelitis optica spectrum disorders. Mult Scler J Exp Transl Clin 2021;7(4). 20552173211052656.
43. Ma X, Kermode AG, Hu X, et al. Risk of relapse in patients with neuromyelitis optica spectrum disorder: Recognition and preventive strategy. Mult Scler Relat Disord 2020;46:102522.
44. Mealy MA, Wingerchuk DM, Greenberg BM, et al. Epidemiology of neuromyelitis optica in the United States: a multicenter analysis. Arch Neurol 2012; 69(9):1176–80.
45. Wingerchuk DM, Hogancamp WF, O'Brien PC, et al. The clinical course of neuromyelitis optica (Devic's syndrome). Neurology 1999;53(5):1107–14.
46. Kleiter I, Gahlen A, Borisow N, et al. Apheresis therapies for NMOSD attacks: A retrospective study of 207 therapeutic interventions. Neurol Neuroimmunol Neuroinflamm 2018;5(6):e504.
47. Bonnan M, Valentino R, Debeugny S, et al. Short delay to initiate plasma exchange is the strongest predictor of outcome in severe attacks of NMO spectrum disorders. J Neurol Neurosurg Psychiatr 2018;89(4):346–51.
48. Mealy MA, Shin K, John G, et al. Bevacizumab is safe in acute relapses of neuromyelitis optica. Clin Exp Neuroimmunol 2015;6(4):413–8.
49. Tahara M, Oeda T, Okada K, et al. Safety and efficacy of rituximab in neuromyelitis optica spectrum disorders (RIN-1 study): a multicentre, randomised, double-blind, placebo-controlled trial. Lancet Neurol 2020;19(4):298–306.
50. Nikoo Z, Badihian S, Shaygannejad V, et al. Comparison of the efficacy of azathioprine and rituximab in neuromyelitis optica spectrum disorder: a randomized clinical trial. J Neurol 2017;264(9):2003–9.
51. Gao F, Chai B, Gu C, et al. Effectiveness of rituximab in neuromyelitis optica: a meta-analysis. BMC Neurol 2019;19(1):36.
52. Giovannelli J, Ciron J, Cohen M, et al. A meta-analysis comparing first-line immunosuppressants in neuromyelitis optica. Ann Clin Transl Neurol 2021; 8(10):2025–37.
53. Cree BAC, Bennett JL, Kim HJ, et al. Inebilizumab for the treatment of neuromyelitis optica spectrum disorder (N-MOmentum): a double-blind, randomised placebo-controlled phase 2/3 trial. Lancet 2019;394(10206):1352–63.
54. Traboulsee A, Greenberg BM, Bennett JL, et al. Safety and efficacy of satralizumab monotherapy in neuromyelitis optica spectrum disorder: a randomised, double-blind, multicentre, placebo-controlled phase 3 trial. Lancet Neurol 2020;19(5):402–12.
55. Yamamura T, Kleiter I, Fujihara K, et al. Trial of satralizumab in neuromyelitis optica spectrum disorder. N Engl J Med 2019;381(22):2114–24.
56. Zhang C, Zhang M, Qiu W, et al. Safety and efficacy of tocilizumab versus azathioprine in highly relapsing neuromyelitis optica spectrum disorder (TANGO): an open-label, multicentre, randomised, phase 2 trial. Lancet Neurol 2020;19(5):391–401.
57. Pittock SJ, Berthele A, Fujihara K, et al. Eculizumab in Aquaporin-4-Positive Neuromyelitis Optica Spectrum Disorder. N Engl J Med 2019;381(7):614–25.
58. Pittock SJ, Barnett M, Bennett JL, et al. Ravulizumab in Aquaporin-4-Positive Neuromyelitis Optica Spectrum Disorder. Ann Neurol 2023;93(6):1053–68.
59. Traub J, Häusser-Kinzel S, Weber MS. Differential Effects of MS Therapeutics on B Cells-Implications for Their Use and Failure in AQP4-Positive NMOSD Patients. Int J Mol Sci 2020;(14):21.
60. Johns TG, Bernard CC. The structure and function of myelin oligodendrocyte glycoprotein. J Neurochem 1999;72(1):1–9.
61. Roth MP, Malfroy L, Offer C, et al. The human myelin oligodendrocyte glycoprotein (MOG) gene: complete nucleotide sequence and structural characterization. Genomics 1995;28(2):241–50.
62. Pi K-S, Sang Y, Straus SK. Viral Proteins with PxxP and PY Motifs May Play a Role in Multiple Sclerosis. Viruses 2022;14(2):281.
63. Corbali O, Chitnis T. Pathophysiology of myelin oligodendrocyte glycoprotein antibody disease. Front Neurol 2023;14:1137998.
64. Sechi E, Cacciaguerra L, Chen JJ, et al. Myelin Oligodendrocyte Glycoprotein Antibody-Associated Disease (MOGAD): A Review of Clinical and MRI Features, Diagnosis, and Management. Front Neurol 2022;13:885218.
65. Banwell B, Bennett JL, Marignier R, et al. Diagnosis of myelin oligodendrocyte glycoprotein antibody-associated disease: International MOGAD Panel proposed criteria. Lancet Neurol 2023;22(3):268–82.
66. Parrotta E, Kister I. The expanding clinical spectrum of myelin oligodendrocyte glycoprotein (MOG) antibody associated disease in children and adults. Front Neurol 2020;11:960.
67. Mariano R, Messina S, Kumar K, et al. Comparison of Clinical Outcomes of Transverse Myelitis Among Adults With Myelin Oligodendrocyte Glycoprotein

Antibody vs Aquaporin-4 Antibody Disease. JAMA Netw Open 2019;2(10):e1912732.
68. Vazquez Do Campo R, Stephens A, Marin Collazo IV, et al. MOG antibodies in combined central and peripheral demyelination syndromes. Neurol Neuroimmunol Neuroinflamm 2018;5(6):e503.
69. Banks SA, Morris PP, Chen JJ, et al. Brainstem and cerebellar involvement in MOG-IgG-associated disorder versus aquaporin-4-IgG and MS. J Neurol Neurosurg Psychiatr 2020. https://doi.org/10.1136/jnnp-2020-325121.
70. López-Chiriboga AS, Majed M, Fryer J, et al. Association of MOG-IgG Serostatus With Relapse After Acute Disseminated Encephalomyelitis and Proposed Diagnostic Criteria for MOG-IgG-Associated Disorders. JAMA Neurol 2018 Nov 1;75(11):1355–63.
71. Elfasi A, Alkabie S, Rodriguez E, et al. Anti-myelin oligodendrocyte glycoprotein (anti-MOG) meningoencephalitis. ACTRIMS Forum; 2023.
72. Montalvo M, Khattak JF, Redenbaugh V, et al. Acute symptomatic seizures secondary to myelin oligodendrocyte glycoprotein antibody-associated disease. Epilepsia 2022;63(12):3180–91.
73. Sechi E, Buciuc M, Pittock SJ, et al. Positive predictive value of myelin oligodendrocyte glycoprotein autoantibody testing. JAMA Neurol 2021;78(6):741–6.
74. Levy M, Yeh EA, Hawkes CH, et al. Implications of Low-Titer MOG Antibodies. Mult Scler Relat Disord 2022;59:103746.
75. Ramanathan S, Mohammad S, Tantsis E, et al. Clinical course, therapeutic responses and outcomes in relapsing MOG antibody-associated demyelination. J Neurol Neurosurg Psychiatr 2018;89(2):127–37.
76. Elfasi A, Alkabie S, Rodriguez E, et al. Treatment Response to Different Immunotherapies in Relapsing Myelin-Oligodendrocyte Glycoprotein Antibody - Associated Disease (MOGAD). ACTRIMS Forum 2023;2023.
77. Satukijchai C, Mariano R, Messina S, et al. Factors Associated With Relapse and Treatment of Myelin Oligodendrocyte Glycoprotein Antibody-Associated Disease in the United Kingdom. JAMA Netw Open 2022;5(1):e2142780.
78. Jurynczyk M, Messina S, Woodhall MR, et al. Clinical presentation and prognosis in MOG-antibody disease: a UK study. Brain 2017;140(12):3128–38.
79. Chen JJ, Flanagan EP, Bhatti MT, et al. Steroid-sparing maintenance immunotherapy for MOG-IgG associated disorder. Neurology 2020;95(2):e111–20.
80. Nagelhus EA, Ottersen OP. Physiological roles of aquaporin-4 in brain. Physiol Rev 2013;93(4):1543–62.

Toxic and Drug-Related White Matter Diseases of the Brain and Spine

Amit Agarwal, MD[a], John H. Rees, MD[b], Shyamsunder Sabat, MD[b,*]

KEYWORDS

• Toxic • Drug • White matter • MR imaging

KEY POINTS

- Wide range of endogenous and exogenous toxins can alter the delicately balanced brain microenvironment.
- Toxic-metabolic leukoencephalopathy can have acute or subacute to chronic course depending on the underlying insult.
- Therapeutic agents form the major category of exogenous toxins with significant increase during the last decade, driven by the new immunotherapeutic agents.
- Classic imaging findings of acute toxic leukoencephalopathy (ATL) include bilateral symmetric white matter restricted diffusion.
- Intramyelinic edema is the most common mechanism for reversible restricted diffusion seen in ATL.

INTRODUCTION

The brain microenvironment is delicately balanced by numerous physiologic mechanisms primarily through the blood–brain barrier. Apart from the main factors including oxygen, carbon dioxide, and the pH level, the physiologic environment also includes metabolic substrates, neurotransmitters, and electrolytes. This can however be disturbed following exposure to diverse endogenous and exogenous toxins, resulting in a wide range of toxic and metabolic encephalopathies. Clinically, these conditions usually present acutely with mental status changes, confusion, delirium, and are frequently seen in an emergency setting. However, the effect of the toxins can be more gradual and long-standing with a subacute to chronic clinical course. Imaging with MRI forms the cornerstone in the evaluation of these entities, both for acute and nonacute presentations, with few entities having classic radiographic features, whereas others being nonspecific. Accurate diagnosis by the radiologist and rapid correction of the underlying abnormality is vital to avoid any long-term neurologic complications.[1] The entire list of endogenous and exogenous toxins is long. In this review, we focus on the imaging abnormalities resulting from exogenous toxins and primarily resulting in white matter toxicity (leukoencephalopathy) and myelopathy. The list of white matter toxins has been broadly classified into 4 categories (**Fig. 1**) of therapeutic agents, drugs of abuse, environmental toxins, and occupational (industrial) exposure. The class with the most significant recent increase in neurologic complications is that of therapeutic agents, driven by the significant increased usage of immunotherapy during the last decade. Although, in this review, we focus on leukoencephalopathies, it is important to note that some imaging overlap with variable involvement of cortical and deep gray matter may occur with some of these toxins.[2,3]

Funding information: None.
[a] Department of Radiology, Mayo Clinic, 4500 San Pablo Road, Jacksonville, FL 32224, USA; [b] Department of Radiology, University of Florida at Gainesville, 1600 Southwest Archer Road, Gainesville, FL 32608, USA
* Corresponding author.
E-mail address: ssab0003@radiology.ufl.edu

Magn Reson Imaging Clin N Am 32 (2024) 253–275
https://doi.org/10.1016/j.mric.2023.12.002
1064-9689/24/

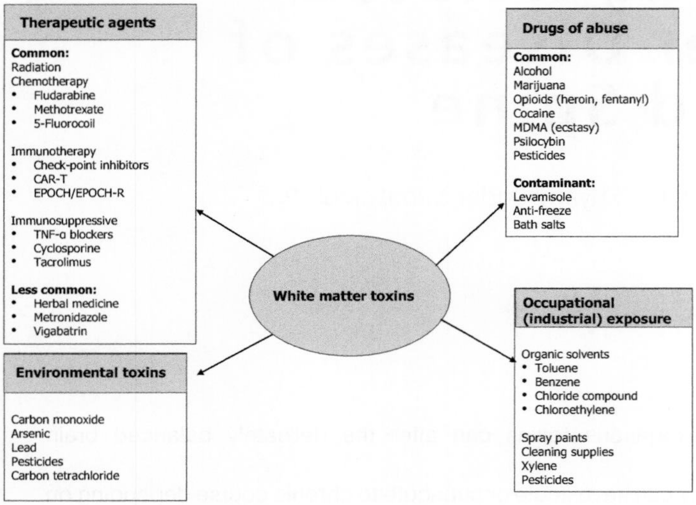
Therapeutic agents
Common:
Radiation
Chemotherapy
• Fludarabine
• Methotrexate
• 5-Fluorocoil
Immunotherapy
• Check-point inhibitors
• CAR-T
• EPOCH/EPOCH-R
Immunosuppressive
• TNF-α blockers
• Cyclosporine
• Tacrolimus
Less common:
• Herbal medicine
• Metronidazole
• Vigabatrin
Drugs of abuse
Common:
Alcohol
Marijuana
Opioids (heroin, fentanyl)
Cocaine
MDMA (ecstasy)
Psilocybin
Pesticides
Contaminant:
Levamisole
Anti-freeze
Bath salts
White matter toxins
Occupational (industrial) exposure
Organic solvents
• Toluene
• Benzene
• Chloride compound
• Chloroethylene
Spray paints
Cleaning supplies
Xylene
Pesticides
Environmental toxins
Carbon monoxide
Arsenic
Lead
Pesticides
Carbon tetrachloride

Fig. 1. This figure outlines the 4 major categories of white matter toxins with the common and uncommon causes. Therapeutic agents (including radiation) and "illicit" drugs of abuse are much more common than the other 2 categories.

CEREBRAL EDEMA

Conventionally, cerebral edema has been divided into cytotoxic edema and vasogenic edema, with the former seen in the context of ischemic insult with restricted diffusion and the latter occurring around space occupying lesions and showing facilitated (increased) diffusion. Cytotoxic edema involves the gray matter and is irreversible, signifying cell death. However, vasogenic edema involves the white matter, spares the cortex, has T2/fluid attenuated inversion recovery (FLAIR) hyperintensity secondary to fluid accumulation in extracellular space and shows increased apparent diffusion coefficient (ADC) values. Although these 2 major categories still form the vast majority of cerebral edema identified, the concepts of excitotoxic injury and intramyelinic edema has gained prominence during the last decade.[4] **Fig. 2** provides a basic illustration of the most important alterations affecting brain tissue in each type of edema. Intramyelinic edema represents nonneurotoxic edema where fluid accumulates within the periaxonal space or spaces between myelin layers. Although this is a potential extracellular space, it is histologically isolated from other extracellular spaces by the zonula occludens (tight junction), and this forms the basis of reversible restricted diffusion. Edema limited to the intramyelinic cleft results in completely reversible restricted diffusion, primarily limited to white matter, and is commonly seen in acute toxic leukoencephalopathies, mimicking ischemic stroke (**Fig. 3**). However, when associated with intracellular edema of astrocytes, oligodendrocytes, and axons, it results in irreversible or partially reversible restricted

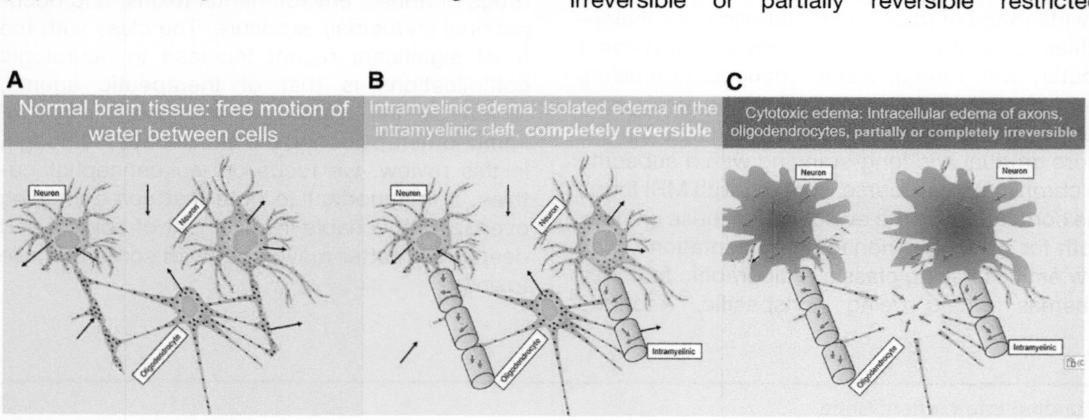

Fig. 2. Types of cerebral edema. (*A*) Free motion of water between cells in normal brain tissue. (*B*) Intramyelinic edema with swollen myelin sheath, with water trapped in the intramyelinic clefts and is completely reversible. Normal diffusion of water between axons, oligodendrocytes, and extracellular space. (*C*) Cytotoxic edema with intracellular edema of axons, oligodendrocytes along with intramyelinic edema. This is partially or completely irreversible.

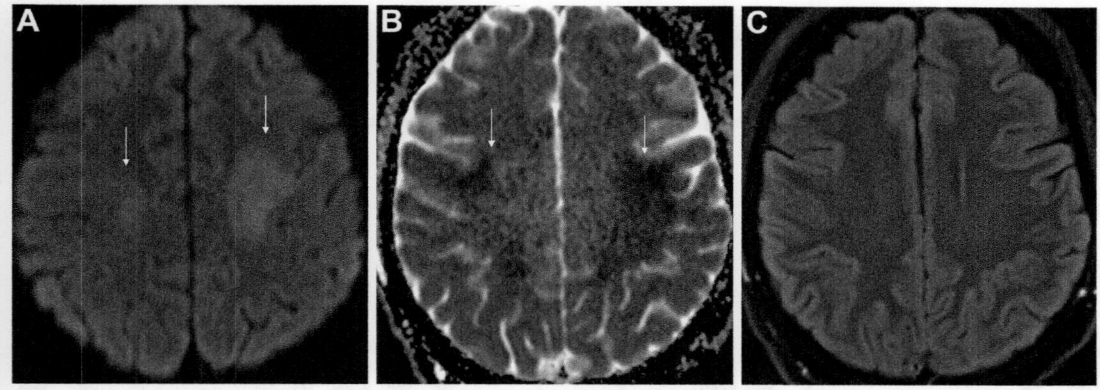

Fig. 3. ATL 3 days after intrathecal methotrexate in a 23-year-old girl with leukemia. Diffusion image (*A*) reveals asymmetric areas of restricted diffusion in bilateral centrum semiovale with corresponding low ADC values (*B*) (*arrows*). No definite signal abnormality noted on T2/FLAIR image (*C*).

diffusion and forms the basis of pathologic conditions such as ischemic stroke. This discussion is relevant in the context of toxic leukoencephalopathies because vast majority of these insults with restricted diffusion is secondary to reversible intramyelinic edema, which may, however, progress to intracellular edema and result in permanent tissue damage.[5]

IMAGING PATTERNS OF NEUROTOXICITY

Glutamate is the dominant and most important excitatory amino acid and is the primary neurotransmitter responsible for important neurologic functions such as cognition, memory, and movement. Neurotoxicity secondary to exogenous or endogenous toxins is primarily driven by excitotoxic brain injury characterized by rapid intense glutamate release setting up the stage for intramyelinic edema with possibility of cascade effect and cell injury. Although the glutamate receptors are widely distributed, some sites are more vulnerable to insult compared with others, resulting in a specific anatomic pattern of brain changes.[4] A great example would be the vulnerability of splenium of corpus callosum to wide range of toxins resulting in the relatively recent proposal of the term "cytotoxic lesion of the corpus callosum" (CLOCC), an umbrella term for all these entities.[6] However, this terminology is erroneous because it is now confirmed that most of these lesions are reversible, and the underlying pattern of edema is more "intramyelinic" rather than true "cytotoxic." Deep gray matter nuclei including the basal ganglia and the dentate nuclei form the most vulnerable structures in excitotoxic brain insult followed by cortical gray matter. However, because we are focusing on white matter changes, in this article, the common patterns would include symmetric periventricular white matter involvement with gray matter sparing. This is a pattern that defines acute toxic leukoencephalopathy (ATL), secondary to intramyelinic edema with high chance of reversibility and better outcomes, following rapid correction.[7] Other patterns include patchy asymmetric white matter changes (demyelination pattern), involvement of the corticospinal tracts, isolated involvement of the corpus callosum, parieto-occipital subcortical vasogenic edema, and central brainstem involvement. **Fig. 4** provides an illustration of common imaging patterns in toxic leukoencephalopathies and highlights the common underlying causes. These patterns of white matter changes may coexist along with or without concomitant involvement of gray matter (**Fig. 5**). Two of the frequent imaging patterns/conditions include posterior reversible encephalopathy syndrome (PRES) with typical imaging findings including vasogenic edema in the parieto-occipital white matter and focal restricted diffusion within the splenium of corpus callosum (CLOCC). Both these entities have a wide range of etiologic differentials and the pathophysiology and vulnerability of these regions to insult is still poorly understood. These might occasionally occur along with other manifestations of toxic leukoencephalopathy (**Fig. 6**). Unlike ATL, chronic persistent diffuse brain injury resulting from cumulative or repeated exposures over months or years results in chronic toxic encephalopathy. This includes occupational (industrial) and environmental exposures to solvents or less frequently heavy metals. These patients usually present with varying degrees of cognitive changes with or without cerebellar symptoms. Finally, cord involvement (myelopathy) in isolation or along with brain involvement can be seen secondary to numerous toxic disorders, such as heroin intake, neurolathyrism, radiation-induced, and nitrous oxide. These usually involve the peripheral white

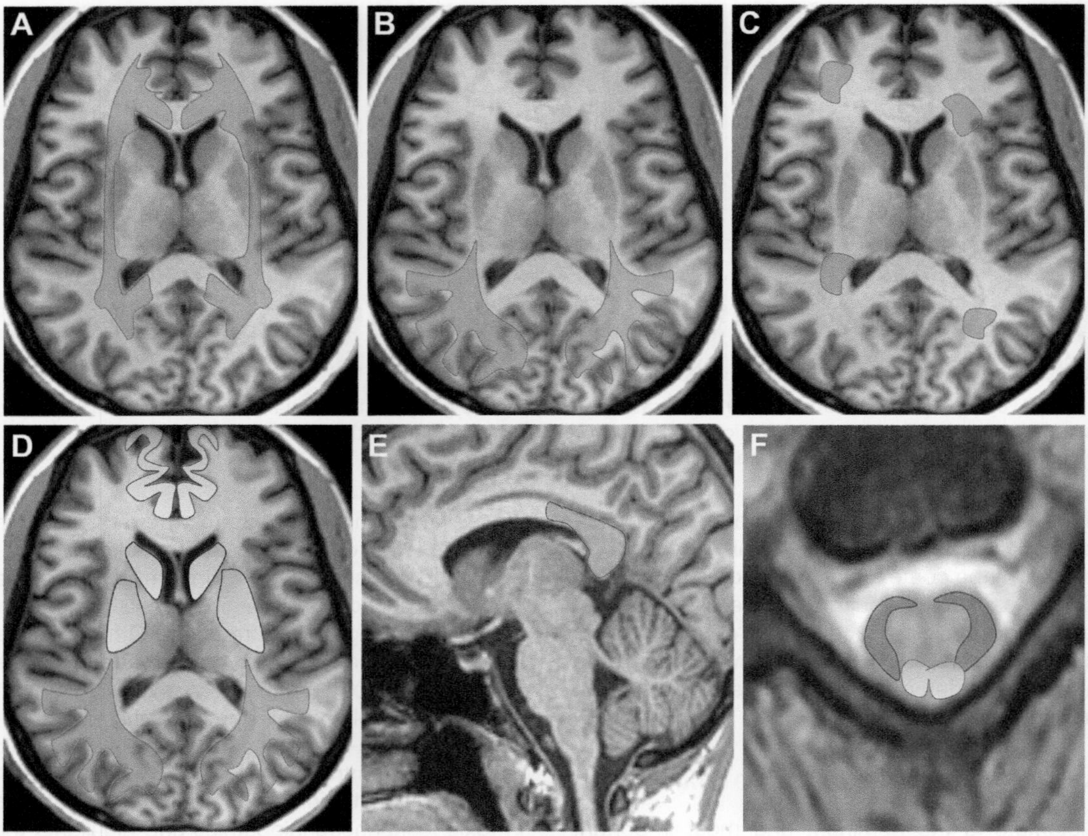

Fig. 4. Common neuroimaging pattern in toxic leukoencephalopathies and myelopathy. (*A*) Periventricular symmetric/near-symmetric white matter signal changes, with or without, restricted diffusion is the classic pattern in wide range of acute and chronic toxic leukoencephalopathies, respectively. (*B*) Subcortical white matter edema is the classic PRES pattern with an exhaustive list of underlying causes including white matter toxins. (*C*) Patchy discrete white matter lesions, mimicking demyelinating lesions, can be seen in conditions such as levamisole toxicity. (*D*) Cortical and deep gray matter is frequently associated with white matter changes in many causes of toxic and metabolic encephalopathies. (*E*) Isolated involvement of the corpus callosum is seen in "cytotoxic lesions of the corpus callosum" or Marchiafava-Bignami disease with the former having a lengthy list of differentials. (*F*) Toxic myelopathies tend to preferentially involve the peripheral white matter tracts including the anterolateral columns or dorsal sensory columns.

matter tracts, often mimicking subacute combined degeneration of the cord.[1,3,8]

DIAGNOSTIC TESTS AND NEUROIMAGING

Most of the patients with acute toxic leukoencephalopathies present in an emergency room (ER) setting, and apart from serological-work up and toxicology screening, neuroimaging studies are also routinely performed. Imaging in the form of noncontrast head computed tomography (CT) is usually the first line of investigation given the widespread availability, short acquisition time, and easy logistics, especially in an acutely ill patient with mental status changes. This does serve as a basic screening tool to rule out hemorrhage, ischemic stroke, and profound areas of vasogenic edemas. However, the role of CT is limited to white matter insults and even in positive cases, findings are nonspecific. MR imaging is the cornerstone for diagnosis and grading of acute and chronic leukoencephalopathies. This may be challenging in the ER or intensive care unit setting given the complex logistics and long scan times. There has been significant optimization in magnetic resonance (MR) protocols during the last few years given the higher dependency on MR imaging for many conditions, most commonly for stroke imaging. "Ultrafast MR imaging" (**Fig. 7**) similar to "quick stroke protocol" with scan times as short as 3 to 4 minutes have been developed, which offers higher diagnostic value compared with noncontrast head CT.[9] ATL should not be diagnosed in the absence of corroborating neuroradiologic

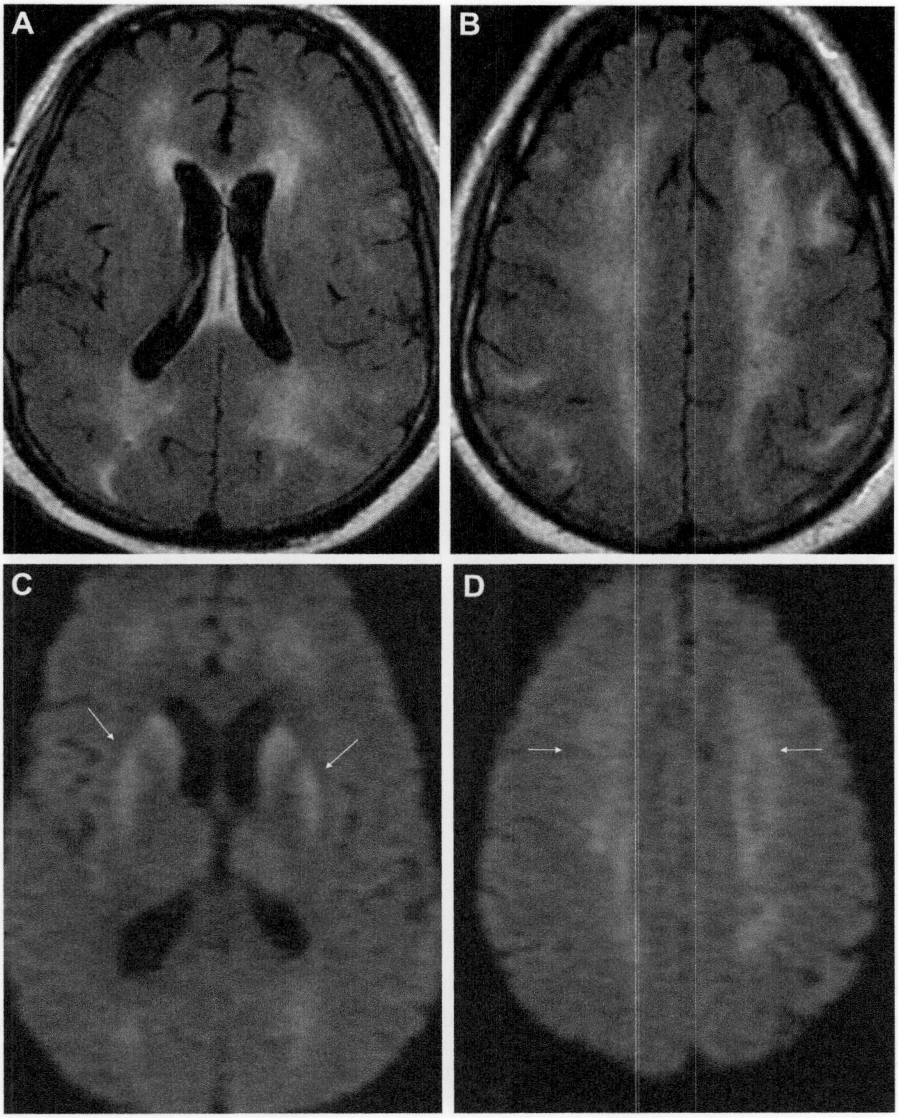

Fig. 5. Concomitant involvement of the deep gray matter nuclei (basal ganglia) with ATL in a patient on "dug cocktail" (Ketamine-MDMA). T2/FLAIR images (*A, B*) show extensive leukoencephalopathy with signal changes in the deep-white matter. DWI reveals mild restricted diffusion in the basal ganglia (*C, D, arrows*) and similar symmetric changes in the white matter. MDMA, 3,4-methylenedioxymethamphetamine (Ecstasy).

evidence. Serologic and urine screening for toxins and illicit drug abuse are increasingly being performed in the ER. Five drugs commonly tested in the United States on urine screen, as targeted for drug screening by the National Institute on Drug Abuse include cocaine, amphetamines, marijuana, phencyclidine (PCP), and opioids. The treatment of ATL is primarily supportive, starting with removal of the exposure with complete recovery possible in most cases. Neuroimaging in chronic toxic encephalopathies relies on routine MR imaging of the brain along with noninvasive vascular studies (such as magnetic resonance angiography [MRA]). Apart from toxins, there are numerous other causes for leukoencephalopathies including metabolic, demyelinating, infectious, vascular, traumatic, and genetic etiologies. A detailed discussion of these leukoencephalopathies is beyond the scope of this article, but it is important to point out that clinical features and MR imaging can together usually lead to the correct diagnosis.[1,2]

The 4 broad classes of agents causing toxic encephalopathies are discussed below.

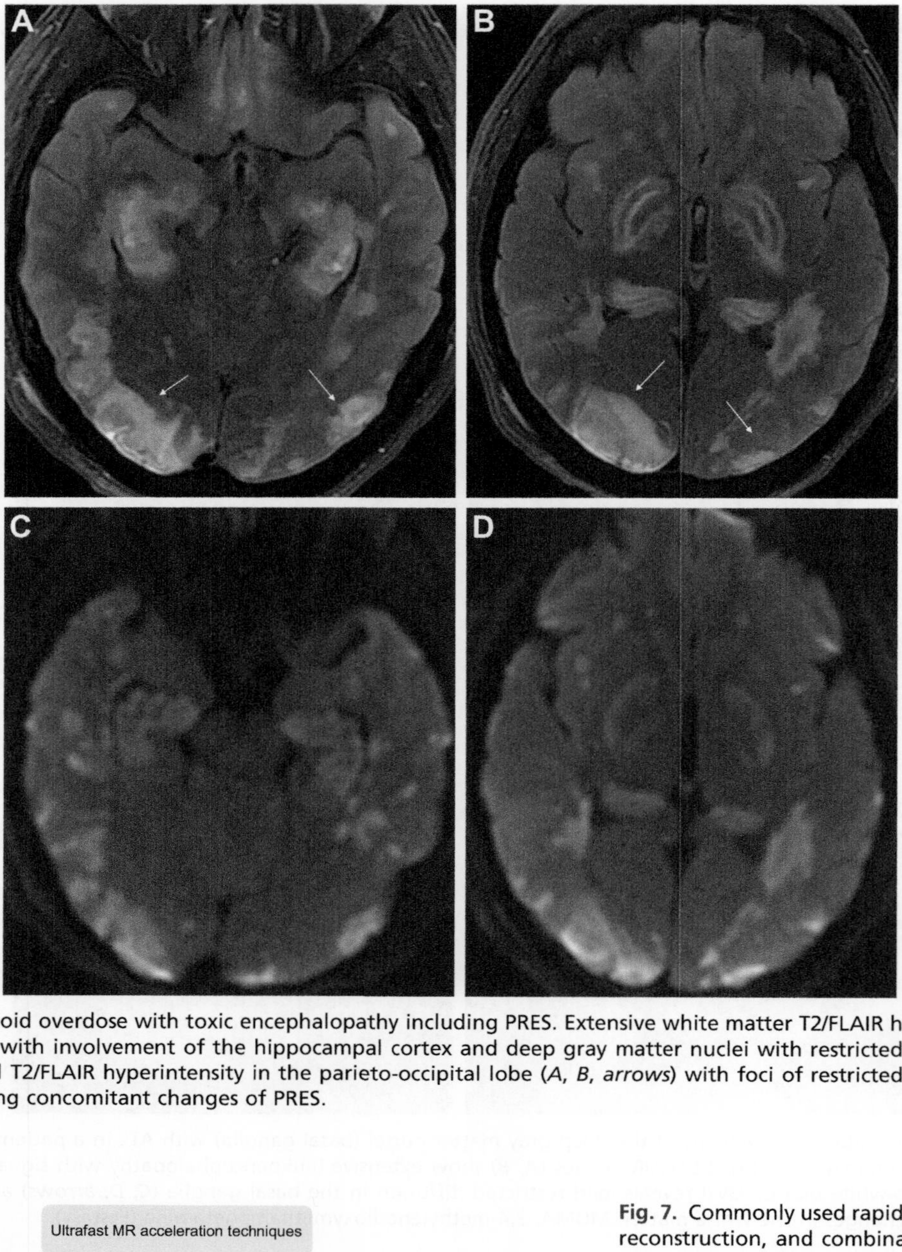

Fig. 6. Opioid overdose with toxic encephalopathy including PRES. Extensive white matter T2/FLAIR hyperintensity along with involvement of the hippocampal cortex and deep gray matter nuclei with restricted diffusion. Subcortical T2/FLAIR hyperintensity in the parieto-occipital lobe (*A, B, arrows*) with foci of restricted diffusion, representing concomitant changes of PRES.

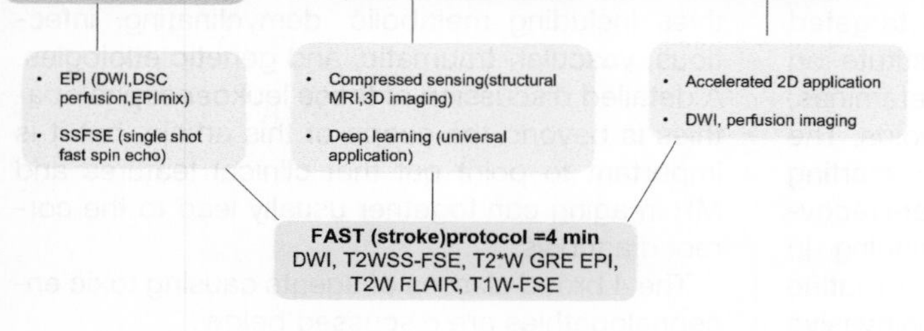

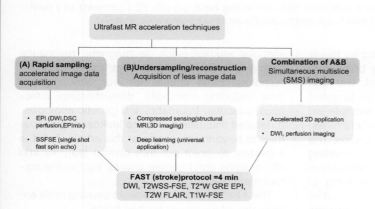

Fig. 7. Commonly used rapid sampling, reconstruction, and combination techniques for "fast" and "ultrafast" MR imaging. "Fast" stroke protocol at our program with scan time of around 4 minutes. DWI, diffusion-weighted imaging; EPI, echoplanar imaging; GRE, gradient echo; SS-FSE, fast-spin echo.

Therapeutic Agents

Radiation-induced white matter changes are one of the most common patterns of toxic leukoencephalopathies, with good direct correlation of degree of neurotoxicity and the total dose received. This is more common with whole brain irradiation and is becoming less frequent due to the usage of stereotactic (targeted) radiosurgery. Moreover, acute radiation-induced white matter changes are rare because these usually have a long-standing chronic course, presenting with cognitive decline secondary to irreversible myelin loss seen as confluent areas of T2/FLAIR hyperintensity without restricted diffusion.[2,10] One of the underreported entities includes "radiation recall reaction," which is an unpredictable phenomenon characterized by an acute inflammatory reaction limited to previously irradiated areas and precipitated by administration of systemic chemotherapeutic agents including alkylating agents, taxanes, and anthracyclines. This usually presents within a few days to weeks after exposure to the agent, most frequently (around two-thirds) presenting as dermatitis, and less frequently involving other organs such as lungs, gastrointestinal system, and the central nervous system (CNS). Imaging reveals rapid development of extensive white matter edema, mass effect, and enhancement in the prior radiation bed with resolution within few weeks after stopping treatment (**Fig. 8**).[11]

Methotrexate (MTX), 5-fluorouracil (5-FU), and carmustine are the most commonly chemotherapeutic agents implicated in toxic leukoencephalopathies. Other agents with significant association with ATL include cisplatin, cytarabine, levamisole, and fludarabine. The immunosuppressive agents such as cyclosporine and tacrolimus, commonly used in transplant patients, and antimicrobial agents such as amphotericin A, may produce similar reversible white matter changes. MTX is an important part of the treatment protocol in pediatric and adult leukemias. It is a cell cycle-specific agent that inhibits

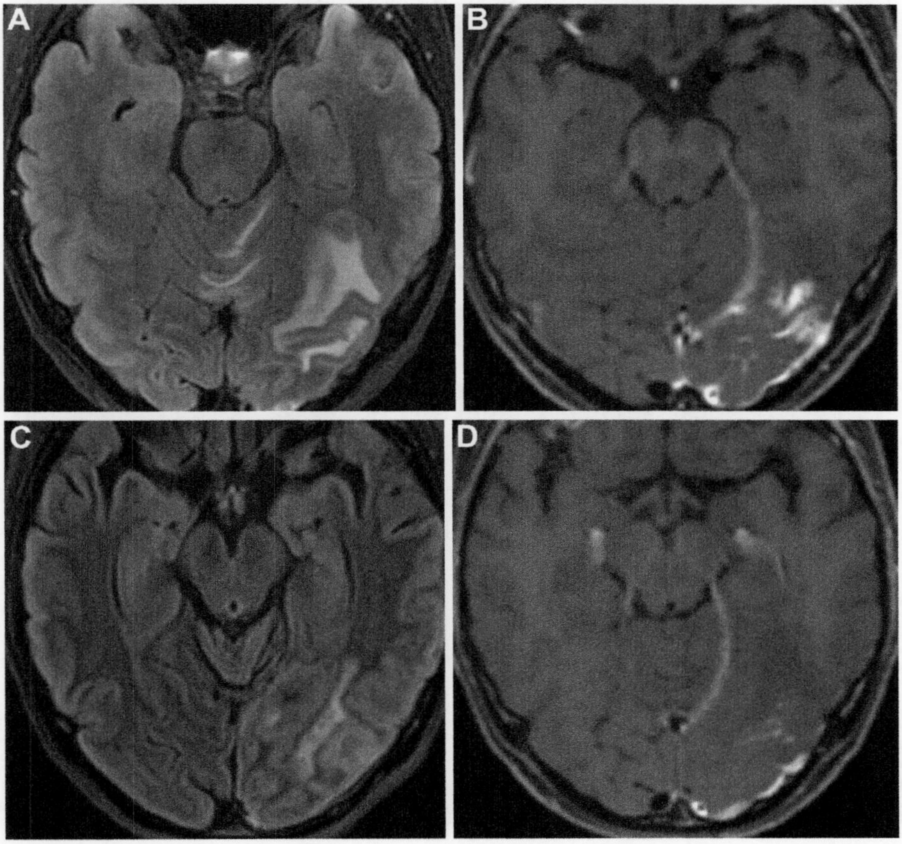

Fig. 8. Development of brain parenchymal edema (*A*) with patchy enhancement (*B*) in the left parietooccipital lobe and cerebellum after administration of trastuzumab in a 28-year-old with history of brain radiation, presumably representing "radiation recall effect." Near complete resolution of edema and enhancement (*C, D*) few weeks after cessation of the targeted monoclonal antibody.

cell replication by suppressing dihydrofolate-reductase, thereby preventing the conversion of folic acid to tetrahydrofolic acid. ATL can be a side effect of both intravenous MTX and intrathecal MTX with the incidence ranging from 3% to 10%, which is aggravated by the presence of various factors such as dose, route of administration (40% in intrathecal, 10% in intravenous [IV] route), young age, and if associated with radiotherapy. Carmustine (BCNU) is an alkylating chemotherapeutic commonly used for gliomas, multiple myeloma, and lymphomas (Hodgkin and non-Hodgkin). 5-FU is a common antineoplastic and antimetabolic agent used in wide range of neoplasm including gastrointestinal, breast, and head and neck cancers. The most common imaging appearance for ATL is symmetric or near-symmetric areas of restricted diffusion in the white matter, classically in the region of centrum semiovale (see **Fig. 3**). Corresponding subtle signal changes may also be seen in T2/FLAIR images, with no enhancement, edema, or mass effect. Clinical and radiographic findings are reversible with complete resolution in a few weeks. Rarely, this may progress to the more severe, typically progressive, and fatal form known as "disseminated necrotizing leukoencephalopathy." This is characterized by solid nodular or confluent areas of enhancement with edema and mass effect, mimicking tumoral enhancement (**Fig. 9**).[3,12–14]

Immunotherapeutic agents

Other categories of therapeutic agents implicated in white matter toxicity include the newly described immunotherapeutic agents such as checkpoint

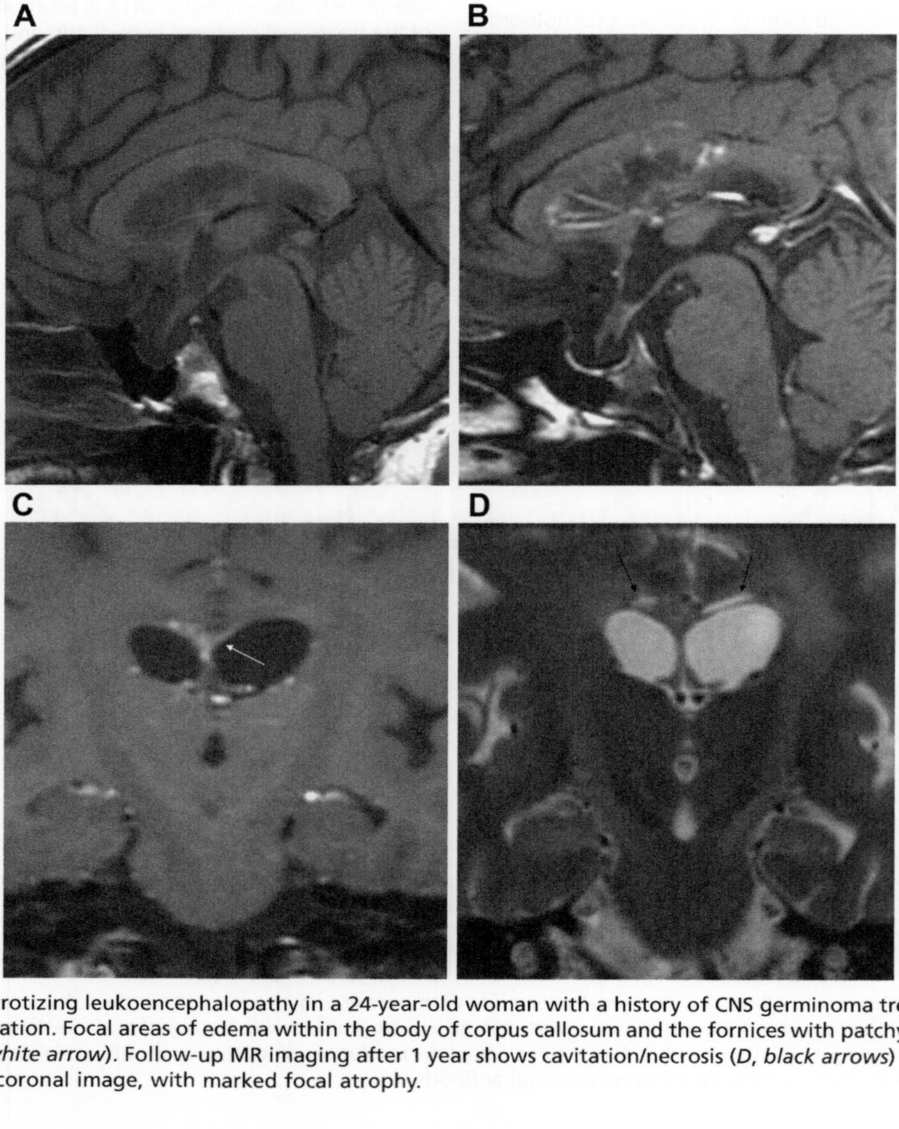

Fig. 9. Necrotizing leukoencephalopathy in a 24-year-old woman with a history of CNS germinoma treated with chemoradiation. Focal areas of edema within the body of corpus callosum and the fornices with patchy enhancement (*C, white arrow*). Follow-up MR imaging after 1 year shows cavitation/necrosis (*D, black arrows*) on the T2-weighted coronal image, with marked focal atrophy.

inhibitors, chimeric antigen receptor T-cell therapy (CAR-T), and etoposide phosphate (EPOCH) treatment regimen. Immune checkpoint inhibitors, known as monoclonal antibodies, work by activating the immune system and include programmed cell death protein 1 and ligand inhibitors, used for a wide range of solid tumors and melanoma. CAR-T is a form of immunotherapy that uses specially altered T cells and is part of treatment protocol for lymphomas, leukemias, and multiple myeloma. EPOCH is an intensive chemotherapy regimen intended for the treatment of aggressive non-Hodgkin lymphoma, frequently combined with rituximab (R-EPOCH or EPOCH-R) with the regimen consisting of etoposide, prednisolone, oncovin, cyclophosphamide (alkylating antineoplastic agent), hydroxydaunorubicin, and rituximab (monoclonal antibody). Neurologic complications of immunotherapy include acute encephalopathy with cortical restricted diffusion, hypophysitis, aseptic meningoencephalitis, ATL, myelopathy, myositis, peripheral radiculopathy, and polyradiculopathy with Guillain-Barre syndrome (GBS) like symptoms (**Figs. 10** and **11**). Two new categories of complication with these agents include immune reconstitution inflammatory syndrome (IRIS) and immune effector cell-associated neurotoxicity syndrome (ICANS). IRIS is paradoxic worsening of symptoms following abrupt improvement in an individual's immune function, classically described in human immunodeficiency virus (HIV)/acquired immunodeficiency syndrome patients on antiretroviral therapy, and of late, increasingly seen with immunomodulatory drugs. Neuroimaging features of IRIS include small punctuate or patchy foci of enhancement with a perivascular distribution and perilesional edema, usually associated with progressive multifocal leukoencephalopathy (**Fig. 12**). The pattern of punctate T2 hyperintensity with or without punctate enhancement is referred to as

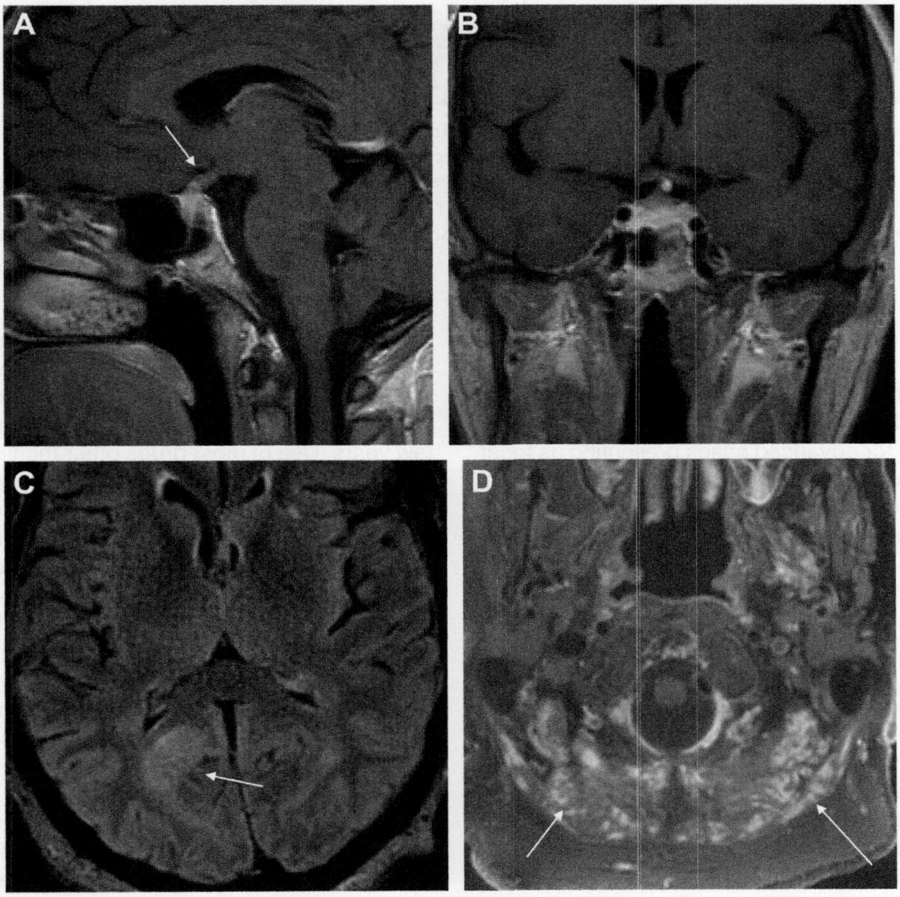

Fig. 10. Neurologic complications of immunotherapeutic agents in different patients. Hypophysitis with thickening and enhancement of the infundibulum (*A, arrow*) represents the most common neurologic complication of immunotherapy. Aseptic meningoencephalitis with subtle T2/FLAIR edema in the right parietal lobe (*C, arrow*) and florid myositis (*D, arrows*) in different patients on immunotherapy.

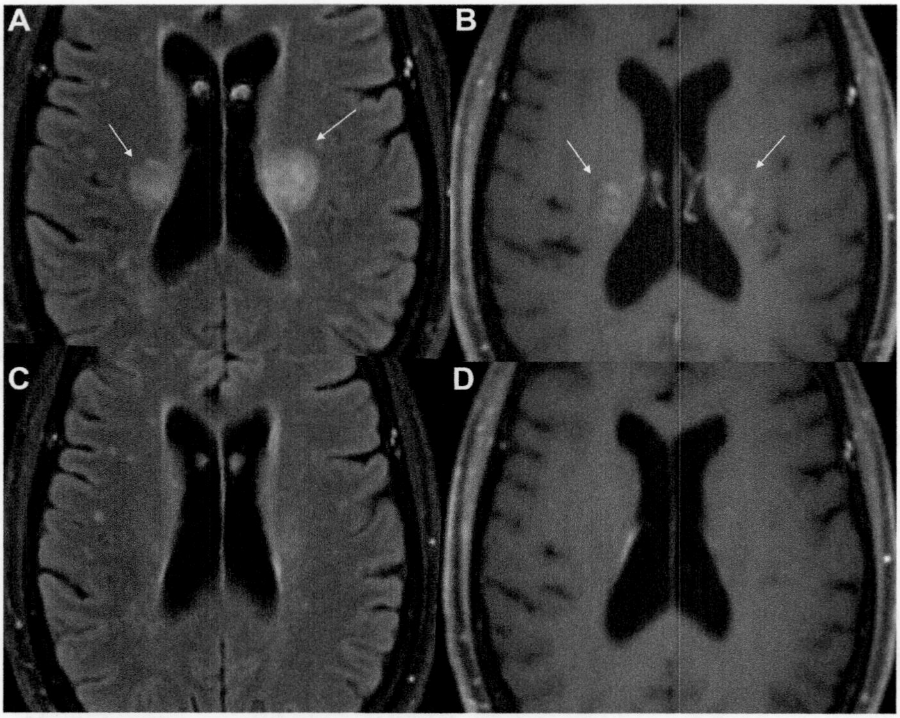

Fig. 11. Granulocyte-macrophage-colony-stimulating-factor (GM-CSF)-related encephalitis in a 64-year-old patient with metastatic breast cancer on clinical trial who received placebo and GM-CSF. MR imaging (*A, B, arrows*) 2 months after initiation of therapy demonstrates symmetric confluent regions of expansile T2 hyperintensity with associated patchy enhancement within the corona radiata. Complete resolution of these changes is seen on follow-up MR imaging (*C, D*) obtained after 5 months. (Case courtesy: Amit Desai MD, Mayo Clinic, Florida.)

"starry sky" pattern. ICANS, previously known as cytokine release encephalopathy syndrome or CAR T-cell-related encephalopathy syndrome, is a neuropsychiatric condition occurring days to weeks following CAR-T therapy. Imaging is usually negative except for advanced cases presenting as focal or diffuse cerebral edema involving the gray and white matter, often with a fulminant fatal course (**Fig. 13**). Finally, posterior reversible encephalopathy syndrome with varying degrees of reversible brain edema can be seen with most of the chemotherapeutic agents listed earlier.[15,16]

Drugs of Abuse (Illicit Drugs)

Illicit drug use in the United States has been increasing with an estimated 25 million Americans aged 12 years or older (around 10%) having used an illicit drug in the past month. "Illicit" refers to use of illegal drugs, including marijuana according to federal law, and misuse of prescription drugs. There has been a continuous increase in the use of illicit drugs, primarily driven by recent increase in use of marijuana (cannabis), secondary to legalization of recreational and/or medicinal usage in many states. After alcohol, marijuana is the most used illicit drug and has the highest rate of dependence or abuse among all drugs. Marijuana and hallucinogen use by young adults aged 19 to 30 years has reached historic highs in the last few years. Use of most drugs other than marijuana has stabilized during the past decade or has declined. The national drug-involved overdose death rate has also continuously increased during the last decade with the biggest spike seen in synthetic opioids (primarily fentanyl) and psychostimulants (primarily methamphetamine). The most common illicit drugs of abuse and drug-involved overdosage deaths are reported by the National Institute on Drug Abuse and are continuously updated. Deaths due to prescription (natural opioids), benzodiazepines, and heroin have either remained stable or declined during the last decade.[17,18]

Neurologic changes from alcohol abuse include Wernicke encephalopathy, hepatic encephalopathy cerebellar degeneration, osmotic demyelination syndrome, and Marchiafava-Bignami disease. The last 2 entities primarily involve the white matter. Osmotic demyelination syndrome

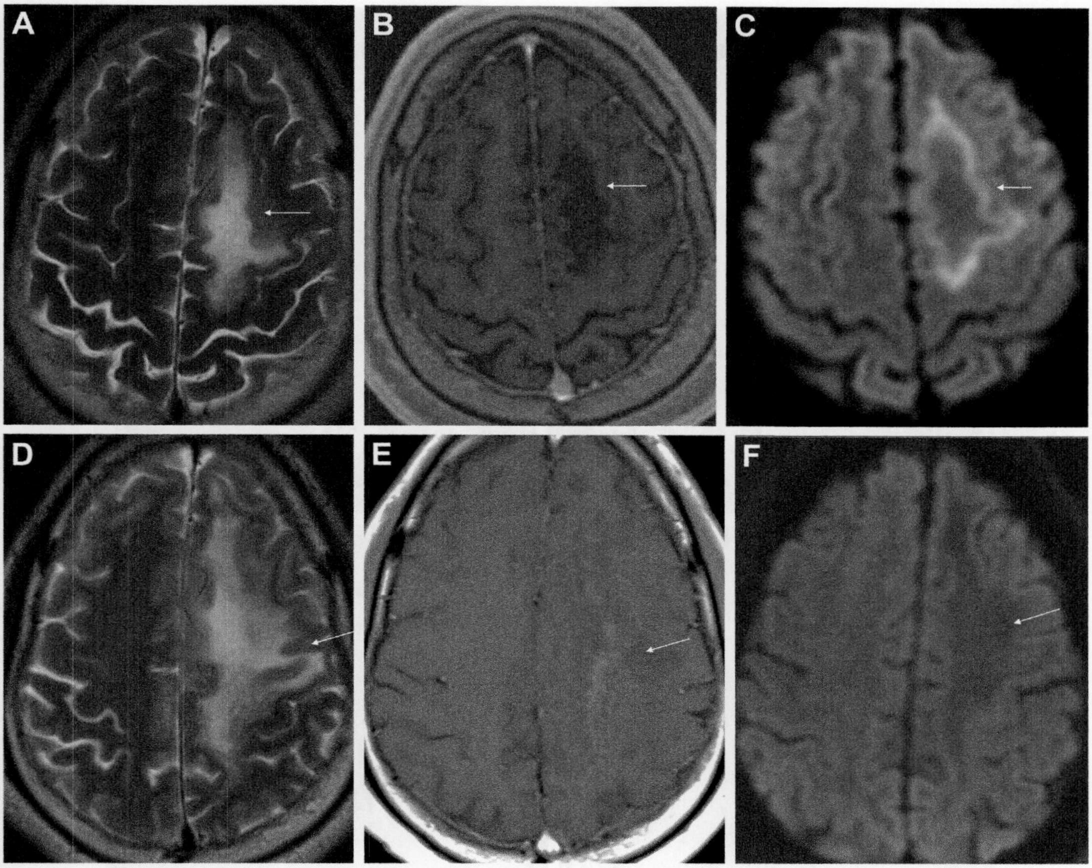

Fig. 12. Progressive multifocal leukoencephalopathy (PML) (top panel) and PML-IRIS complex (bottom panel) in an HIV patient. MR imaging reveals a large area of white matter T2 hyperintensity (*A*) with low T1 signal (*B*) and peripheral restricted diffusion in the left frontal lobe (*arrows*) consistent with PML. Low T1 signal is characteristic of PML, and restricted diffusion (*C*) represents active demyelination. Follow-up MR imaging, 4 weeks after initiation of retroviral (HAART) therapy reveals paradoxic worsening of white matter changes (*D*) with resolution of restricted diffusion (*F*). New patchy foci of enhancement ("starry-sky" pattern) seen in the subcortical region representing immune-reactivation (*E*). HAART, highly active anti-retroviral treatment.

refers to acute demyelination seen in the setting of osmotic changes, classically seen with the rapid correction of hyponatremia, seen in chronic alcoholics and debilitated patients. Traditionally known as central pontine myelinolysis, it is now recognized that extrapontine structures such as deep gray nuclei can also be involved. Marchiafava-Bignami disease is a rare neurologic disorder usually seen in the context of chronic alcoholism and malnutrition with necrosis and demyelination of the corpus callosum, classically in the medial lamina. Corpus callosum may seem edematous in the acute phase and atrophic in the chronic phase (**Fig. 14**).

No definite imaging changes have been reported with occasional marijuana usage. Studies have however shown that chronic heavy cannabis use during adolescence and young adulthood alters ongoing development of white matter microstructure, contributing to functional impairment. Although findings are not conclusive, early studies have shown lower axonal connectivity and fractional anisotropy in corpus callosum and superior longitudinal fasciculi in subjects with long-standing cannabis usage. Neurologic manifestations are however common when cannabis is combined with contaminants such as heavy metals, pesticides, bath salt, and antifreeze.[2,7,19]

Toxic leukoencephalopathy is a known risk with excessive use of many different substances of abuse. **Table 1** provides an outline of the commonly used drugs in United States and their neuroimaging manifestations. Opiates, such as morphine and codeine, are natural opioids found in the opium poppy, whereas synthetic opioids, such as methadone, are chemically made. Heroin

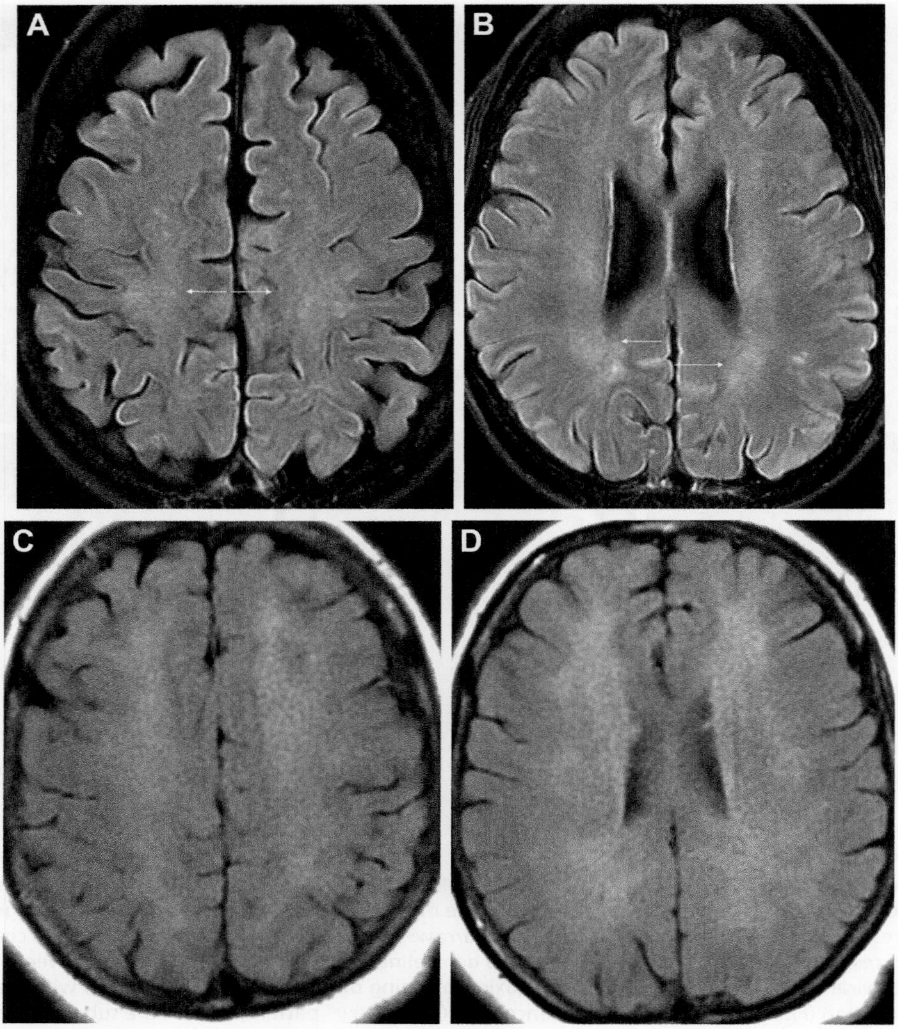

Fig. 13. ICANS in 2 different patients; first with multiple myeloma (*A, B*) and second with leukemia (*C, D*), both presenting with neuropsychiatric symptoms a few weeks after initiation of CAR-T therapy. Multiple axial FLAIR images reveal subtle T2/FLAIR hyperintensity in the centrum semiovale (*A, arrows*) and the periventricular white matter (*B, arrows*). More prominent similar changes with diffuse edema noted in the second patient (*C, D*).

is a semisynthetic opioid made with chemically processed morphine. These synthetic/semisynthetic compounds enter the brain quickly and produce a more immediate effect with elevated risk for neurologic complications. Fentanyl is a prescription opioid that is 100 times more powerful than morphine and is the leading cause for overdosage deaths in the country. Numerous overdoses have occurred because people did not know what they were taking was contaminated with fentanyl. Heroin-induced leukoencephalopathy (HLE) is a rare but important condition in chronic heroin abusers. Although initial reports suggested HLE is associated with such inhalational abuse, a large 2018 study suggested that although a majority of about 60% of heroin patients with TLE were abusers by the inhalation route, IV abuse constituted 30%, and snorting comprised 10%. The predominant hypothesis is that some impurity mixed with heroin, which produces a toxic chemical on combustion, including (although less likely) possibly aluminum in the foil are responsible for the toxicity. The clinical syndrome passes through 3 stages during weeks to months—the first stage being cerebellar with ataxia and dysarthria, the second stage with myoclonic jerks, choreoathetoid movements, spastic paresis, and 25% progressing to the third

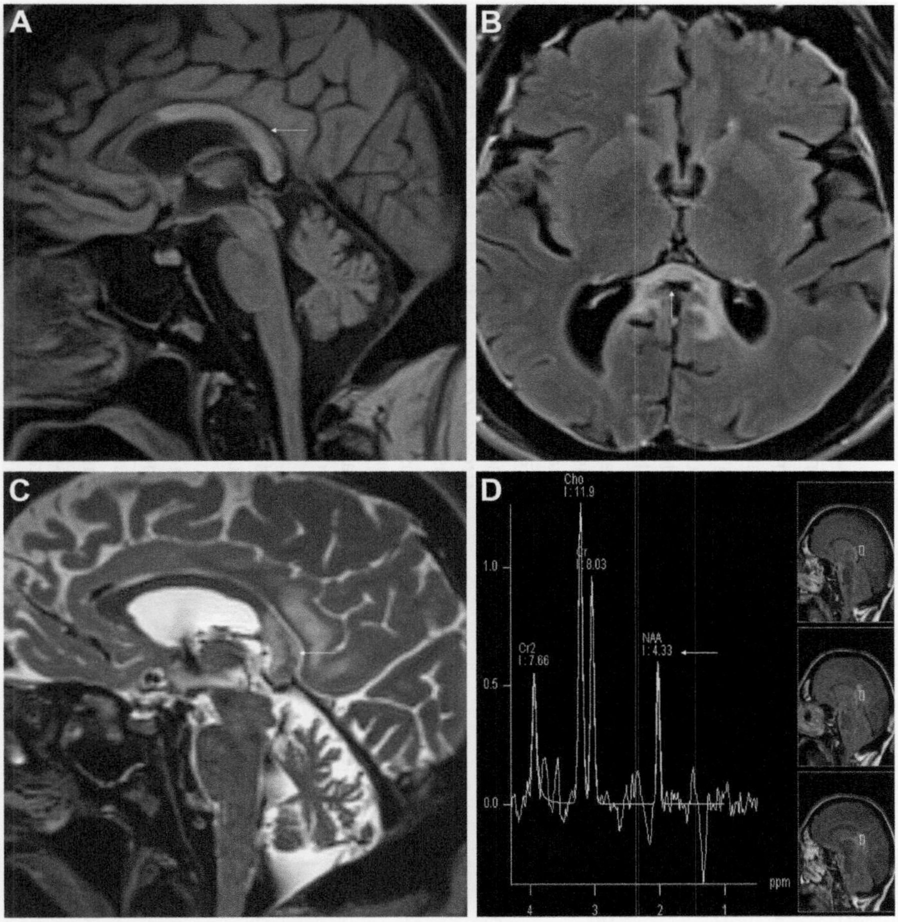

Fig. 14. Marchiafava-Bignami disease in a chronic alcoholic presenting with cognitive decline and hemialexia. Multiple T2/FLAIR sagittal (*A, C*) and axial (*B*) images reveal hyperintensity with atrophic changes involving the posterior body and splenium of corpus callosum (*arrows*), along with similar signal changes in the pericallosal white matter. MR spectroscopy (*D*) reveals decrease in NAA values (*arrow*) and reversal of NAA/Cr ratio. NAA, N-acetylaspartate.

stage of akinetic mutism, extensor posturing, central pyrexia, and eventual death. The clinical course progresses despite removal of initial toxin, due to continued release of toxin from lipid-rich myelin deposits. The toxicity is dose dependent. MR imaging shows diffuse, nonenhancing, symmetric T2/FLAIR hyperintensities in the periventricular and deep cerebral white matter with a posterior to anterior gradient with more severe cases involving the frontal lobe too. Signal abnormalities are also very commonly seen in the cerebellum, posterior limbs of internal capsule extending inferiorly into the corticospinal tracts, splenium of corpus callosum, lemniscal pathways of the brainstem, and hippocampus. Heroin taken via routes such as IV injection, sniffing, snorting produces signal abnormality in the subcortical U fibers, whereas U fibers tend to be spared in "chasing the dragon" (heroin heated vapor) abuse (**Fig. 15**). MR spectroscopy shows elevated lactate and decreased NAA levels. Histologic changes show widespread, confluent spongiform (vacuolar) degeneration of the white matter.[1,2,20]

The most common form of cocaine brain injury is vascular injury causing ischemic and hemorrhagic stroke caused by vascular mechanisms. A second mechanism of cocaine neurotoxicity is metabolic in nature and called cocaine-induced leukoencephalopathy (CLE). CLE is an acute to subacute leukoencephalopathy with MR imaging findings similar to HLE showing bihemispheric white matter T2 and FLAIR hyperintensity, absent restricted diffusion, lack of contrast enhancement and sparing of U fibers like seen with chasing the dragon type toxicity. A notable difference is lack of occipital, cerebellar, and brainstem

Table 1
Most common used illicit drugs in United States, along with their street names and neurologic complications (National Institute on Drug Abuse)

Commonly Abused Drugs (National Institute of Health)		
Substance	Commercial/street name	Neuroimaging findings
Alcohol (ethyl alcohol)	Wine, beer, and liquor	Wernicke encephalopathy, cerebellar degeneration, Marchiafava-Bignami disease
Cannabinoids (marijuana, hashish)	Dope, ganja, herb, joint, weed, hash oil, and hemp	Rare with pure cannabinoids. Toxic leukoencephalopathy and deep-gray matter edema when combined with antifreeze, bath salts
Opioids (heroin, opium)	Smack, brown sugar, dope, and white horse	Ischemia, reversible vasospasm (most common), vasculitis, toxic leukoencephalopathy, HLE, exclusively after heroin inhalation (chasing the dragon)
Stimulants (cocaine, amphetamine, and methamphetamine)	Coke, crack, meth, chalk, crystal, and rock	Hemorrhagic (SAH, parenchymal) >> ischemic strokes (cocaine-induced vasoconstriction, vasculitis)
Club drugs (Flunitrazepam, MDMA: methylenedioxymethamphetamine)	Ecstasy, Adam, roofies, roofinol, and roofies	Vasospasm and parenchymal necrosis (most common occipital cortex and globus pallidus)
Dissociative drugs (ketamine, PCP, and dextromethorphan)	Valium, special K, angel dust, and magic mint	Usually unremarkable routine MR imaging, small incidence of toxic leukoencephalopathy
Hallucinogens (LSD, mescaline, and psilocybin)	Blue heaven, magic mushroom, and purple passion	Usually unremarkable, small incidence of toxic leukoencephalopathy
Inhalants	Solvents, paint thinners, and laughing gas	Acute stage: leukoencephalopathy; Chronic abusers: cerebellar and cerebral white matter demyelination and gliosis
Contaminants (levamisole, fentanyl)	Fentanyl: China Town, Dance Fever	Levamisole: Multifocal inflammatory leukoencephalopathy Fentanyl: Ischemia, vasculitis, and toxic leukoencephalopathy

Abbreviations: LSD, lysergic acid diethylamide; SAH, subarachnoid hemorrhage.

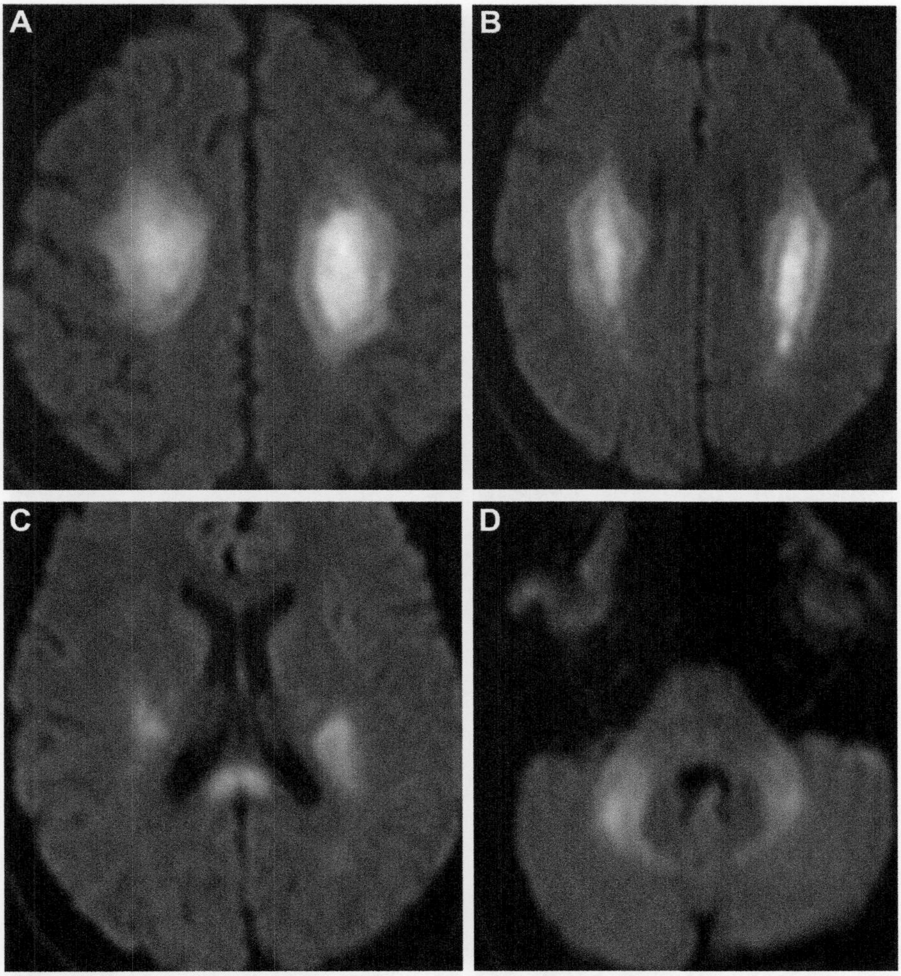

Fig. 15. HLE (heroin-associated spongiform leukoencephalopathy secondary to inhalation of heroin fumes (chasing the dragon). Multiple axial DW images reveal widespread symmetric areas of restricted diffusion in the supratentorial and infratentorial white matter with the involvement of the centrum semiovale (*A*), posterior corona radiata and posterior limb of internal capsules, (*B, C*) symmetric involvement of middle cerebellar peduncles (*D*). There is sparing of adjacent gray matter structures and subcortical U-fibers.

involvement, seen typically with HLE. More recently, another type of cocaine leukoencephalopathy has been seen caused by the common adulterant levamisole. Originally introduced as a human and animal anthelminthic agent, levamisole has immunomodulatory properties and has been used in rheumatoid arthritis, inflammatory bowel disease (IBD), nephrotic syndrome, and aphthous ulcers. However, its usage has been discontinued due to serious side effects such as leukopenia, tissue necrosis, and encephalopathy. It is colorless, tasteless, and odorless and hence can be a common adulterant in cocaine in various regions of the world. Moreover, its metabolism produces aminorex, which is an independent neurostimulant, allowing cheaper effective substitution. However, levamisole can cause a multifocal inflammatory leukoencephalopathy (**Fig. 16**). Mechanism is thought to be immune mediated and includes transient autoimmune response toward myelin or other proteins via molecular mimicry or nonspecific activation of T cell clones. MR imaging findings include multifocal enhancing white matter lesions in the supratentorial brain or additionally in the infratentorial region. Pure infratentorial lesions are usually not seen. Open ring pattern of enhancement is seen in about one-fourth of cases. Radiologic differentiation from multiple sclerosis (MS) and acute disseminated encephalo-myelitis (ADEM) may be difficult. Biopsy shows active demyelination with perivascular lymphocytes. Good response is seen with

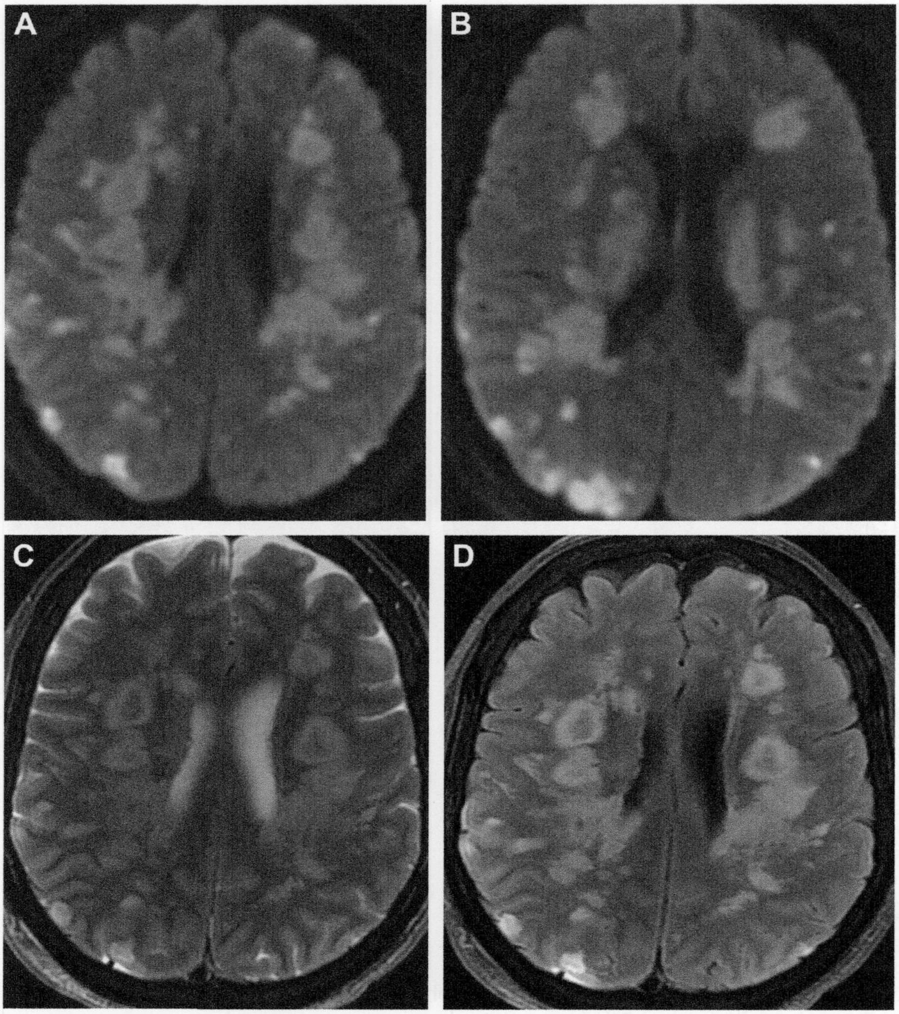

Fig. 16. Overdose of opioid contaminated with levamisole. Extensive multifocal white matter lesions with restricted diffusion (*A, B*) seen scattered throughout the supratentorial brain consistent with multifocal inflammatory leukoencephalopathy. T2/FLAIR images (*C, D*) reveal lamellated appearance representing varying stages of toxic demyelination.

steroids, immunoglobulins, and plasmapheresis, if treated early.[21–24]

Environmental and Occupational (Industrial) Toxins

Workers in various industries may be exposed to leukotoxins ranging from manufacturing, construction, agriculture, military service, and several others. In the occupational and environmental domains, chronic toxic leukoencephalopathy (CTL) is more relevant than acute changes. CTL is characterized by chronic neurobehavioral morbidity and slowly progressive white matter abnormality on brain MR imaging. Organic solvents constitute a large group of volatile hydrocarbons and their derivatives and exposure to these is a major problem is occupations dealing with it such as paints, adhesives, dry cleaning, surface cleaning, printing, plastics, pesticides, and chemicals. Toluene is a major component of organic solvents. Routes of entry into the body include inhalation of vapor and skin absorption, and imaging findings typically develop after 4 years of chronic exposure. MR imaging features include focal or diffuse white matter T2 hyperintensity affecting the centrum semiovale, cerebellum, internal capsule, and brainstem. Progressive increase in T2 hypointensity of the thalami, red nuclei, substantia nigra, and dentate nuclei is also seen along with global brain atrophy and thinning of corpus callosum, depending on duration and severity.[25,26]

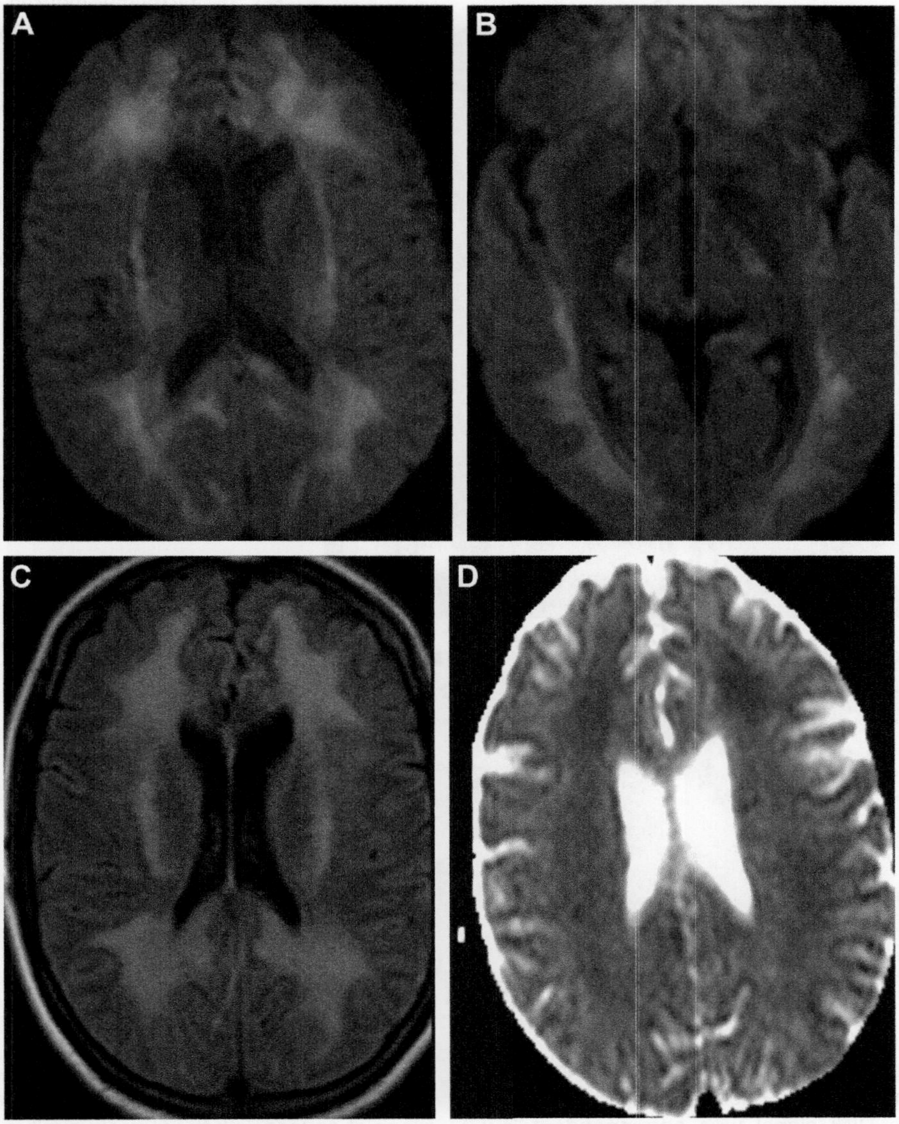

Fig. 17. Delayed hypoxic leukoencephalopathy secondary to CO poisoning. Initial MR imaging study was normal with clinical return to baseline followed by severe neurologic deterioration and new neurologic symptoms. Follow-up MR imaging after 2-week reveals extensive diffuse white matter restricted diffusion (*A, B*) with low ADC values (*D*) and corresponding T2/FLAIR hyperintensity (*C*). Patient had profound long-term neurologic complications and deficits.

Carbon monoxide (CO) is an important environmental toxin and has been implicated in delayed posthypoxic leukoencephalopathy (DPHL) after recovery from acute CO poisoning. Although rare, the condition is potentially devastating. DPHL is a rare consequence of global hypoxia with ischemic demyelination occurring days to weeks after recovery from coma and a period of prolonged cerebral hypo-oxygenation seen in CO poisoning and heroin overdose (**Fig. 17**). Myelin secretion occurs every 19 to 22 days thereby explaining the delayed onset of symptoms. It is characterized by acute neuropsychiatric symptoms and is diagnosed by ruling out potential causes of delirium in a setup of post-CO poisoning or another global hypoxic event. Imaging findings are similar to that of DPHL from other causes and includes confluent, symmetric involvement of the periventricular white matter and centrum semiovale with restricted diffusion. Restricted diffusion can persist for months due to intramyelinic edema and helps in differentiation from cytotoxic edema, which usually resolves within few weeks. These areas exhibit high signal on T2/FLAIR sequences with no mass effect or contrast

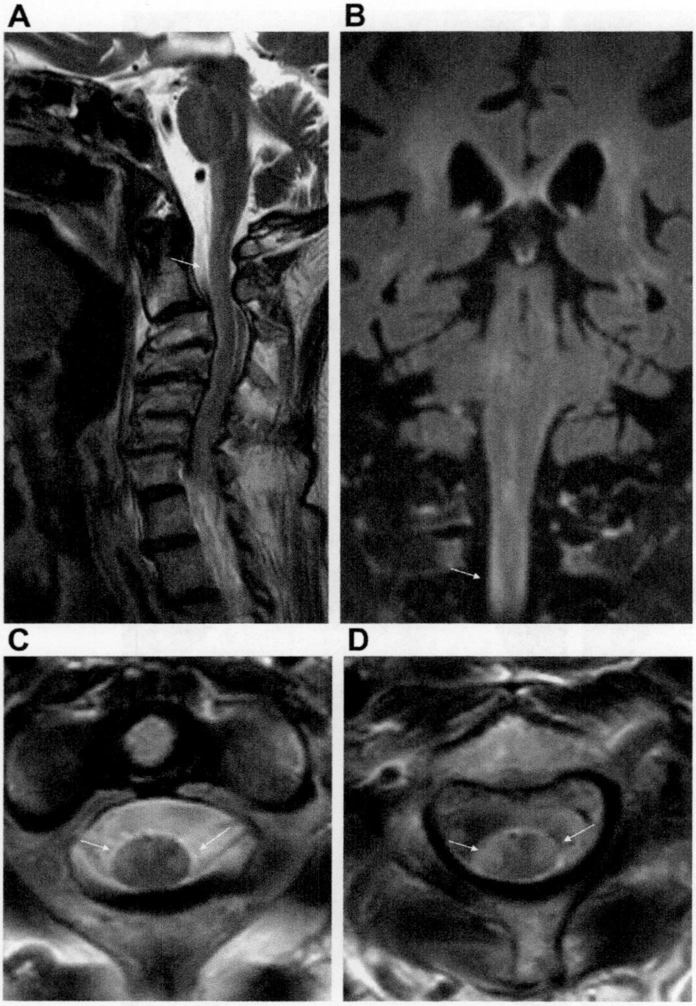

Fig. 18. Tacrolimus-induced toxic leukoencephalopathy and myelopathy. MR imaging study reveals long segment T2 hyperintensity within the cervical cord and lower brainstem (*A, arrow*) along with leukoencephalopathy (*B, arrow*). Axial T2-weighted images through the cervical cord shows preferential involvement of the peripheral columns with sparing of the central gray matter (*C, D, arrows*).

enhancement. Diffusion-weighted imaging (DWI) plays an important role because it has been shown that a high DWI signal with correspondent low ADC persisting for months is typically associated with this condition. This feature allows the differentiation between DPHL and white matter infarcts with the latter progressing into gliosis with resolution of DWI changes in few weeks.[22,26]

Toxic (spongiform) leukoencephalopathy with intramyelinic fluid accumulation can also be caused by numerous other industrial agents such as ethidium bromide, triethyltin, methyl bromide, hexachlorophene, and cycloleucine. The list of these toxins is exhaustive and beyond the scope of this article. However, in the absence of the commoner therapeutic and illicit-drug-related causes of leukoencephalopathy, a careful evaluation for these underlying factors should be considered by the clinical team because many of these toxins are clinically occult.[27]

Toxic myelopathies

Metabolic and toxic myelopathies have a wide range of causes with the former usually secondary to nutritional deficiency (similar to Vitamin B12) and the latter secondary to the exposure to an external toxic agent. There is significant clinical and imaging overlap between these entities and other noncompressive myelopathies. However, because these are amenable to treatment, recognition of the underlying toxin and corrections results in clinical and radiological normalization. One major imaging distinction between toxic/metabolic myelopathy and other causes such as paraneoplastic myelitis and idiopathic transverse myelitis is the preferential involvement of the white matter tracts including the dorsal columns and corticospinal tracts, in the former category (**Fig. 18**). Clinical presentation of myelopathy includes gait abnormalities, varying degree of upper and lower extremity sensorimotor changes with hyperreflexia,

Table 2
Common causes of toxic myelopathies and their neuroimaging manifestations

No Geographic Predilection		Geographic Predilection (Rare)	
Chemotherapy-related (methotrexate, doxorubicin, vincristine, cytarabine, and newer immunotherapy agents)	History of chemotherapy, preferential involvement of the peripheral columns, similar to that of subacute combine degeneration. Often associated with acute or chronic leukoencephalopathy	Cassava (African countries)	Consumption of insufficiently processed cassava root (*Manihot esculenta*) that contains cyanogens. Motor neuron damage with spastic paraparesis or quadriparesis along with optic neuropathy
Radiation-induced	When dosage exceeds 45 Gy, sharply demarcated long-segment area of cord signal changes, fatty marrow changes in adjacent spine	Lathyrism (South Asia and Africa)	Irreversible and nonprogressive optic atrophy, degeneration of motor cortex, and pyramidal tracts
Nitrous-dioxide toxicity	Findings similar to Vitamin B12 related subacute spinal degeneration which with reversible swelling of myelin sheaths in the posterior and lateral columns	Fluorosis (India, China, and Japan)	Excessive levels of fluoride ions in the blood from unprocessed groundwater (deep borewell). Ossification of posterior longitudinal ligament, ligamentum flavum with compressive myelopathy
Heroin-induced myelopathy	Inhalation (chasing the dragon) or intravenous use. Progressive with preferential involvement of the ventral pons and lateral and posterior spinal columns	Clioquinol (antifungal, used in Japan)	Subacute Myelo-Optico Neuropathy. Long-segment signal changes in the cord columns along with optic atrophy
Organophosphate toxicity (pesticides)	Secondary to cholinergic crisis. Spinal cord atrophy that can persists long after the cholinergic effects have subsided	Spinal Sea Stroke (North Carolina, Virginia)	Spinal and brainstem infarctions caused by contact with toxic marine animals while swimming

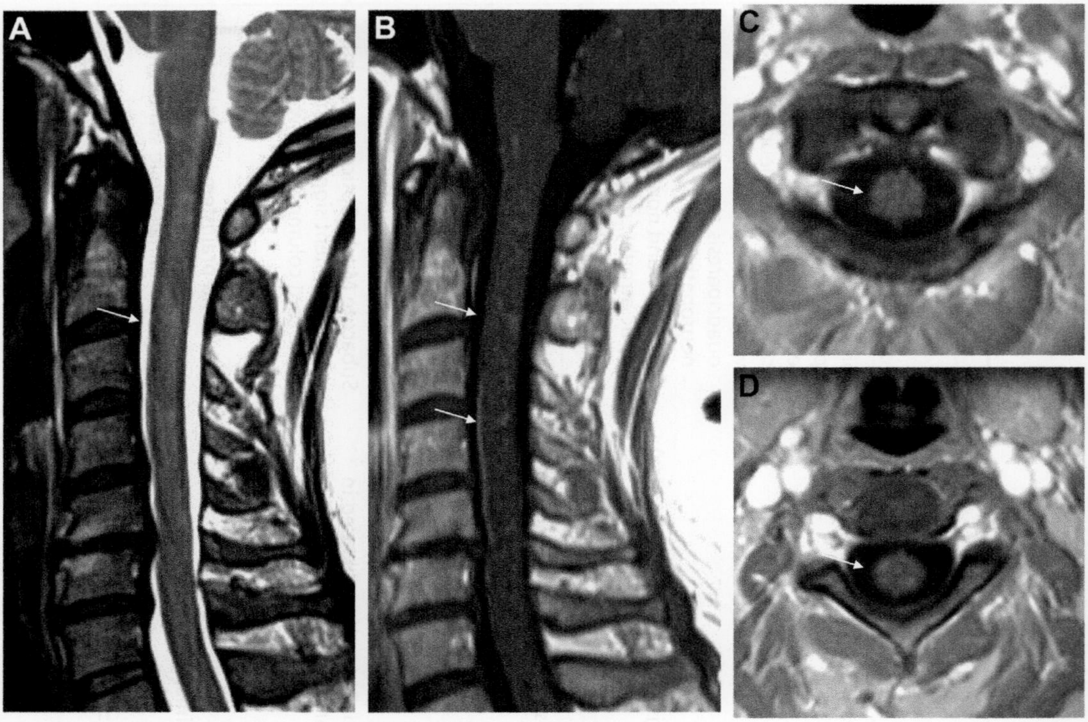

Fig. 19. Ipilimumab-induced myelitis. A 43-year-old patient with metastatic melanoma treated with ipilimumab (Yervoy). After initiation of therapy, patient developed Lhermitte's symptoms, myoclonic jerking, and gait. MR imaging demonstrates longitudinally extensive expansile intramedullary T2 hyperintensity (*A, arrow*) and associated patchy enhancement within the cervical and upper thoracic spinal cord (*B–D, arrows*). (Case courtesy: Amit Desai MD, Mayo Clinic, Florida.)

spasticity, and autonomic dysfunction noted on physical examination. Toxic myelopathies can be broadly categorized into those with geographic predilection and those without. **Table 2** outlines the common causes of toxic myelopathies and their neuroimaging manifestations. Common causes of myelopathies without geographic prediction include chemotherapy-related myelopathies and radiation-induced myelopathy. Numerous chemotherapeutic agents have been reported to cause myelopathy, such as methotrexate, doxorubicin, vincristine, cytarabine with higher risk in patients with prior spinal irradiation. Myelitis with patchy cord edema and enhancement is also occasionally seen as an adverse effect of newer immunotherapeutic agents such as ipilimumab (**Fig. 19**). These are diagnostically challenging because the clinical onset is variable ranging from 48 hours to months after treatment presenting with either transient, flaccid, and are flexic paraparesis or progressive spastic-ataxic paraparesis. Given the rarity of these conditions, it should be a diagnosis of exclusion after ruling out neoplasm, infection, and paraneoplastic myelopathy.[8,28,29]

Radiation myelopathy occurs secondary to radiation of spinal cord, vertebral neoplasm, or adjacent structures such as head and neck, lungs, and mediastinum. The incidence depends on total radiation dose, radiation dose per fraction, and factors in limiting the volume and dose with most centers limiting the total dose to the cord to 45 Gy in 1.8-Gy to 2-Gy fractions. Radiation-induced cord changes could be acute transient myelopathy or chronic progressive. The former occurs within the first 6 months after exposure, more frequently seen in the cervical region and is due to transient demyelination. Chronic progressive radiation myelopathy presents several months to a couple of years following the exposure secondary to death of vascular endothelial cells with demyelination and tissue necrosis. Patchy multifocal or long-segment changes can be seen on MR imaging; however, these changes have the unique feature of being sharply demarcated by the radiation field (**Fig. 20**). This can also be recognized by the presence of fatty bone marrow changes in the adjacent vertebral bodies.

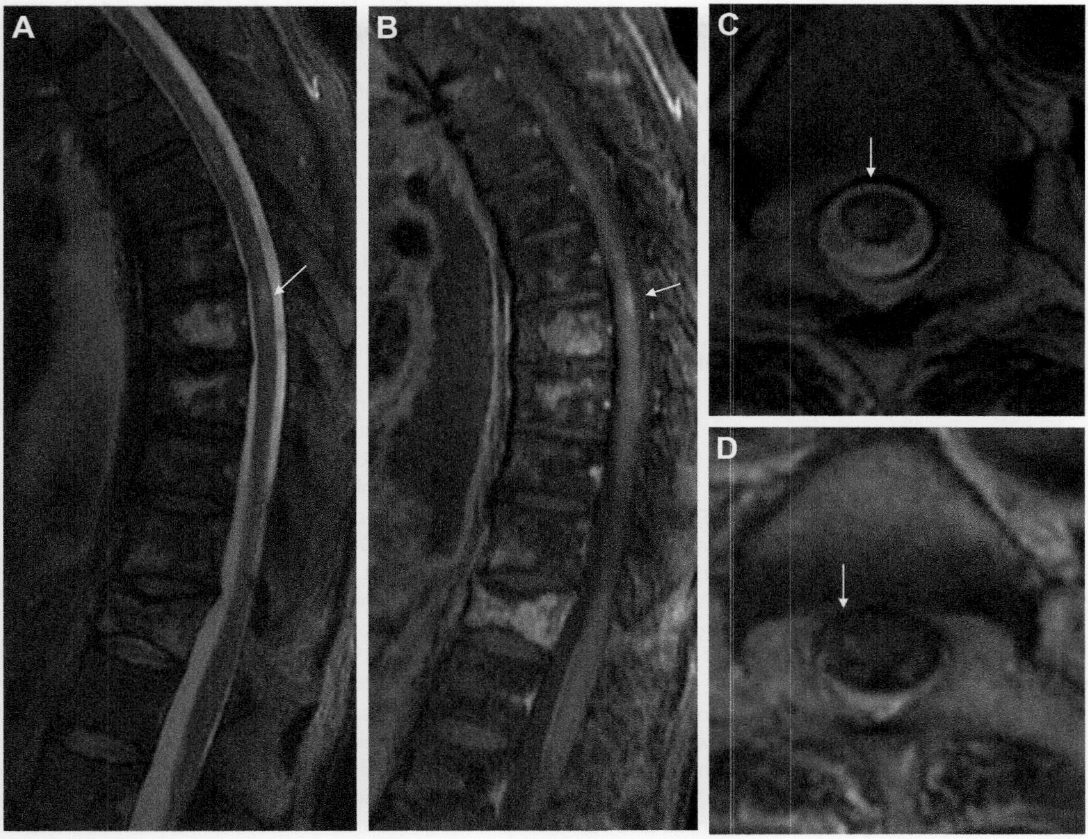

Fig. 20. Radiation-induced myelopathy in a 67-year-old patient with metastatic esophageal carcinoma. Multiple MR imaging images include T2-TSE sagittal and axial (*A, C*), T1-fat saturated postcontrast (*B, D*). Study reveals long segment cord T2 hyperintensity (*A, C, arrows*) within the radiation-field with patchy enhancement (*B, D, arrows*). Osseous metastasis with multiple pathologic fractures is also noted in the thoracic spine.

Less common causes include nitrous oxide toxicity, heroin-induced myelopathy, and organophosphate toxicity. Nitrous oxide is used as an analgesic and anesthetic in surgical and dental procedures and causes irreversible inactivation of vitamin B12 producing a clinico-radiological presentation similar to vitamin B12 deficiency and may occur after a single or multiple exposure. Imaging features are similar to that seen in vitamin B12 deficiency with long segment T2 hyperintense signal in the posterior and lateral columns of the spinal cord on T2-weighted imaging, with or without contrast enhancement. The other category of toxic myelopathies without geographic predilection is rare with causes including cassava, lathyrism, fluorosis, or clioquinol toxicity. The diagnosis in these conditions is made based on history of exposure and toxicology screening, more than specific radiological features. These entities, although common in certain geographic locations, are rare in the United States.[8,30]

SUMMARY

Neurotoxic side effects of therapeutic agents and illicit drug usage are increasingly being reported. Neurologic complications of immunotherapeutic agents are also increasingly being recognized. Neuroradiologic and neuropathological studies are the primary means of identifying toxins that target cerebral white matter. Radiologists should be aware of these various toxins and their complications because many of the toxic leukoencephalopathies can rapidly be corrected.

CLINICS CARE POINTS

- MR imaging is the preferred imaging modality in clinical suspicion of ATL.
- Restricted diffusion in toxic leukoencephalopathy is secondary to intramyelinic edema and is amenable to rapid correction.

- Knowledge about the new immunotherapeutic agents and their complications is important for the radiologist.
- Neuroimaging features of toxic leukoencephalopathies can mimic stroke, demyelination, and cancer progression in many cases.

DISCLOSURE

No commercial or financial conflicts of interest for any authors.

REFERENCES

1. de Oliveira AM, Paulino MV, Vieira APF, et al. Imaging patterns of toxic and metabolic brain disorders. Radiographics 2019 Oct;39(6):1672–95.
2. Filley CM, Kleinschmidt-DeMasters BK. Toxic leukoencephalopathy. N Engl J Med 2001;345:425–32.
3. McKinney AM, Kieffer SA, Paylor RT, et al. Acute toxic leukoencephalopathy: potential for reversibility clinically and on MRI with diffusion-weighted and FLAIR imaging. AJR Am J Roentgenol 2009;193:192–206.
4. Lipton SA, Rosenberg PA. Excitatory amino acids as a final common pathway for neurologic disorders. N Engl J Med 1994;330(9):613–22.
5. Moritani T, Smoker WRK, Sato Y, et al. Diffusion-weighted imaging of acute excitotoxic brain injury. AJNR Am J Neuroradiol 2005;26(2):216–28.
6. Takanashi J, Barkovich AJ, Sihara T, et al. Widening spectrum of a reversible splenial lesion with transiently reduced diffusion. AJNR Am J Neuroradiol 2006 Apr;27(4):836–8.
7. Özütemiz C, Roshan SK, Kroll NJ, et al. Acute toxic leukoencephalopathy: etiologies, imaging findings, and outcomes in 101 patients. AJNR Am J Neuroradiol 2019 Feb;40(2):267–75.
8. Ramalho J, Nunes RH, da Rocha AJ, et al. Toxic and metabolic myelopathies. Semin Ultrasound CT MR 2016 Oct;37(5):448–65.
9. Kazmierczak PM, Dührsen M, Forbrig R, et al. Ultrafast brain magnetic resonance imaging in acute neurological emergencies: diagnostic accuracy and impact on patient management. Invest Radiol 2020 Mar;55(3):181–9.
10. Katsura M, Sato J, Akahane M, et al. Recognizing radiation-induced changes in the central nervous system: where to look and what to look for. Radiographics 2021 Jan-Feb;41(1):224–48.
11. Burris HA, Hurtig J. Radiation recall with anticancer agents. Oncol 2010;15(11):1227–37.
12. Rimkus Cde M, Andrade CS, Leite Cda C, et al. Toxic leukoencephalopathies, including drug, medication, environmental, and radiation-induced encephalopathic syndromes. Semin Ultrasound CT MR 2014;35:97–117.
13. Schroyen G, Meylaers M, Deprez S, et al. Prevalence of leukoencephalopathy and its potential cognitive sequelae in cancer patients. J Chemother 2020 Nov;32(7):327–43.
14. Strati P, Nastoupil LJ, Westin J, et al. Clinical and radiologic correlates of neurotoxicity after axicabtagene ciloleucel in large B-cell lymphoma. Blood Adv 2020 Aug 25;4(16):3943–51.
15. Dunham SR, Schmidt R, Clifford DB. Treatment of progressive multifocal leukoencephalopathy using immune restoration. Neurotherapeutics 2020 Jul;17(3):955–65.
16. Yoon JG, Smith DA, Tirumani SH, et al. CAR T-cell therapy: an update for radiologists. AJR Am J Roentgenol 2021 Dec;217(6):1461–74.
17. Peacock A, Leung J, Larney S, et al. Global statistics on alcohol, tobacco and illicit drug use: 2017 status report. Addiction 2018 Oct;113(10):1905–26.
18. Sloboda Z. Changing patterns of "drug abuse" in the United States: connecting findings from macro- and microepidemiologic studies. Subst Use Misuse 2002 Jun-Aug;37(8–10):1229–51.
19. Zuccoli G, Siddiqui N, Cravo I, et al. Neuroimaging findings in alcohol-related encephalopathies. AJR Am J Roentgenol 2010 Dec;195(6):1378–84.
20. Keogh CF, Andrews GT, Spacey SD, et al. Neuroimaging features of heroin inhalation toxicity: "chasing the dragon". AJR Am J Roentgenol 2003 Mar;180(3):847–50.
21. González-Duarte A, Williams R. Cocaine-induced recurrent leukoencephalopathy. NeuroRadiol J 2013 Oct;26(5):511–3.
22. Vosoughi R, Schmidt BJ. Multifocal leukoencephalopathy in cocaine users: a report of two cases and review of the literature. BMC Neurol 2015;15:208.
23. Gilbert JW, Xu N, Zhou W, Shuy L, et al. Clinical and MRI characteristics of levamisole-induced leukoencephalopathy in 16 patients. J Neuroimaging 2011;21:e188.
24. Tollens N, Post P, Martins D, et al. Multifocal leukoencephalopathy associated with intensive use of cocaine and the adulterant levamisole in a 29-year-old patient. Neurol Res Pract 2022 Aug 1;4(1):38.
25. Filley CM. Occupation and the risk of chronic toxic leukoencephalopathy. Handb Clin Neurol 2015;131:73–91.
26. Filley CM. Toluene abuse and white matter: a model of toxic leukoencephalopathy. Psychiatr Clin 2013 Jun;36(2):293–302.
27. Zemina K, Piña Y, Malafronte P, et al. Spongiform leukoencephalopathy: a unique case of biopsy

confirmed leukoencephalopathy secondary to toxic, non-inflammatory exposure. SAGE Open Med Case Rep 2021;9. 2050313X211042984.

28. Schwendimann RN. Metabolic and toxic myelopathies. Continuum 2018 Apr;24(2):427–40.
29. Khan M, Ambady P, Kimbrough D S, et al. Radiation-induced myelitis: initial and follow-up MRI and clinical features in patients at a single tertiary care institution during 20 years. AJNR Am J Neuroradiol 2018 Aug;39(8):1576–81.
30. Corrêa DG, da Cruz LCH Jr, da Rocha AJ, Pacheco FT. Imaging Aspects of Toxic and Metabolic Myelopathies. Semin Ultrasound CT MR 2023;44(5):452–63.

Uncommon and Miscellaneous Inflammatory Disorders of the Brain and Spine

John D. Comer, MD, PhD*, Aristides A. Capizzano, MD, MSc

KEYWORDS

• Neuroinflammatory disorders • Autoimmune • Vasculitis • Encephalitis

KEY POINTS

- Inflammatory disorders of the brain and spine demonstrate variable imaging abnormalities with significant overlap, posing a significant diagnostic challenge particularly for the more uncommon neuroinflammatory entities.
- Synthesis of the salient clinical presentation and any apparent geographic predilection of signal alteration on MRI may aid in guiding to the underlying diagnosis or suggestion of an underlying neuroinflammatory disorder.
- Increased awareness of the more uncommon neuroinflammatory entities among radiologists will also assist in the consideration of these diagnoses when evaluating MRI examinations.

INTRODUCTION

Inflammatory disorders of the brain and spine have highly variable imaging appearances on MRI, often involving the brain parenchymal white matter in conjunction with spinal cord intramedullary lesions. As discussed in the accompanying articles regarding the more common neuroinflammatory disorders, the morphologic and geographic distribution of these lesions can provide clues to the underlying diagnosis or spectrum of diseases that should be considered. Diagnostic consideration of the more uncommon neuroinflammatory disorders is hampered by both their rarity and the high degree of overlap in their imaging appearances. Narrowing of the differential diagnostic possibilities requires the integration of the salient clinical data, as well as the morphologic traits, geographic distribution, and other signal alterations observed on diagnostic imaging. In this article, many of the less commonly encountered neuroinflammatory disorders will be reviewed with the aim of improving awareness of these more rare conditions and providing a degree of guidance when considering these entities as a diagnostic possibility.

NEUROSARCOIDOSIS

Clinical Findings

Sarcoidosis is an idiopathic multisystem inflammatory disorder characterized histopathologically by epithelioid noncaseating granulomas, with the greatest predilection for the pulmonary system in 90% to 95% of patients.[1,2] In the setting of systemic disease, symptomatic central nervous system (CNS) involvement has been reported in up to 5% of patients, though imaging findings may be present in up to 10% of cases with postmortem studies demonstrating evidence of disease in up to 25% of patients, indicating a higher percentage of subclinical disease.[3,4] Isolated CNS involvement is less common, present in up to 1% of patients.[4,5] Cranial neuropathies, including

Division of Neuroradiology, Department of Radiology, University of Michigan Health System, 1500 East Medical Center Drive, B2-A209 UH, Ann Arbor, MI 48109, USA
* Corresponding author.
E-mail address: comerjo@med.umich.edu

Magn Reson Imaging Clin N Am 32 (2024) 277–287
https://doi.org/10.1016/j.mric.2024.01.006
1064-9689/24/

facial nerve paralysis and vision loss, headache, seizure, and meningism, are among the most frequent clinical presentations, with more uncommon clinical symptoms related to hypothalamic/pituitary dysfunction and hydrocephalus, as well as lower extremity weakness related to spinal cord involvement.[3,4] Clinical diagnosis of definite neurosarcoidosis requires tissue biopsy. However, CNS biopsy is often not feasible secondary to the lack of a biopsy-appropriate site, and diagnosis of probable neurosarcoidosis may rely on tissue pathology outside the CNS, as well as additional findings including chest radiography, gallium scan, and serum angiotensin-converting enzyme.[2,4] In the setting of isolated CNS involvement, a high degree of clinical suspicion, as well as compatible clinical presentation and the exclusion of other etiologies, is needed.[2] Cerebrospinal fluid (CSF) studies have been suggested to parallel disease severity but otherwise demonstrate nonspecific findings.[1,3,4]

Imaging Findings

MRI findings in neurosarcoidosis are highly variable, reflecting the variety of clinical presentations in the setting of the disease (**Fig. 1**). Neurosarcoidosis demonstrates a predilection for basal leptomeningeal enhancement, with involvement of the parenchyma thought to be secondary to spread of inflammation along the perivascular spaces.[3,5,6] Parenchymal involvement may present as multiple or solitary variably enhancing lesions, with periventricular T2 hyperintense white matter lesions a common finding.[5,6] Pachymeningeal thickening/enhancement may also be seen, often within the posterior fossa.[5,6] Hydrocephalus is more rarely associated, reported in 5% to 12% of patients.[6] Cranial nerve involvement may also be seen, with the optic, trigeminal, and facial/vestibulocochlear nerve complexes most often involved.[5,6] The hypothalamic-pituitary axis may also be involved, which is thought to be secondary to anatomic proximity to the basal meninges.[5,6] Variably enhancing, T2 hyperintense intramedullary lesions of the spinal cord may also be seen, with associated fusiform enlargement of the affected spinal cord segments.[5,6] Finally, engorgement of the deep medullary veins has also been described on susceptibility-weighted imaging (SWI) sequences with additional findings of cortical vein vessel wall enhancement, which may be related to an underlying component of vascular inflammation.[7–9] Given the variable imaging appearance of neurosarcoidosis, differential considerations must always be included, with differential entities including infectious and neoplastic etiologies.

NEURO-BEHCET'S DISEASE

Clinical Findings

Behcet's disease is an inflammatory disorder, classically diagnosed with the concurrent clinical presentation of uveitis and aphthous oral and genital ulcerations, now known to demonstrate multisystem involvement, including the pulmonary, gastrointestinal, vascular, and nervous systems.[10] Although vasculitis is considered a core pathologic component, within the CNS, a contributing vasculitic process is not usually demonstrated.[10,11] Neurologic involvement has been reported in 4% to 49%, and clinical presentations may be divided into 2 groups according to CNS parenchymal or non-parenchymal involvement.[10–12] In the setting of CNS parenchymal involvement, pyramidal signs, hemiparesis, behavioral changes, sphincter dysfunction, and headache are most commonly observed, with less prominent clinical findings including brainstem signs, such as ophthalmoplegia and bulbar signs, pyramidocerebellar syndrome, sensory disturbance, and fever.[10] CNS non-parenchymal involvement accounts for approximately 20% of cases and often presents with symptoms of increased intracranial pressure, with the most common clinical presentations including papilledema, headache, sixth cranial nerve palsy, and pyramidal signs.[10] Less common clinical presentations of CNS parenchymal and non-parenchymal involvement have been described elsewhere.[10] Importantly, clinically, neuro-Behcet's disease may present similarly to multiple sclerosis, with a variable progressive or relapsing-remitting course.[12]

Imaging Findings

During an acute presentation of neuro-Behcet's disease, T2/fluid-attenuated inversion recovery (FLAIR) signal alteration with possible superimposed enhancement is most commonly observed within the basal ganglia, diencephalon, and brainstem regions, and less commonly within the spinal cord[11,12] (**Fig. 2**). This signal alteration is most often secondary to vasogenic edema, although atypical lesions may demonstrate areas of restricted diffusion.[13,14] In the acute setting, signal alteration involving the internal capsule may also be seen.[11,15] Spinal cord lesions have also been observed to extend longitudinally 2 or more segments, with involvement of the posterolateral cord.[12] The observed time course of lesions is also critical in suggesting the diagnosis, as patients in clinical remission may demonstrate smaller lesions within the prior area of involvement or may demonstrate interval resolution of signal alteration.[11] Importantly, this emphasizes the

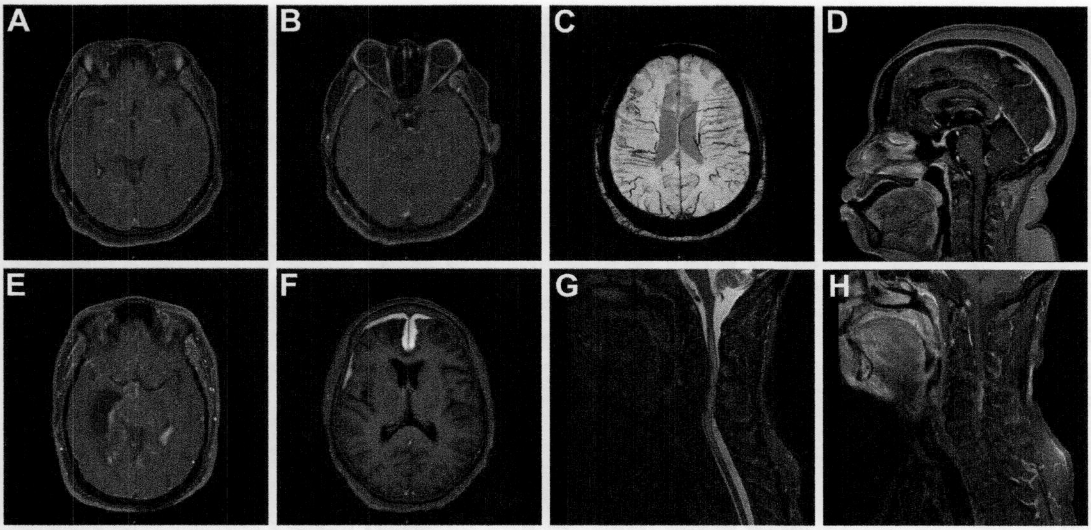

Fig. 1. Neurosarcoidosis. (*A–D*) A patient with a history of neurosarcoidosis and limited responsiveness to multiple immunosuppressive regimens presenting with severe headache and right-sided facial pain. T1 postcontrast imaging demonstrated diffuse leptomeningeal enhancement (*A, B*) with additional involvement of the cisternal segment of the right oculomotor nerve (*B*). Enhancement at the right Meckel's cave was additionally observed (not shown). Susceptibility-weighted imaging (SWI) imaging (*C*) demonstrated medullary vein engorgement. Sagittal T1 postcontrast imaging (*D*) demonstrated nodularity of the pituitary infundibulum. (*E*) T1 postcontrast imaging in a patient with a history of neurosarcoidosis and obstructive hydrocephalus status post-VP shunt presenting with seizures and mental status change in the setting of missed immunosuppressive therapy. Imaging demonstrated diffuse leptomeningeal and pial enhancement with enlargement of the right temporal horn. (*F*) T1 postcontrast imaging in a patient with a history of neurosarcoidosis presenting with seizures and severe headache. Imaging demonstrated significant pachymeningeal thickening and enhancement along the bifrontal convexities. (*G, H*) A patient with neurosarcoidosis presenting with severe pain and weakness of the bilateral upper extremities. Short tau inversion recovery (STIR) imaging (*G*) demonstrated long segment cervical cord edema with superimposed areas of patchy enhancement (*H*). Confluent periventricular cerebral white matter signal alteration was additionally present (not shown). Cervical cord enhancement resolved with immunosuppressive therapy.

importance of review of clinical history in the setting of a normal examination, as this does not necessarily exclude the diagnosis.[16] Chronically, brainstem atrophy may be seen and is thought to be specific for the diagnosis in cases where there is isolated brainstem volume loss.[11,17] CNS parenchymal and CNS non-parenchymal presentations must also be considered, as parenchymal signal alteration is rarely seen in the latter presentation with dural venous sinus occlusion being a more common finding.[11] Differential considerations include multiple sclerosis, infection, cerebrovascular disease, neoplasm, and compressive myelopathy.[10] Distinction from multiple sclerosis can be challenging in cases where the predominant lesion is not located within the brainstem and is instead limited to the periventricular region. Although more uncommon, in such cases, a careful review of the clinical presentation may provide guidance to arrive at the correct diagnosis. In many cases, however, a differential diagnosis must still be provided.

CENTRAL NERVOUS SYSTEM VASCULITIS

Clinical and Imaging Findings

Vasculitis is a generic pathologic entity encompassing the inflammation of blood vessel walls and the clinical sequela secondary to alterations in vascular flow due to luminal narrowing or obstruction and changes in vascular tone, which lead to a wide variety of systemic effects depending on the vasculature involved.[18] Because there is a high degree of overlap in clinical presentations and imaging findings, both will be combined within this section.

CNS vasculitis may occur as a component of systemic vasculitis, may be related to connective tissue disorders, infection, malignancy, drug abuse, or treatment-related effects, or it may present in isolation with only neurologic clinical manifestations.[18] Clinical manifestations are greatly diverse, with clinical suspicion dependent on patient presentation as well as rheumatologic laboratory studies. Vasculitis is generally classified

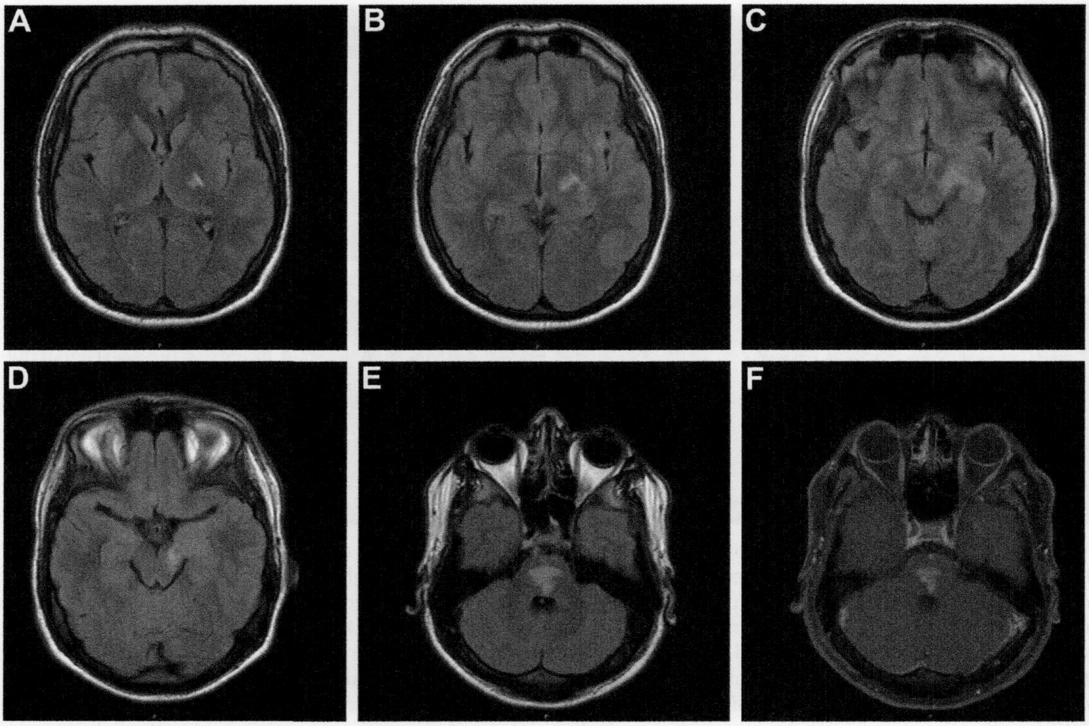

Fig. 2. Neuro-Behcet's disease. A patient with a history of recurrent aphthous ulcers and prior admission with presumed aseptic meningitis presenting with severe headache, neck pain, and gait difficulties. Cerebrospinal fluid (CSF) demonstrated pleocytosis without a causative organism. Fluid-attenuated inversion recovery (FLAIR) imaging (*A–D*) demonstrated signal alteration involving the posterior limb of the left internal capsule, left thalamus, left cerebral peduncle, and adjacent left midbrain, as well as the medial left temporal lobe. Patient symptoms improved following intravenous steroid administration. Patient then presented again with diffuse facial numbness and right eye blurriness, with imaging demonstrating a new enhancing, FLAIR hyperintense pontine lesion (*E, F*). As patient workup had thus far been negative, although there was no history of genital ulcers or uveitis, the patient was treated for presumed Neuro-Behcet's disease with immunosuppressive therapy, resulting in gradual improvement in symptoms.

according to the size of the arteries involved and associated pathologic lesions.[18] Accordingly, imaging findings depend on the caliber of vessels involved, with T2/FLAIR, diffusion-weighted imaging, and SWI sequences assisting in detecting associated ischemic change and hemorrhage, as well as leptomeningeal and pachymeningeal enhancement on postcontrast sequences.[18,19] Imaging analysis of vessels may reveal a variety of pathology, including vessel wall thickening, luminal narrowing or occlusion, aneurysm formation, and venous sinus thrombosis.[18] Imaging findings are generally nonspecific but are helpful in combination with clinical findings to suggest CNS vasculitis as a generic diagnostic possibility as part of a broader differential diagnosis (**Fig. 3**). Beyond clinical and imaging findings, vessel wall biopsy is required for definitive diagnosis.[18]

The large-vessel vasculitides, including Takayasu arteritis and giant cell arteritis, generally do not demonstrate intracranial involvement, while the medium-vessel and small-vessel vasculitides demonstrate increasing CNS involvement.[18] Polyarteritis nodosa may present with CNS findings in approximately 10% of patients, including vessel wall thickening resulting in luminal narrowing or occlusion and aneurysm formation.[18] In the pediatric population, Kawasaki disease may present with CNS findings in up to 30% of patients, with findings including subdural effusions, cerebral infarctions, subcortical lesions, corpus callosum lesions, and imaging findings of posterior reversible encephalopathy syndrome.[18,20] In the small-vessel vasculitides, CNS involvement is more common, with microscopic polyangiitis CNS involvement estimated in 37% to 72% of patients, and in 35% of patients with granulomatosis with polyangiitis.[18] CNS involvement is also common with eosinophilic granulomatosis with polyangiitis.[18,21] Vessel pathology limited to the CNS may

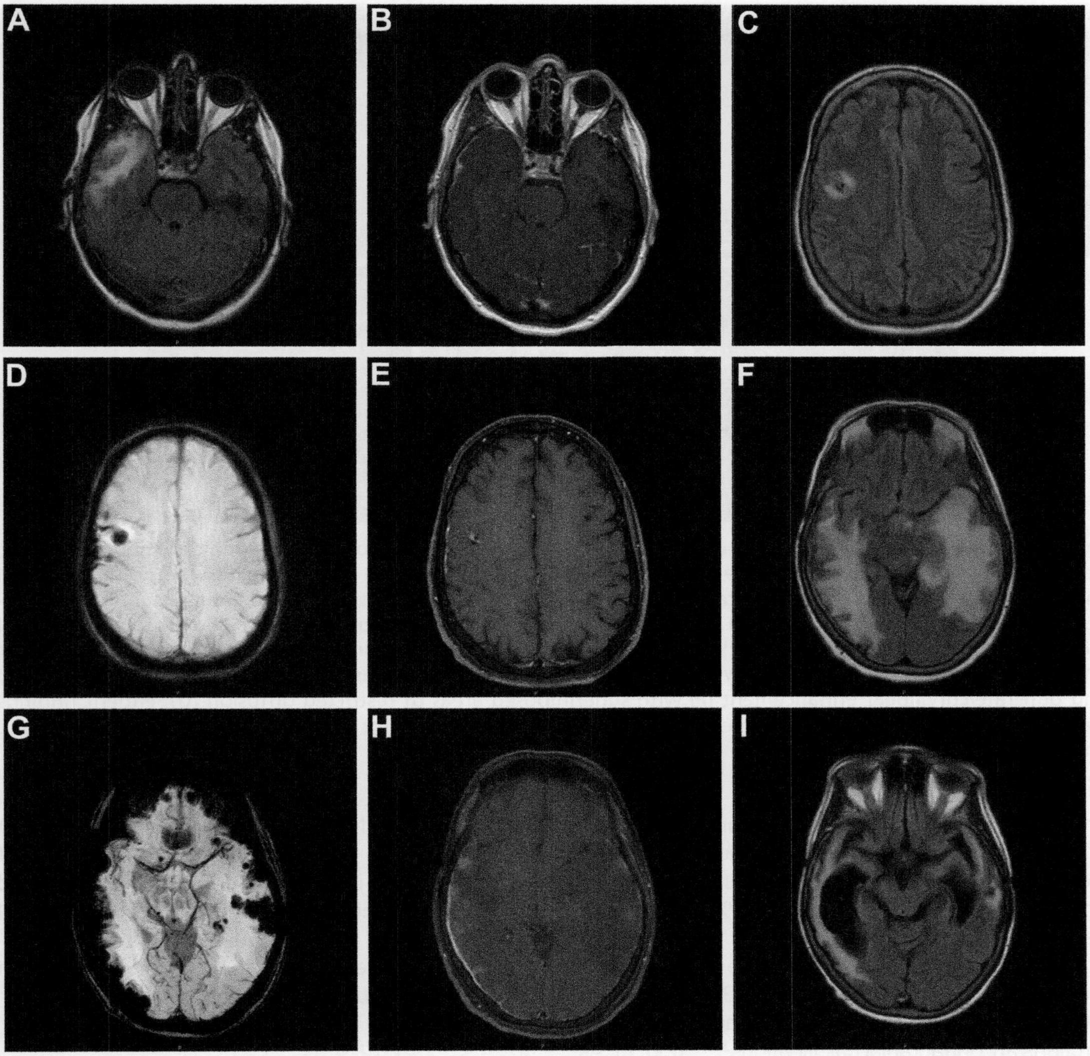

Fig. 3. Central nervous system (CNS) vasculitis. A patient initially presented with severe headache, seizures, and right facial pain. Initial imaging demonstrated right anterior temporal fluid-attenuated inversion recovery (FLAIR) hyperintensity (*A*) with adjacent right middle cranial fossa dural enhancement (*B*). Biopsy was performed with pathology demonstrating atypical vasculitis. Multiple immunosuppressive regimens were attempted with a relapsing disease course. A relapsing episode resulted in new right frontal FLAIR hyperintensity (*C*) with superimposed hemorrhage (*D*) and punctate/curvilinear enhancement (*E*). A more severe relapse later in the disease course resulted in extensive bitemporal FLAIR hyperintensity (*F*) again with superimposed hemorrhage (*G*) and patchy parenchymal and pachymeningeal and leptomeningeal enhancement (*H*). Repeat biopsy again demonstrated CNS vasculitis with acute necrotizing and lymphocytic features. Long-term sequela of disease resulted in extensive gliosis and encephalomalacia (*I*).

be seen in primary angiitis of the CNS, including the hemorrhagic and pseudotumoral forms, reversible cerebral vasoconstriction syndrome, and moyamoya disease.[18]

Systemic disease entities with a CNS vasculitic component will be further discussed here, including systemic lupus erythematosus and Sjogren's syndrome.[18] Infectious, drug abuse–related, and treatment-related etiologies also demonstrate CNS vessel involvement and have been reviewed in detail elsewhere.[18]

Systemic Lupus Erythematosus

Systemic lupus erythematosus (SLE) is a systemic autoimmune disease associated with a vasculitis

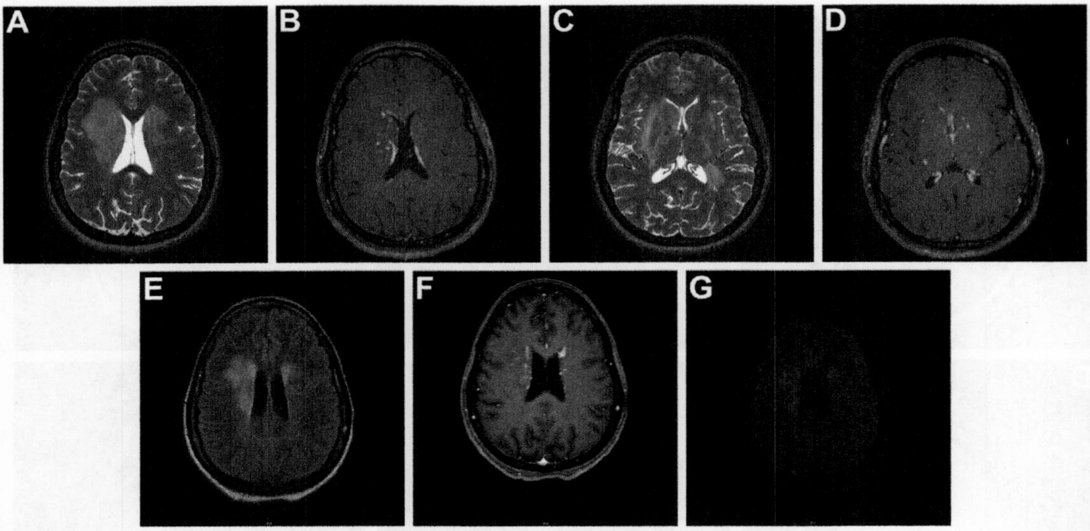

Fig. 4. Systemic lupus erythematosus (SLE). A patient with a history of combined variable immunodeficiency, neuropsychiatric SLE with visual and auditory hallucinations, and possible Sjogren's syndrome presenting with chronic arthralgias and acute mental status change following abrupt discontinuation of immunosuppressive therapy. Imaging demonstrated extensive T2 signal alteration involving periventricular, deep, and subcortical cerebral white matter (*A*), as well as at the level of the basal ganglia (*C*), with superimposed areas of punctate/curvilinear enhancement (*B, D*). Short-term follow-up imaging demonstrated similar distribution of FLAIR hyperintensity (*E*) and punctate/curvilinear enhancement (*F*) with superimposed areas of restricted diffusion (*G*). Patient findings were compatible with a lupus cerebritis with possible etiologies including vasculitis and autoimmune encephalitis.

and vasculopathy of medium and small arterioles and capillaries, with neuropsychiatric components including stroke, psychosis, epilepsy, and neurocognitive defects occurring in 14% to 75% of patients.[18,22,23]

Imaging findings commonly include cerebral white matter lesions, reported in 60% to 86% of patients, and brain atrophy, with additional findings including infarctions and intracranial calcifications[18,23] (**Fig. 4**). As with the other vasculitides, intracranial hemorrhage may be an additional feature with variable involvement of the intracranial compartments.[18,23] Signal alteration in the spinal cord is less common, reported in 1% to 3% of patients, manifesting as multilevel signal alteration with possible superimposed contrast enhancement.[18,22–25]

A secondary antiphospholipid antibody (APLA) syndrome is common in the setting of SLE, reported in 30% to 50% of patients, presenting with vascular thrombosis, thrombocytopenia, and miscarriages.[18,19,23,26] While imaging findings are nonspecific, variably demonstrating cerebral white matter signal alteration, infarction, and microhemorrhages, abnormal imaging findings are more commonly observed in patients with SLE alone.[18,27,28] Moreover, the additional associated clinical history may aid in raising suspicion for SLE with secondary APLA syndrome. Notably, anti-N-methyl-d-aspartate receptor (anti-NMDAr) antibodies are also common in the setting of SLE, reported in 30% to 40% of patients, and are likely associated with more advanced clinical symptoms.[23,29] Anti-NMDAr antibodies will be discussed in greater detail in the following sections in the setting of autoimmune encephalitis.

Sjogren's Syndrome

Sjogren's syndrome is a systemic autoimmune disease with glandular involvement most commonly preceding neurologic disease.[18] Neurologic manifestations most commonly affect the peripheral nervous system secondary to small vessel vasculitis, with CNS involvement reported in 10% to 60% of patients.[30,31] Imaging findings include periventricular and subcortical white matter lesions, as well as infarctions and microhemorrhages.[18,30] In the spinal cord, multilevel transverse myelitis has been described with possible predilection for the longitudinal spinal cord tracts.[32,33]

AUTOIMMUNE ENCEPHALITIS

Clinical and Imaging Findings

Autoimmune encephalitis is a generic pathologic entity encompassing a highly variable clinical and imaging presentation depending on the antibody eliciting an immune-mediated inflammatory response, as well as the involved CNS anatomy.[34–38] The various autoimmune encephalitides may be classified as paraneoplastic or nonparaneoplastic according to the concurrent presence of malignancy, or as group I or group II according to the intracellular or cell surface location of the antigen driving the immune-mediated response, with group I entities demonstrating overlap with paraneoplastic disease.[34,36,39,40] A third group may also be considered involving synaptic antigens that are variably intracellular or at the cell surface depending on vesicular recycling.[35] Clinically, the group I encephalitides demonstrate poorer clinical outcomes with decreased therapeutic benefit of associated immunotherapies, while the group II encephalitides demonstrate improved responsiveness to immunotherapy treatment.[36] While clinical presentation depends on the CNS anatomy involved, the autoimmune encephalitides commonly affect the limbic system, often resulting in clinical presentations associated with limbic encephalitis including memory changes, confusion, psychiatric symptoms, and seizure.[36] However, because the involved CNS anatomy can be highly variable, clinical features are generally nonspecific, overlapping with other inflammatory, infectious, and toxic-metabolic encephalitides.[36] CSF findings are generally nonspecific, variably demonstrating pleocytosis, elevated protein concentration, and the presence of oligoclonal bands.[37,41,42] Imaging findings are also generally nonspecific, though particular group I and group II entities demonstrate some predilection for particular CNS anatomic locations.[36] Despite these limitations, however, increased awareness among radiologists of these entities will aid in guiding clinicians to the correct diagnosis. Once clinical suspicion is established, CSF and serum laboratory analysis for the presence of autoantibodies may confirm the diagnosis.[36] A number of antibodies have been identified as playing a role in autoimmune encephalitis and have been reviewed elsewhere, with the more common entities discussed here.[34–38]

Anti-Hu Encephalitis

Anti-Hu (anti-neuronal nuclear antibody 1) encephalitis is the most common paraneoplastic, group I entity, preceding a diagnosis of small-cell lung cancer in more than 70% of patient cases.[34,36,43] Large fiber sensory neuropathy is the most frequently presenting clinical feature, with CNS symptoms including cerebellar and brainstem disorders as well as limbic encephalitis.[36,42–45] As with other group I autoimmune encephalitides, this subtype does not respond well to immunotherapy and carries the most severe prognosis among group I entities.[36] Imaging findings include T2/FLAIR hyperintensity involving the medial temporal lobes, cerebellar edema, or atrophy, as well as signal alteration within the brainstem and spinal cord[34,35,37] (**Fig. 5**).

Anti-N-Methyl-D-Aspartate Receptor Encephalitis

Anti-NMDAr encephalitis is one of the most common nonparaneoplastic, group II entities, with clinical features often involving a viral prodrome followed by behavioral and psychiatric symptoms, memory changes, central hypoventilation, and

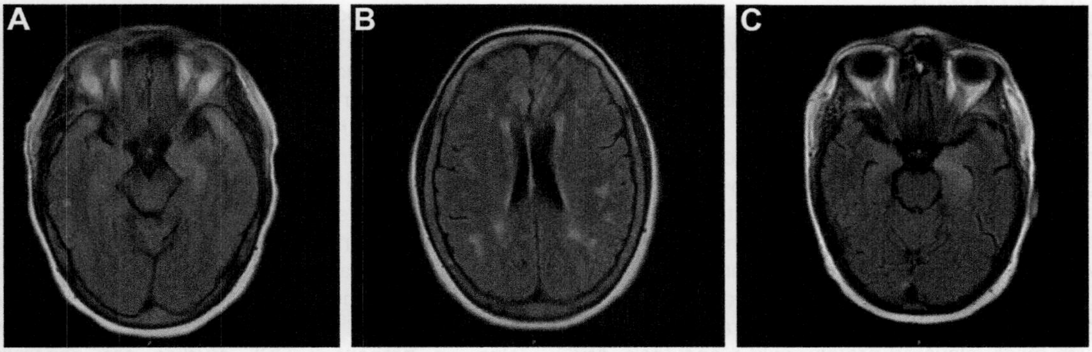

Fig. 5. Anti-Hu autoimmune encephalitis. A patient with a history of breast cancer presenting with seizures and altered mental status. Cerebrospinal fluid (CSF) was notably negative for infection and negative for herpes simplex virus (HSV). A paraneoplastic/autoimmune encephalitis was considered as a possibility, and the patient was empirically treated with intravenous immunoglobulin (IVIG). An encephalopathy panel returned positive for anti-Hu antibodies. Imaging demonstrated FLAIR hyperintensity involving the bilateral medial temporal lobes (*A*), as well as the periventricular and subcortical cerebral white matter (*B*). Additional imaging example of FLAIR hyperintensity within the bilateral medial temporal lobes in a different patient diagnosed with anti-Hu autoimmune encephalitis (*C*).

movement disorders.[34,41,46,47] Importantly, although anti-NMDAr encephalitis is categorized as a nonparaneoplastic encephalitis and has been associated with ovarian teratomas, underlying or concurrent malignancy has also been demonstrated and must always be considered as a component of the diagnostic workup.[34,41,46] As such, medical treatment consists of immunotherapy with concurrent neoplasm assessment and treatment.[40,46] Imaging findings are generally nonspecific and may include T2/FLAIR hyperintensities involving the bilateral medial temporal lobes, patchy involvement of the supratentorial and infratentorial parenchyma, as well as the brainstem and spinal cord.[41] Interestingly, normal MRI brain examinations are also commonly observed and do not exclude the diagnosis, underscoring the importance of correlation with the clinical presentation.[41,46]

Voltage-gated Potassium Channel Encephalitis

Voltage-gated potassium channel encephalitis is a more common group II entity clinically presenting with intractable epilepsy in addition to features of limbic encephalitis.[34,48] Although imaging findings may be absent, T2/FLAIR signal alteration involving the medial temporal lobes with variable partially superimposed restricted diffusion and postcontrast enhancement may be observed, with the additional finding of increased association with the development of mesial temporal sclerosis on follow-up imaging examination.[34,35,48]

CHRONIC LYMPHOCYTIC INFLAMMATION WITH PONTINE PERIVASCULAR ENHANCEMENT RESPONSIVE TO STEROIDS

Clinical Findings

Chronic lymphocytic inflammation with pontine perivascular enhancement responsive to steroids (CLIPPERS) is a CNS inflammatory disease primarily involving the perivascular areas of the pons, midbrain, and cerebellum, with lesions of the basal ganglia and spinal cord as well as meningeal inflammation also described.[49] Clinical features depend on the location and distribution of parenchymal lesions, with clinical presentation most commonly including gait ataxia, dysarthria, diplopia, and facial sensory changes.[49,50] CSF studies are generally nonspecific, with mildly elevated protein, mild pleocytosis, and possible oligoclonal bands.[50,51] Although CLIPPERS etiology remains largely unknown, histopathologically, the disease appears mediated by perivascular lymphocytic infiltration, and the medical treatment includes high-dose corticosteroids.[49] Although clinical features typically resolve following corticosteroid administration, symptom recurrence frequently occurs, demonstrating a relapse-remitting course, and requiring repeat or chronic immunosuppressive therapy.[49,52] Because the etiology of CLIPPERS remains largely unexplained, clinical criteria for definitive diagnosis are not well defined though various criteria have been proposed, requiring assessment of differential diagnoses including neoplastic, paraneoplastic, infectious, and other inflammatory CNS etiologies.[50,52,53]

Imaging Findings

Imaging features of CLIPPERS most commonly demonstrate areas of T2/FLAIR hyperintensity predominantly involving the midbrain, pons, and cerebellum, with involvement of the supratentorial subcortical white matter and spinal cord also described, without significant findings of mass effect[49,50,52] (**Fig. 6**). Moreover, the margins of T2/FLAIR hyperintensity closely approximate areas of superimposed punctate/curvilinear enhancement.[49,50,52] Lesions are also noted to be responsive to corticosteroid therapy, with complete/near complete resolution of parenchymal signal alteration and postcontrast enhancement following treatment.[49,50,52] Recurrence of signal alteration and postcontrast enhancement mirrors clinical relapse, with radiologic findings again responsive to corticosteroid treatment.

SUSAC'S SYNDROME

Clinical Findings

Susac's syndrome presents with the clinical triad of encephalopathy, branch retinal artery occlusions, and hearing loss, with each component demonstrating variable severity and temporal onset, and thought to be secondary to an immune-mediate inflammatory response.[54–56] Clinical presentation of the associated encephalopathy includes headache, memory loss and confusion, behavioral changes, ataxia, and dysarthria.[54,55] Branch retinal artery occlusions result in visual impairment that is most commonly bilateral, though unilateral visual change may also occur.[55] Finally, hearing loss is also most commonly bilateral, with sensorineural hearing loss predominantly within the low-frequency to mid-frequency range which is thought to manifest secondary to microangiopathic infarction of the cochlear apex.[55,57,58] Tinnitus and vertigo may also be present.[55] CSF studies are generally nonspecific, with case studies demonstrating elevated protein levels, mild pleocytosis, and with oligoclonal bands not commonly seen.[56,59] The overall clinical course is self-limiting, resulting in variable degrees of morbidity depending on disease severity.[55,60] While this clinical triad is considered specific for Susac's syndrome, the variability in

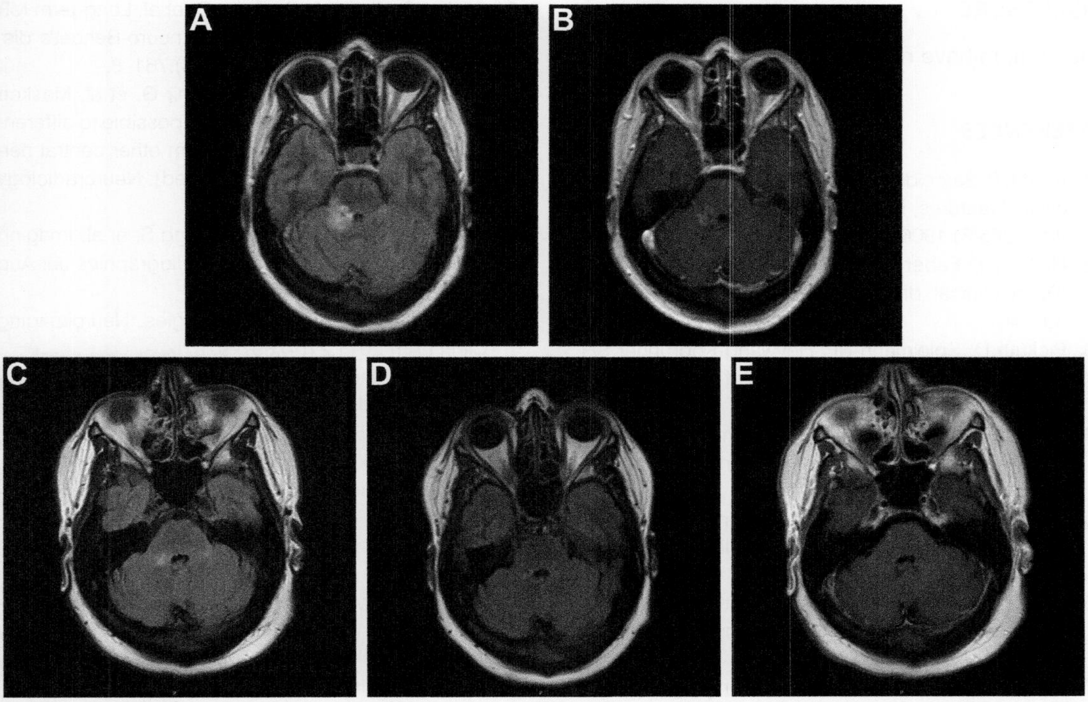

Fig. 6. Chronic lymphocytic inflammation with pontine perivascular enhancement responsive to steroids (CLIPPERS). A patient presented with right hemibody numbness followed by left hemibody numbness, gait difficulties, and hand clumsiness. Initial workup was negative for infectious etiology, negative for paraneoplastic syndrome, negative for extractable nuclear antigen (ENA) panel, and negative for fluorescent treponemal antibody (FTA). Imaging demonstrated fluid-attenuated inversion recovery (FLAIR) hyperintensity involving the right middle cerebellar peduncle and anterior pons (*A*) with superimposed enhancement (*B*). Steroid therapy was initiated, resulting in significant improvement in clinical symptoms and with resolution of right middle cerebellar peduncle enhancement (*E*) and decreased FLAIR hyperintensity (*C*). FLAIR hyperintensity and enhancement within the anterior pons were also no longer appreciated (*C, E*). Follow-up examination demonstrated near complete resolution of FLAIR hyperintensity within the right middle cerebellar peduncle (*D*). Initial negative workup and clinical and imaging responsiveness to steroid therapy strongly suggested a diagnosis of CLIPPERS.

temporal onset of the syndrome components and limited visual and hearing assessment secondary to encephalopathy may greatly increase the challenge of establishing the diagnosis, with estimates of less than 20% of patients demonstrating the clinical triad at disease onset.[54,55,59] This clinical challenge underscores the importance of radiologic findings in this syndrome.

Imaging Findings

Imaging features of Susac's syndrome predominantly demonstrate T2/FLAIR hyperintensities within the central portion of the body and splenium of the corpus callosum.[54,55] This central location of the corpus callosal lesions as well as the absence of callosal atrophy aid in distinguishing Susac's syndrome from other inflammatory disorders such as multiple sclerosis and acute disseminated encephalomyelitis.[54] T2/FLAIR signal alteration may also be seen within the centrum semiovale, internal capsule, and periventricular white matter, as well as within the basal ganglia, thalamus, and brainstem.[54,55,60] Superimposed enhancement may be seen in the acute setting, with leptomeningeal enhancement less common.[54,55,61]

SUMMARY

Inflammatory disorders of the brain and spine demonstrate a high degree of overlap on imaging examination, requiring a deep synthesis of clinical presentation and radiologic examination to suggest this particular category of disease, as well more specific neuroinflammatory entities. Consideration of the more uncommon neuroinflammatory diseases is further hampered by their overall rarity. By increasing awareness of the clinical and imaging features of these less common neuroinflammatory entities, arrival at the correct underlying diagnosis and administration of associated medical treatment may be greatly supported.

DISCLOSURE

The authors have nothing to disclose.

REFERENCES

1. Kidd DP. Sarcoidosis of the central nervous system: clinical features, imaging, and CSF results. J Neurol 2018;265(8):1906–15.
2. Hoitsma E, Faber CG, Drent M, et al. Neurosarcoidosis: a clinical dilemma. Lancet Neurol 2004;3(7): 397–407.
3. Pickuth D, Spielmann RP, Heywang-Kobrunner SH. Role of radiology in the diagnosis of neurosarcoidosis. Eur Radiol 2000;10(6):941–4.
4. Smith JK, Matheus MG, Castillo M. Imaging manifestations of neurosarcoidosis. AJR Am J Roentgenol 2004;182(2):289–95.
5. Ginat DT, Dhillon G, Almast J. Magnetic resonance imaging of neurosarcoidosis. J Clin Imaging Sci 2011;1:15.
6. Bathla G, Singh AK, Policeni B, et al. Imaging of neurosarcoidosis: common, uncommon, and rare. Clin Radiol 2016;71(1):96–106.
7. Bathla G, Soni N, Moritani T, et al. Engorged Medullary Veins in Neurosarcoidosis: A Reflection of Underlying Phlebitis? AJNR Am J Neuroradiol 2019; 40(3):E14–5.
8. Zamora C, Hung SC, Tomingas C, et al. Engorgement of Deep Medullary Veins in Neurosarcoidosis: A Common-Yet-Underrecognized Cerebrovascular Finding on SWI. AJNR Am J Neuroradiol 2018; 39(11):2045–50.
9. Bathla G, Watal P, Gupta S, et al. Cerebrovascular manifestations in neurosarcoidosis: how common are they and does perivascular enhancement matter? Clin Radiol 2018;73(10):907 e15–e907 e23.
10. Akman-Demir G, Serdaroglu P, Tasci B. Clinical patterns of neurological involvement in Behcet's disease: evaluation of 200 patients. The Neuro-Behcet Study Group. Brain 1999;122(Pt 11):2171–82.
11. Akman-Demir G, Bahar S, Coban O, et al. Cranial MRI in Behcet's disease: 134 examinations of 98 patients. Neuroradiology 2003;45(12):851–9.
12. Kocer N, Islak C, Siva A, et al. CNS involvement in neuro-Behcet syndrome: an MR study. AJNR Am J Neuroradiol 1999;20(6):1015–24.
13. Borhani-Haghighi A, Kardeh B, Banerjee S, et al. Neuro-Behcet's disease: An update on diagnosis, differential diagnoses, and treatment. Mult Scler Relat Disord 2020;39:101906.
14. Kang DW, Chu K, Cho JY, et al. Diffusion weighted magnetic resonance imaging in Neuro-Behcet's disease. J Neurol Neurosurg Psychiatry 2001;70(3): 412–3.
15. Tali ET, Atilla S, Keskin T, et al. MRI in neuro-Behcet's disease. Neuroradiology 1997;39(1):2–6.
16. Gerber S, Biondi A, Dormont D, et al. Long-term MR follow-up of cerebral lesions in neuro-Behcet's disease. Neuroradiology 1996;38(8):761–8.
17. Coban O, Bahar S, Akman-Demir G, et al. Masked assessment of MRI findings: is it possible to differentiate neuro-Behcet's disease from other central nervous system diseases? [corrected]. Neuroradiology 1999;41(4):255–60.
18. Abdel Razek AA, Alvarez H, Bagg S, et al. Imaging spectrum of CNS vasculitis. Radiographics Jul-Aug 2014;34(4):873–94.
19. Garg A. Vascular brain pathologies. Neuroimaging Clin N Am 2011;21(4):897–926, ix.
20. Alves NR, Magalhaes CM, Almeida Rde F, et al. Prospective study of Kawasaki disease complications: review of 115 cases. Rev Assoc Med Bras 2011; 57(3):295–300.
21. Wolf J, Bergner R, Mutallib S, et al. Neurologic complications of Churg-Strauss syndrome–a prospective monocentric study. Eur J Neurol 2010;17(4): 582–8.
22. Sibbitt WL Jr, Brooks WM, Kornfeld M, et al. Magnetic resonance imaging and brain histopathology in neuropsychiatric systemic lupus erythematosus. Semin Arthritis Rheum 2010;40(1):32–52.
23. Ota Y, Srinivasan A, Capizzano AA, et al. Central Nervous System Systemic Lupus Erythematosus: Pathophysiologic, Clinical, and Imaging Features. Radiographics 2022;42(1):212–32.
24. Goh YP, Naidoo P, Ngian GS. Imaging of systemic lupus erythematosus. Part I: CNS, cardiovascular, and thoracic manifestations. Clin Radiol 2013; 68(2):181–91.
25. Costallat BL, Ferreira DM, Costallat LT, et al. Myelopathy in systemic lupus erythematosus: clinical, laboratory, radiological and progression findings in a cohort of 1,193 patients. Rev Bras Reumatol Engl Ed 2016;56(3):240–51.
26. Schreiber K, Sciascia S, de Groot PG, et al. Antiphospholipid syndrome. Nat Rev Dis Primers 2018; 4:17103.
27. Muscal E, Brey RL. Antiphospholipid syndrome and the brain in pediatric and adult patients. Lupus 2010;19(4):406–11.
28. Kaichi Y, Kakeda S, Moriya J, et al. Brain MR findings in patients with systemic lupus erythematosus with and without antiphospholipid antibody syndrome. AJNR Am J Neuroradiol 2014;35(1): 100–5.
29. Gerosa M, Poletti B, Pregnolato F, et al. Antiglutamate Receptor Antibodies and Cognitive Impairment in Primary Antiphospholipid Syndrome and Systemic Lupus Erythematosus. Front Immunol 2016;7:5.
30. Tzarouchi LC, Tsifetaki N, Konitsiotis S, et al. CNS involvement in primary Sjogren Syndrome: assessment of gray and white matter changes with MRI

and voxel-based morphometry. AJR Am J Roentgenol 2011;197(5):1207–12.
31. Ging K, Mono ML, Sturzenegger M, et al. Peripheral and central nervous system involvement in a patient with primary Sjogren's syndrome: a case report. J Med Case Rep 2019;13(1):165.
32. Butryn M, Neumann J, Rolfes L, et al. Clinical, Radiological, and Laboratory Features of Spinal Cord Involvement in Primary Sjogren's Syndrome. J Clin Med 2020;9(5).
33. Kahlenberg JM. Neuromyelitis optica spectrum disorder as an initial presentation of primary Sjogren's syndrome. Semin Arthritis Rheum 2011;40(4):343–8.
34. Kelley BP, Patel SC, Marin HL, et al. Autoimmune Encephalitis: Pathophysiology and Imaging Review of an Overlooked Diagnosis. AJNR Am J Neuroradiol 2017;38(6):1070–8.
35. Ball C, Fisicaro R, Morris L 3rd, et al. Brain on fire: an imaging-based review of autoimmune encephalitis. Clin Imaging 2022;84:1–30.
36. Liang C, Chu E, Kuoy E, et al. Autoimmune-mediated encephalitis and mimics: A neuroimaging review. J Neuroimaging 2023;33(1):19–34.
37. da Rocha AJ, Nunes RH, Maia AC Jr, et al. Recognizing Autoimmune-Mediated Encephalitis in the Differential Diagnosis of Limbic Disorders. AJNR Am J Neuroradiol 2015;36(12):2196–205.
38. Dalmau J, Graus F. Antibody-Mediated Encephalitis. N Engl J Med 2018;378(9):840–51.
39. Graus F, Saiz A, Dalmau J. Antibodies and neuronal autoimmune disorders of the CNS. J Neurol 2010; 257(4):509–17.
40. Gultekin SH, Rosenfeld MR, Voltz R, et al. Paraneoplastic limbic encephalitis: neurological symptoms, immunological findings and tumour association in 50 patients. Brain 2000;123(Pt 7):1481–94.
41. Dalmau J, Tuzun E, Wu HY, et al. Paraneoplastic anti-N-methyl-D-aspartate receptor encephalitis associated with ovarian teratoma. Ann Neurol 2007;61(1):25–36.
42. Dalmau J, Graus F, Rosenblum MK, et al. Anti-Hu–associated paraneoplastic encephalomyelitis/sensory neuronopathy. A clinical study of 71 patients. Medicine (Baltimore). Mar 1992;71(2):59–72.
43. Graus F, Keime-Guibert F, Rene R, et al. Anti-Hu-associated paraneoplastic encephalomyelitis: analysis of 200 patients. Brain 2001;124(Pt 6):1138–48.
44. Alamowitch S, Graus F, Uchuya M, et al. Limbic encephalitis and small cell lung cancer. Clinical and immunological features. Brain 1997;120(Pt 6):923–8.
45. Mason WP, Graus F, Lang B, et al. Small-cell lung cancer, paraneoplastic cerebellar degeneration and the Lambert-Eaton myasthenic syndrome. Brain 1997;120(Pt 8):1279–300.
46. Zhang T, Duan Y, Ye J, et al. Brain MRI Characteristics of Patients with Anti-N-Methyl-D-Aspartate Receptor Encephalitis and Their Associations with 2-Year Clinical Outcome. AJNR Am J Neuroradiol 2018;39(5):824–9.
47. Varley JA, Strippel C, Handel A, et al. Autoimmune encephalitis: recent clinical and biological advances. J Neurol 2023.
48. Kotsenas AL, Watson RE, Pittock SJ, et al. MRI findings in autoimmune voltage-gated potassium channel complex encephalitis with seizures: one potential etiology for mesial temporal sclerosis. AJNR Am J Neuroradiol 2014;35(1):84–9.
49. Zhang L, Zhao D, Li J, et al. A case report of CLIPPERS syndrome and literature review. Medicine (Baltim) 2021;100(22):e26090.
50. Tobin WO, Guo Y, Krecke KN, et al. Diagnostic criteria for chronic lymphocytic inflammation with pontine perivascular enhancement responsive to steroids (CLIPPERS). Brain 2017;140(9):2415–25.
51. Dudesek A, Rimmele F, Tesar S, et al. CLIPPERS: chronic lymphocytic inflammation with pontine perivascular enhancement responsive to steroids. Review of an increasingly recognized entity within the spectrum of inflammatory central nervous system disorders. Clin Exp Immunol 2014;175(3):385–96.
52. Zhuang E, Shane L, Ramezan N, et al. Chronic lymphocytic inflammation with pontine perivascular enhancement responsive to steroids, a mimicker of malignancy: a case report and review of the literature. J Med Case Rep 2021;15(1):246.
53. Simon NG, Parratt JD, Barnett MH, et al. Expanding the clinical, radiological and neuropathological phenotype of chronic lymphocytic inflammation with pontine perivascular enhancement responsive to steroids (CLIPPERS). J Neurol Neurosurg Psychiatry 2012;83(1): 15–22.
54. Saenz R, Quan AW, Magalhaes A, et al. MRI of Susac's syndrome. AJR Am J Roentgenol 2005;184(5): 1688–90.
55. Susac JO, Murtagh FR, Egan RA, et al. MRI findings in Susac's syndrome. Neurology 2003;61(12):1783–7.
56. Jarius S, Kleffner I, Dorr JM, et al. Clinical, paraclinical and serological findings in Susac syndrome: an international multicenter study. J Neuroinflammation 2014;11:46.
57. Monteiro ML, Swanson RA, Coppeto JR, et al. A microangiopathic syndrome of encephalopathy, hearing loss, and retinal arteriolar occlusions. Neurology 1985;35(8):1113–21.
58. Petty GW, Engel AG, Younge BR, et al. Retinocochleocerebral vasculopathy. Medicine (Baltimore) 1998;77(1):12–40.
59. Wilf-Yarkoni A, Elkayam O, Aizenstein O, et al. Increased incidence of Susac syndrome: a case series study. BMC Neurol 2020;20(1):332.
60. Demir MK. Case 142: Susac syndrome. Radiology 2009;250(2):598–602.
61. Susac JO. Susac's syndrome. AJNR Am J Neuroradiol 2004;25(3):351–2.

Bacterial, Viral, and Prion Infectious Diseases of the Brain

Amy M. Condos, MD[a,*], Pattana Wangaryattawanich, MD[b], Tanya J. Rath, MD[c]

KEYWORDS

• Prion • Meningitis • Encephalitis • Cerebritis • Empyema • Abscess • Ventriculitis

KEY POINTS

- Bacterial central nervous system (CNS) infection encompasses a range of conditions such as meningitis, cerebritis, brain abscesses, empyemas, and ventriculitis. The imaging features of these infections vary by the anatomic compartment affected. Classic MR imaging features of bacterial abscesses are a ring-enhancing mass with dual rim on T2 fluid-attenuated inversion recovery (FLAIR) imaging and marked central restricted diffusion.
- Tuberculous infection in the CNS can present in 2 main forms: meningitis or intraparenchymal forms like tuberculomas and tuberculous abscesses. Tubercular meningitis is characterized by thick nodular leptomeningeal enhancement in the basal cisterns, which distinguishes it from pyogenic bacterial meningitis and viral meningitis where thin leptomeningeal enhancement is observed.
- Viral CNS infections trigger a host inflammatory response that can result in meningitis or encephalitis. Viral CSF testing and serology tests are crucial for diagnosing these infections. In herpes simplex virus encephalitis, MR imaging usually shows temporal lobe involvement with restricted diffusion and increased T2 FLAIR signal. Identifying these MR imaging features early is vital for prompt treatment with acyclovir to reduce neurologic complications.
- In sporadic Creutzfeldt-Jakob disease (CJD), characteristic imaging includes symmetric restricted diffusion in the cerebral cortices and basal ganglia, commonly affecting the insula, cingulate gyrus, superior frontal gyrus, caudate nucleus, and putamen. Variant CJD typically presents as restricted diffusion in the bilateral pulvinar nucleus of the thalamus known as the pulvinar and hockey stick signs. Early recognition of these imaging features of CJD is critical for patient counseling and ruling out treatable conditions.

INTRODUCTION

Brain infections caused by bacteria and viruses are a significant health concern worldwide. Imaging is an essential diagnostic tool in the evaluation of brain infections, providing detailed information on the location, extent, and severity of the infection. This review article summarizes the characteristic imaging features of bacterial, viral, and prion brain infections, which when interpreted in conjunction with clinical information are critical to arriving at the appropriate diagnosis and guiding therapy.

PATHOPHYSIOLOGY AND ROUTE OF SPREAD OF BACTERIAL AND VIRAL INFECTION

Traditionally, the brain was considered immunologically privileged due to the structural and

[a] Department of Radiology, University of Washington School of Medicine, Seattle, WA, USA; [b] Department of Radiology, University of Washington School of Medicine, 1959 Northeast Pacific Street, Seattle, WA 98195-7115, USA; [c] Neuroradiology Section, Department of Radiology, Mayo Clinic Arizona, 5777 East Mayo Boulevard, Phoenix, AZ 85054, USA
* Corresponding author. 2545 Northeast 85th Street, Seattle, WA 98115.
E-mail address: acondos@uw.edu

Magn Reson Imaging Clin N Am 32 (2024) 289–311
https://doi.org/10.1016/j.mric.2023.11.001
1064-9689/24/

functional blood-brain barrier, but the recent discovery of the glymphatic system by Dr Maiken Nedergaard has challenged that theory. The glymphatic system is a lymphatic system for the brain, which removes waste from the central nervous system (CNS) via lymphatic channels.[1] The glymphatic system establishes that there is communication between the cerebrospinal fluid (CSF) compartment and the interstitium, consequently, the brain is not "immunologically privileged," but rather actively monitored and guarded by lymphocytes.

There are multiple potential routes of spread of brain infection, with the most common being (1) hematogenous spread from an extracranial infection (2) local extension (ie, dental disease, sinusitis, or otomastoiditis), commonly along valveless emissary veins, (3) direct extension from trauma or surgery, and (4) transsynaptic spread from the peripheral nervous system, for example, in the setting of herpes and rabies infection. Despite undergoing typical work up, 20% to 30% of infections have no identifiable source and are considered cryptogenic.[2]

BACTERIAL INFECTION OF THE BRAIN

Bacterial brain infections encompass a range of conditions including meningitis, cerebritis, brain abscesses, empyemas, and ventriculitis. The imaging features of these infections are variable based on the specific anatomic compartment affected, which are discussed in detail with key teaching points emphasized.

Meningitis

Infectious meningitis is characterized by inflammation of the meninges and can be bacterial, viral, tuberculous, and less commonly fungal, parasitic, or amebic in etiology.[3] Given its high prevalence, with 2.51 million reported cases globally in 2019, radiologists commonly encounter cases of meningitis.[4] The common etiologies for bacterial meningitis vary by age (**Table 1**).[5] Patients with meningitis can present with fever, neck stiffness, headache, and altered mental status. Patients typically experience at least one of these symptoms though all symptoms may not be present.[6] CSF analysis and clinical presentation are critical to confirm the diagnosis as imaging is normal in up to 50% of cases. Complicated meningitis may manifest with symptoms due to increased intracranial pressure, such as enlarging head size in children, persistent headache, nausea, vomiting, papilledema, and cranial neuropathies.[7] Meningitis is considered a medical emergency. Prompt recognition and management of meningitis are vital as the high mortality rate of up to 50% without treatment is reduced to 15% to 25% with treatment.[8] Empiric antibiotic therapy, chosen based on age, should be started immediately and not be delayed for lumbar puncture or imaging. In patients without a history of immunodeficiency, neurologic disease, recent seizure, altered mentation, or focal neurologic deficits, a lumbar puncture can be safely performed without first undergoing a head computed tomography (CT).[9]

Table 1
Common bacterial causes of meningitis by age group

Age	Pathogen
Newborns	Group B streptococcus *Escherichia coli* *Streptococcus pneumoniae* *Listeria monocytogenes*
Older infants and young children	Group B streptococcus *E coli* *S pneumoniae* *Neisseria meningitidis* *Haemophilus influenzae* *Mycobacterium tuberculosis*
Teens and young adults	*S pneumoniae* *N meningitidis*
Older adults	Group B streptococcus *S pneumoniae* *N meningitidis* *H influenzae* *L monocytogenes*

Infectious meningitis usually affects the pia-arachnoid membrane along the surface of the brain, referred to as leptomeninges, causing abnormal leptomeningeal enhancement on postcontrast imaging. The areas of enhancement may extend from the cortical surface into the sulci or basal cisterns or have a gyriform appearance on imaging.[10] MR imaging and CT are not highly sensitive or specific for diagnosing meningitis. In one study, 76% of patients with suspected meningitis had negative head CT results (**Fig. 1**A–H).[9] Therefore, the primary role of imaging is to exclude other potential causes of symptoms and assess for complications. In early meningitis, mild hydrocephalus is often the initial and sole finding. Noncontrast head CT may show subtle sulcal effacement and sulcal hyperattenuation due to alterations in CSF contents.[11] Complications that can arise from meningitis include hydrocephalus, venous thrombosis, vasculitis, infarction, and parenchymal, ventricular, or subdural spread of the disease. Given its excellent soft tissue contrast and higher sensitivity compared to CT, MR

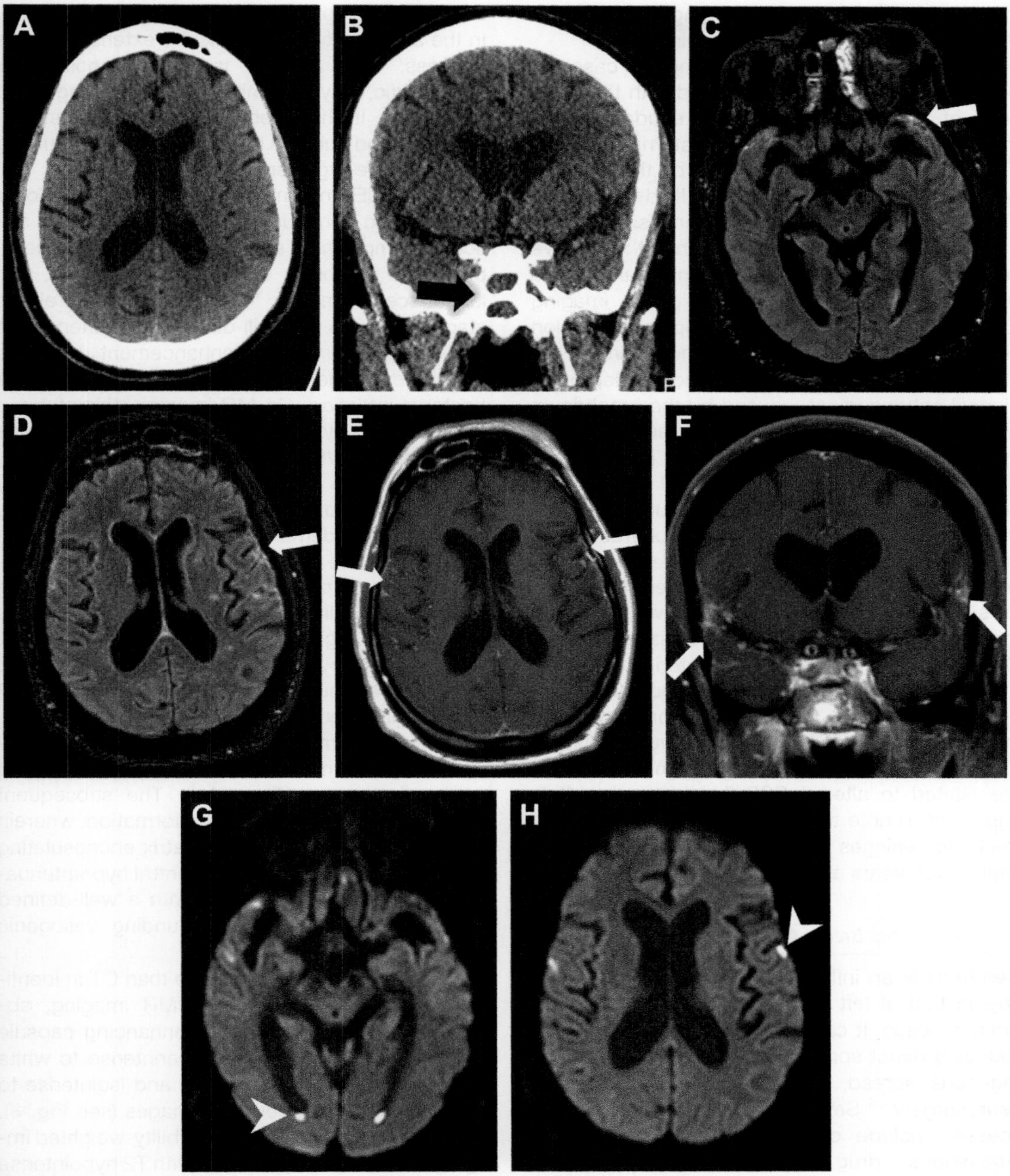

Fig. 1. Bacterial meningitis. A 67-year-old man with type 2 diabetes and acute sinusitis complicated by orbital cellulitis, skull base osteomyelitis, and bacterial meningitis. Blood culture grew *Streptococcus intermedius*. Initial axial (*A*) and coronal (*B*) noncontrast CT show age-related brain volume loss, with no acute intracranial abnormalities. Note sphenoid sinus opacification (*black arrow*) in figure B. Axial FLAIR (*C, D*), axial (*E*), and coronal (*F*) post-contrast T1-weighted images show abnormal FLAIR hyperintense signal in the subarachnoid space with leptomeningeal enhancement, most notable in the bilateral sylvian fissures (*arrows*), compatible with meningitis. Axial DWI (*G,H*) show focal restricted diffusion within the occipital horns of the lateral ventricles as well as within the sylvian fissures (*arrowheads*), secondary to purulent debris. CT, computed tomography; DWI, diffusion-weighted imaging; FLAIR, fluid-attenuated inversion recovery.

imaging is the preferred imaging modality for defining the complications of meningitis.[12]

Many of the MR imaging findings in cases of bacterial meningitis are associated with the presence of pus and proteinaceous exudates filling the CSF subarachnoid and cisternal spaces. These findings are characterized by the nonsuppression of CSF signal on T2 fluid-attenuated inversion recovery (FLAIR) sequences. Postcontrast FLAIR imaging is the most sensitive sequence for detecting leptomeningeal disease (see **Fig. 1**).[13] On diffusion-weighted imaging (DWI), there may be foci of low apparent diffusion coefficient (ADC) signal within the brain parenchyma, sulci, and cisterns.[14] Abnormal leptomeningeal enhancement, caused by the breakdown of the blood-brain barrier, is observed in approximately 50% of patients with acute meningitis.[10] Thin linear enhancement is typical of bacterial and viral meningitis, while thick nodular enhancement is more common in cases of tuberculous or carcinomatous meningitis. In acute meningitis, leptomeningeal enhancement preferentially occurs over the cerebral convexities, while chronic meningitis tends to involve the basal cisterns.[10] Other MR imaging findings in bacterial meningitis may include enlarged CSF spaces, poor visualization of the basal cisterns, cerebral swelling, increased perivascular spaces, hydrocephalus, and subdural effusions. Many of these findings are related to altered CSF flow dynamics. It is important to note that abnormal enhancement of the leptomeninges may persist with chronic meningitis even years after the initial presentation.[10]

Cerebritis and Brain Abscesses

Cerebritis is an inflammation of the brain parenchyma that, if left untreated, can progress to a brain abscess. It can arise from various sources, including direct spread of local infections, hematogenous spread, trauma, or complications of neurosurgery.[15] Several risk factors for brain abscesses include diabetes mellitus, alcoholism, intravenous drug use, immunosuppression, congenital cyanotic heart disease, and arteriovenous shunts.[16] Improvement in treatment of otitis media and early surgical repair of cyanotic heart disease has led to a significant decrease in brain abscesses in developed countries.[16] However, brain abscesses due to trauma or neurosurgical complication have increased due to an increase in surgical volume.[17] Patients commonly present with headache, fever, focal neurologic deficit, nausea, vomiting, or seizure. Unlike meningitis, laboratory findings have limited diagnostic value, and lumbar puncture may be contraindicated due to the risk of increased intracranial pressure. In the absence of intraventricular extension of the abscess, CSF analysis is typically normal or nonspecific, playing a minor role in the diagnostic evaluation. If the infection spreads hematogenously, blood cultures may be useful in identifying the causative organism.

Britt and Enzmann have outlined a pathologic and imaging continuum from cerebritis to an abscess, comprising 4 sequential stages: early cerebritis, late cerebritis, early abscess capsule, and late abscess capsule.[18] During the early cerebritis stage, CT scans reveal ill-defined hypoattenuation with absent or variable enhancement, which is attributed to the inflammatory response to the bacterial infection. On MR imaging, this stage is characterized by a poorly defined T2 hyperintense signal, and DWI may show restricted diffusion, believed to be related to increased cellularity from inflammatory cell migration, brain ischemia, or cytotoxic edema.[19] As the continuum progresses to late cerebritis, central necrosis advances and fibroblasts accumulate at the margin with early reticulin deposition.[18] On CT, this results in a larger region of central hypoattenuation, accompanied by irregular rim enhancement and increased surrounding hypoattenuation. On MR imaging, late cerebritis is depicted by T2 hyperintense signal centrally with central restricted diffusion, irregular rim enhancement, and surrounding vasogenic edema (**Fig. 2**A–I). The subsequent stage is early abscess capsule formation, wherein fibroblasts create a reticulin matrix encapsulating the necrotic material. On CT, central hypoattenuation necrotic debris is seen, with a well-defined enhancing capsule and surrounding vasogenic edema (**Fig. 3**A–G).

MR imaging is more sensitive than CT in identifying brain abscesses.[12] On MR imaging, abscesses typically show a rim-enhancing capsule that appears isointense to hyperintense to white matter on T1-weighted images and isointense to hypointense on T2-weighted images (see **Fig. 3**). Additionally, on T2 and susceptibility-weighted imaging, a dual rim may be seen with T2 hypointense outer rim and T2 hyperintense inner rim.[20] The T2 hypointense capsule signal characteristics are attributed to paramagnetic bactericidal–free radicals generated by active macrophages.[21] This dual rim maybe helpful in differentiating abscesses from necrotic glioblastomas as it is not typically seen with necrotic glioblastomas.[20] Thin (2–7 mm) smooth rim enhancement is characteristic of brain abscesses but can be seen with other lesions.[22] The capsule wall is thinner medially due to reduced migration of fibroblasts, which may result in the formation of daughter abscesses or

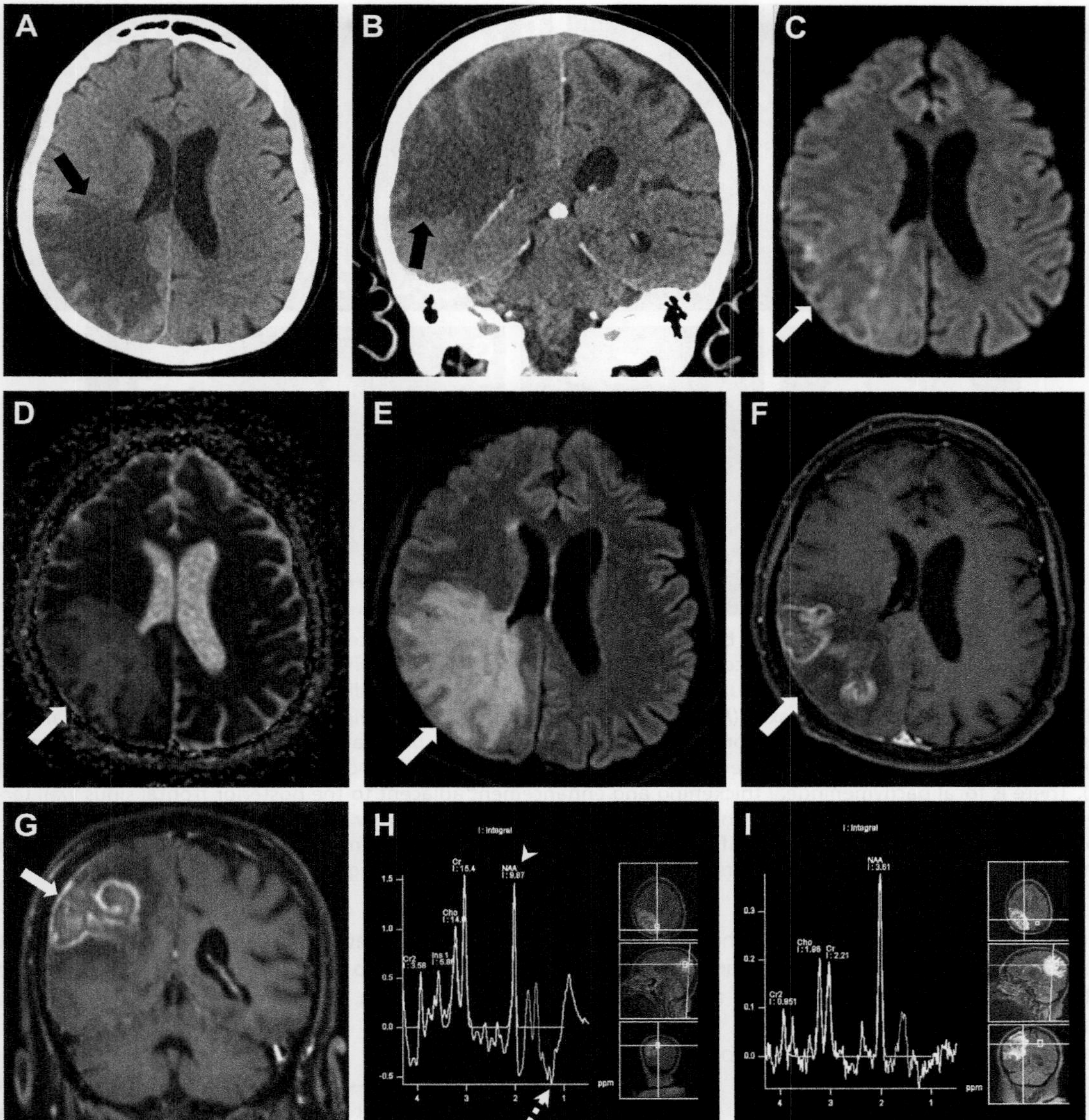

Fig. 2. Cerebritis. A 70-year-old woman with type 2 diabetes and septic shock with arm amputation for *Clostridium septicum* necrotizing soft tissue infection develops cerebritis. Axial (*A*) and coronal (*B*) noncontrast CT images show a large patchy area of brain edema in the right frontoparietal region (*black arrows*), causing mass effect and effacement of the right lateral ventricle. Axial DWI (*C*), ADC map (*D*), FLAIR (*E*), axial (*F*), and coronal (*G*) postcontrast T1-weighted images show a large area of vasogenic edema with scattered foci of restricted diffusion, and heterogeneous enhancement (*arrows*). MRS (single 3D voxel technique, echo time [TE] = 144 ms) of the right superior parietal lobule (*H*) reveals diminished NAA (*arrowhead*) and elevated lactate peaks (*dashed arrow*), consistent with tissue necrosis. Note normal comparison spectral waveform of the contralateral normal brain (*I*). Brain biopsy showed necrotic brain tissue with areas of dense macrophages. ADC, apparent diffusion coefficient; CT, computed tomography; DWI, diffusion-weighted imaging; FLAIR, fluid-attenuated inversion recovery; MRS, magnetic resonance spectroscopy; NAA, N-acetylaspartate.

intraventricular extension (**Fig.** 4A–D).[22] On DWI, bacterial abscesses demonstrate strong central restricted diffusion, likely due to the high viscosity of pus. This finding is particularly helpful in differentiating abscesses from necrotic tumors (**Fig.** 5A–E) and demyelinating lesions, as these conditions typically show peripheral intermediate restricted diffusion. However, it is worth noting that strong central restricted diffusion can occasionally be observed with hematomas or

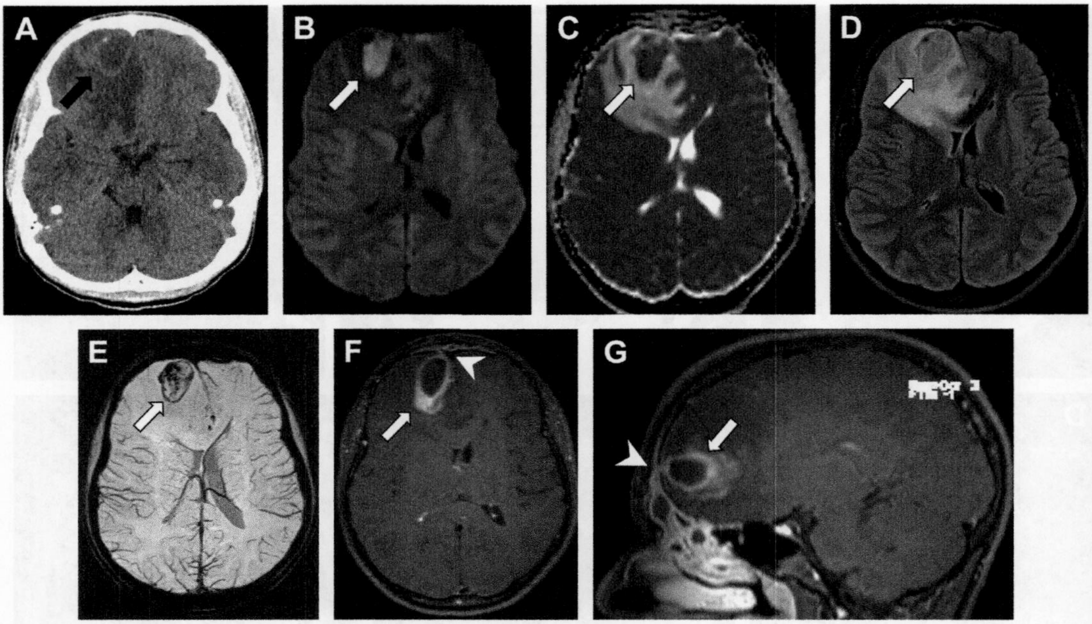

Fig. 3. A brain abscess. A 14-year-old boy with vomiting, lethargy, and acute pansinusitis complicated by a right frontal lobe abscess. Initial axial noncontrast CT (*A*) shows an oval right frontal lobe lesion with central hypoattenuation and peripheral hyperattenuating rim (*black arrow*) with surrounding vasogenic edema. Axial DWI (*B*), ADC map (*C*), FLAIR (*D*), SWI (*E*), axial (*F*), and sagittal (*G*) postcontrast T1-weighted images show a rim-enhancing lesion with central restricted diffusion (*arrows*), characteristic of a brain abscess. Note "dual rim" with inner hyperintense rim and outer hypointense signal on FLAIR image (*D*) with corresponding susceptibility on SWI (*E*). There is focal pachymeningeal thickening and enhancement adjacent to the posterior frontal sinus wall (*arrowheads* in figure *F* and *G*). Following surgical evacuation, cultures grew *Streptococci viridian* and *Staphylococcus epidermidis*. ADC, apparent diffusion coefficient; CT, computed tomography; DWI, diffusion-weighted imaging; FLAIR, fluid-attenuated inversion recovery; SWI, susceptibility-weighted imaging.

metastases.[23] Over 2 to 4 weeks, the matrix transitions from reticulin to collagen, marking the transition to the late capsular phase as the cavity shrinks and the capsule thickens.[18] Please see **Table 2** for a summary of cerebritis to brain abscess continuum.

Advanced imaging techniques, although not frequently used in clinical practice, may add value in diagnosis and treatment monitoring of brain abscesses. High b-value (3000) DWI has shown promise in evaluating the response to therapy, as persistent or increasing restricted diffusion correlates with residual or recurrent abscess.[24] Microstructural evaluation with diffusion tensor imaging (DTI) may be useful in differentiating abscess cavity from other cystic intracranial lesions.[25] Furthermore, perfusion imaging of abscesses shows low cerebral blood volume, whereas neoplasms typically exhibit increased cerebral blood volume. Lastly, magnetic resonance spectroscopy (MRS) may also aid in the diagnosis of brain abscesses. The presence of cytosolic amino acids is sensitive but not a specific marker of bacterial abscesses, with a sensitivity of 0.72 and specificity of 0.3.[26] The elevated amino acid peak is thought to be related to proteolytic enzymes associated with neutrophils.

Empyemas

Empyemas refer to the collection of pus within the subdural or epidural space. It can develop as a complication of meningitis or through direct spread from infections inside or outside the cranial cavity, such as sinusitis or mastoiditis. Epidural empyema generally follows a more benign and chronic course compared to subdural empyema, as the dura acts as a barrier between the infection and the brain parenchyma.[27] Subdural empyema is a relatively rare neurosurgical emergency as it can be rapidly progressive and become life-threatening. Patients typically present with fever and headache. On MR imaging, empyemas appear T2 FLAIR hyperintense and may demonstrate enhancing encapsulating membranes. DWI can help distinguish subdural empyemas from effusion (another complication of meningitis), as empyemas shows restricted diffusion while

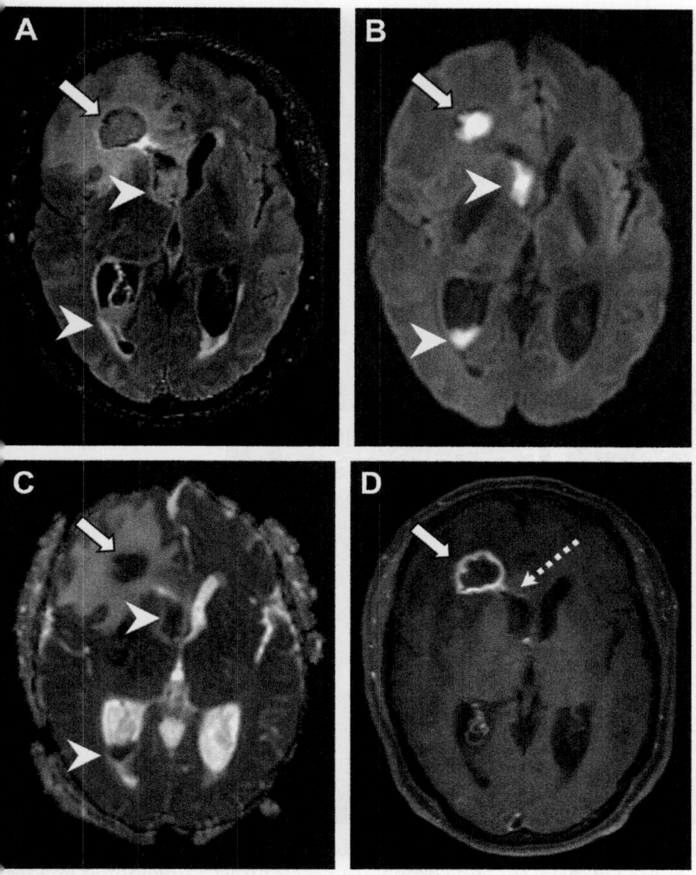

Fig. 4. A brain abscess with intraventricular extension. A 63-year-old woman with acute fever, headaches, and confusion. Axial FLAIR (*A*), DWI (*B*), ADC map (*C*), and postcontrast T1-weighted (*D*) images demonstrate a rim-enhancing lesion with central restricted diffusion and extensive vasogenic edema within the right frontal lobe (*arrows*), consistent with brain abscess. Posteromedially, the abscess ruptures into right lateral ventricle, with layering debris with restricted diffusion within the right frontal horn and occipital horn (*arrowheads* in figures *A–C*). Note thin ependymal enhancement along the frontal horn of the right lateral ventricle (*dashed arrow* in figure *D*), compatible with ventriculitis. Following surgical evacuation of the abscess, cultures grew *Streptococcus milleri* and *Aggregatibacter aphrophilus*. ADC, apparent diffusion coefficient; DWI, diffusion-weighted imaging; FLAIR, fluid-attenuated inversion recovery.

effusion does not (**Figs.** 6A–G and 7A–E).[28] DWI findings of epidural empyema are more variable, with some cases showing low ADC values and others displaying a more mixed ADC signal.[29] This mixed signal is theorized to be related to a decrease in the viscosity and protein content of chronic pus. Additionally, hematomas can exhibit similar restricted diffusion, but they should also demonstrate susceptibility, which serves as a useful feature for differentiation. The typical treatment for empyemas is surgical drainage to alleviate the accumulation of pus and manage the infection.

Ventriculitis

Ventriculitis is an infectious and inflammatory condition that affects the ventricular ependymal lining, with or without layering of pus. It is more commonly observed in infants with meningitis, while relatively rare in adults. The most common organisms associated with ventriculitis are *Staphylococcus* and gram-negative bacteria.[30] For infants, cranial ultrasound is a valuable imaging modality for evaluating ventriculitis, typically revealing echogenic and irregular ependyma with intraventricular debris. However, MR imaging is considered more sensitive than CT in the evaluation of ventriculitis. The most common and possibly the only imaging finding of ventriculitis on MR imaging is the presence of intraventricular debris with restricted diffusion.[31] Less frequently observed imaging findings include ventriculomegaly, T2 hyperintense ependymal wall, and ependymal enhancement (**Fig.** 8A–D). Ependymal wall enhancement is seen in approximately 60% of cases. During the course of ventriculitis, intraventricular adhesions and septations may develop, leading to partial entrapment of CSF. Unlike viral meningitis, periventricular calcifications are uncommon in cases of ventriculitis. Ventriculitis is a severe infection and has a high mortality rate, especially in infants. Early identification of ventriculitis through appropriate imaging studies is crucial to initiate prompt management and treatment. This early intervention may significantly improve survival rates and reduce the risk of long-term complications and morbidity.

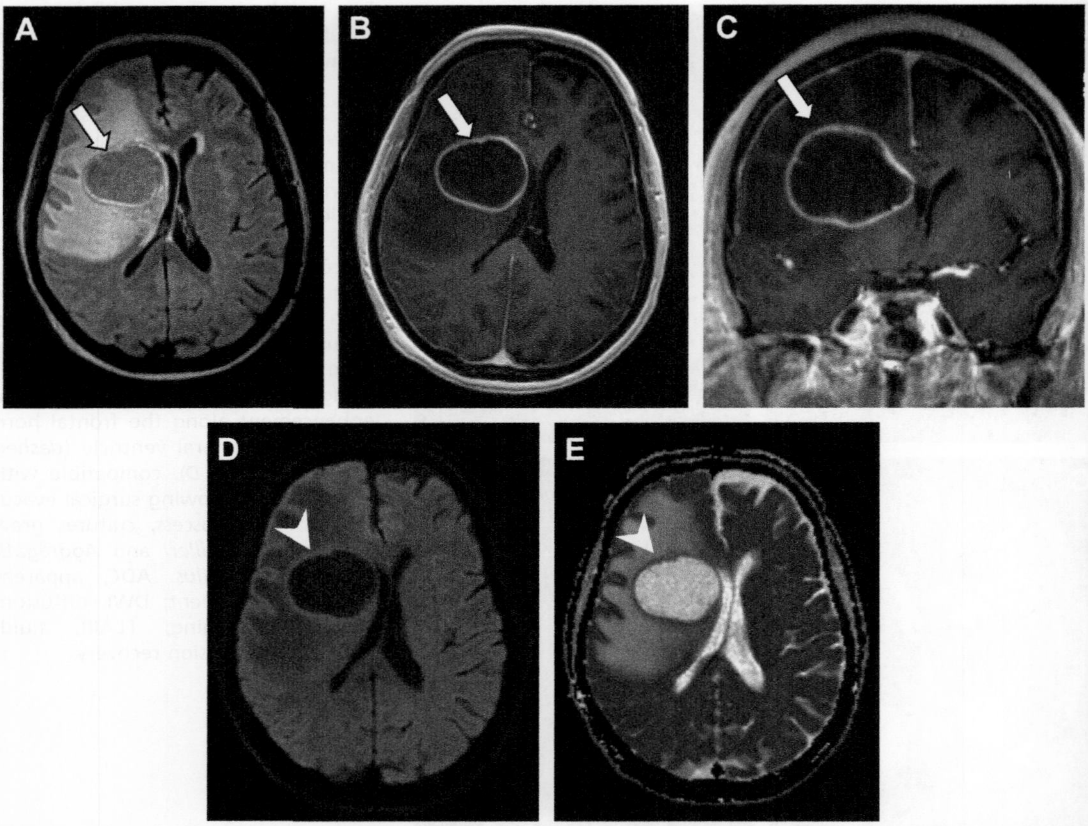

Fig. 5. A necrotic tumor mimicking brain abscess. A 76-year-old woman presents with 2 weeks of left facial droop, headaches, and increasing confusion. Axial FLAIR (*A*), axial (*B*) and coronal (*C*) postcontrast T1-weighted images show a large rim-enhancing lesion with extensive vasogenic edema in the right frontal lobe (*arrows*). Axial DWI (*D*) and ADC map (*E*) show no evidence of central restricted diffusion (*arrowheads*), atypical for abscesses and a raising concern for necrotic tumor. Additional imaging including CT chest (not shown) demonstrated a right upper lobe lung mass. Following craniotomy, final pathology was consistent with metastatic nonsmall cell lung cancer. ADC, apparent diffusion coefficient; DWI, diffusion-weighted imaging; FLAIR, fluid-attenuated inversion recovery.

Tuberculous Brain Infections

Mycobacterium tuberculosis is an atypical bacterium with a high–mycolic acid cell wall which allows the bacteria to evade the normal immune response and contribute to drug resistance. The high–mycolic acid content is responsible for many of the imaging findings.[32] For example, it correlates with the elevated lipid levels on MRS. As a result, the immune system attempts to block and confine the infection, resulting in caseating granulomatous inflammation. Intracranial tubercular granulomas, also known as Rich foci, can be found in various locations within the brain, including the cortical, subpial, or subependymal regions. If these granulomas rupture into the subarachnoid space, it results in tuberculous meningitis.[33]

Classic imaging findings of tuberculous meningitis include thick nodular enhancement within the basal cisterns which can also be observed in other granulomatous infections or neoplastic processes (**Fig. 9**A–D). Leptomeningeal enhancement is typically observed within the Sylvian fissure and cistern on T1-weighted contrast-enhanced images.[34] Additionally, associated vasculitis may occur, most commonly involving the middle cerebral artery and the lenticulostriate arteries. On vessel wall imaging, this vasculitis manifests as concentric vessel wall thickening and enhancement, which can lead to basal ganglia infarctions.[35] Other complications that may arise from tuberculous meningitis include communicating hydrocephalus, cranial neuropathy, or pachymeningitis.

Intraparenchymal localized forms of tuberculosis can manifest as tuberculomas, abscesses, or cerebritis, with these conditions being more prevalent in immunocompromised patients. Tubercular

Table 2
Summary of cerebritis to abscess continuum

Stage	Pathophysiology	Computed Tomography	MR
Early cerebritis	Poorly defined inflammatory response	Ill-defined region of hypoattenuation	Ill-defined T2 hyperintense mass, ± patchy enhancement, ± central restricted diffusion
Late cerebritis	• Marginal fibroblasts appear and begin to lie down reticulin • Central necrosis increases	Core: hypoattenuation increases Rim: irregular enhancement surrounding vasogenic edema	Core: T2 hyperintense, restricted diffusion Rim: T2 hypointense with irregular enhancement surrounding vasogenic edema
Early abscess capsule	• Well-defined capsule of fibroblasts • Increased reticulin and early collagen deposition • Increased new blood vessels surround necrotic center	Hypoattenuation with thin rim enhancement and surrounding vasogenic edema	Core: T2 hyperintense, marked restricted diffusion Rim: Double rim T2 hypointense outer rim with T2 hyperintense inner rim, well-defined thin rim enhancement surrounding vasogenic edema
Late abscess capsule	• Collagen capsule with shrinking necrotic cavity • Gliosis forms around capsule	Cavity shrinks, rim enhancement thickens	Cavity shrinks, rim enhancement thickens, vasogenic edema decreases

abscesses are extremely rare and differ from tuberculomas in their presentation. Abscesses contain pus centrally and are surrounded by a granulation capsule, while tuberculomas represent an intraparenchymal form of the granulomatous reaction to tuberculosis. Tuberculomas are identifiable on MR imaging as well-defined T2 hypointense lesions with solid or rimlike enhancement (**Fig. 10**A–D). Depending on the degree of liquefactive necrosis or caseation, there can be central T2 hyperintense signal (**Fig. 11**A–D).[36] Occasionally, a central calcification or focus of enhancement can result in a targetoid appearance.

Differentiating tuberculomas from tuberculous abscesses can be difficult with imaging alone. Tubercular abscesses tend to exhibit more surrounding vasogenic edema than tuberculomas.[36] MRS may be helpful in differentiating tubercular abscesses from bacterial abscesses. The characteristic magnetic resonance (MR) spectra associated with tubercular abscesses typically show lipid and lactate peaks, in contrast to bacterial abscesses, which commonly display an amino acid peak.[37] This distinction is critical from a clinical perspective since the management approach varies for bacterial and tubercular abscesses. Bacterial abscesses are usually treated with both medical therapy and surgical aspiration, while tubercular abscesses necessitate surgical excision.

VIRAL INFECTION OF THE BRAIN

Viral CNS infections trigger a host inflammatory response that can affect either the meninges or the brain parenchyma, resulting in meningitis or encephalitis, respectively. There are 15 viral families comprising over 100 different viruses that can result in viral CNS infection.[38] Among the numerous viruses capable of causing viral CNS infections, we will focus on the common etiologies: enterovirus (EV), human herpes virus (HHV), human immunodeficiency virus (HIV), and West Nile virus (WNV). A summary table including more viral infections with characteristic imaging features is also provided (**Table 3**). Acute viral meningitis shares similar symptoms with bacterial meningitis, such as headache, fever, and neck pain, but the symptoms are generally less severe. CSF sampling typically shows lymphocytic pleocytosis, moderate protein levels, and normal glucose. In diagnosing viral CNS infections, viral CSF testing can be the single most crucial test. Neuroimaging findings for viral meningitis are usually normal, while viral encephalitis may show areas of nonspecific T2-hyperintense cortical and subcortical

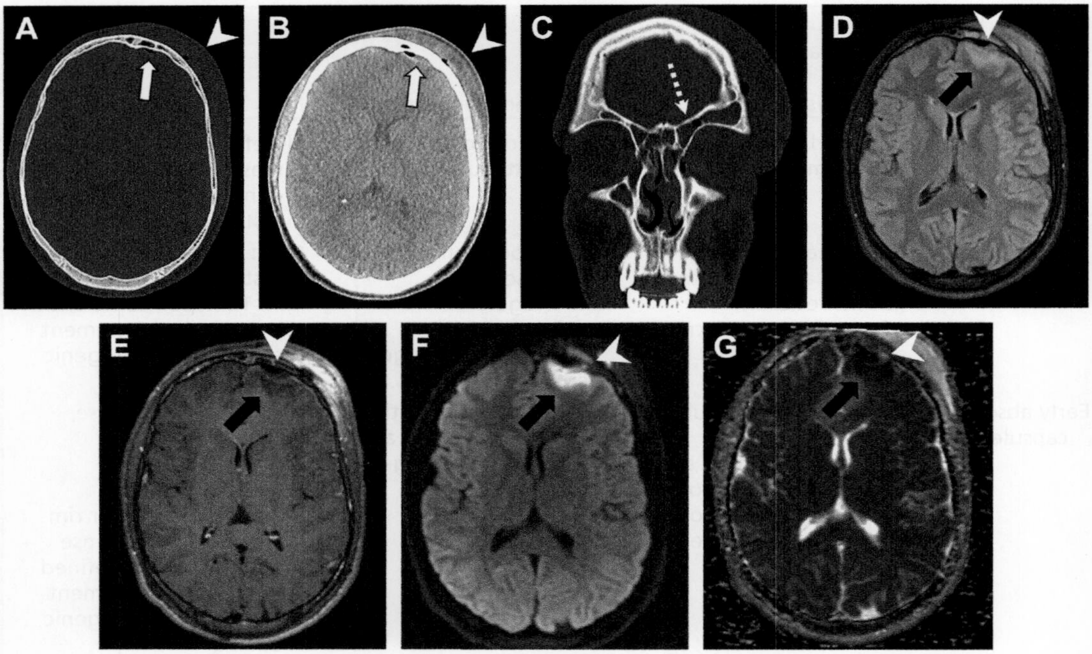

Fig. 6. An epidural empyema. A 19-year-old boy with complicated rhinosinusitis with preseptal cellulitis and epidural empyema with associated frontal lobe cerebritis admitted for seizures and unresponsiveness. Axial CT in bone (*A*) and soft tissue (*B*) windows show a small epidural gas and fluid collection along the left anterior frontal convexity (*arrows*), consistent with epidural empyema. There is marked left frontal scalp swelling containing a small focus of air (*arrowheads*). Coronal CT in bone window (*C*) shows pansinusitis with frontal sinus opacification (*dashed arrow*). Axial FLAIR (*D*), postcontrast T1-weighted image (*E*), DWI (*F*), and ADC map (*G*) show a small rim-enhancing epidural gas and fluid collection with restricted diffusion (*arrowheads*) in the area of known epidural empyema. The subjacent left frontal lobe shows an area of T2 FLAIR hyperintensity with mild enhancement and restricted diffusion (*black arrows*), consistent with focal cerebritis. Following surgical evacuation, cultures were positive for *Niallia circulans* group and *Peribacillus butanolivorans*. ADC, apparent diffusion coefficient; CT, computed tomography; DWI, diffusion-weighted imaging; FLAIR, fluid-attenuated inversion recovery.

white matter signal alteration. Neuroimaging can be valuable in assessing the extent of the disease and monitoring the response to treatment. In terms of treatment, except for herpes encephalitis, which is treated with acyclovir, most viral CNS infections are managed with supportive care.

Enterovirus

EVs are single-stranded ribonucleic acid (RNA) viruses belonging to the Picornaviral family, which includes viral causes of hand, foot, and mouth disease. EV is known to cause epidemic outbreaks in Southeast Asia and the Western Pacific. The most significant EV71 epidemic occurred in China in 2008, resulting in approximately 490,000 infections, with a notable number of severe cases showing neurologic manifestations.[39] EV71 spreads through contact with saliva, respiratory secretions, or oral contact with fecal infections. In affected young children, initial symptoms often involve the upper respiratory or gastrointestinal tract, and a distinctive maculopapular rash may appear on the hands, feet, and mouth. CNS involvement can occur in 10% to 20% of patients.[40] The exact mechanisms underlying CNS infection by EV are not fully understood, but proposed pathways include viral spread across the blood-brain barrier or retrograde axonal transport along peripheral nerves.[41] The viral infection triggers an inflammatory response that can lead to conditions such as meningitis, meningoencephalitis, or myelitis-related acute flaccid paralysis. Typically, CT imaging results for EV CNS infections are normal, and MR imaging findings may be normal or display nonspecific features, such as T2 hyperintense signal in the cortex and subcortical white matter (**Fig. 12**A–F). When EV causes rhombencephalitis, MR imaging demonstrates ill-defined T2 hyperintense lesions in the brainstem and cerebellum, with a relative sparing of the supratentorial brain.[42] The lesions typically involve the posterior brain stem, substantia nigra, dentate nucleus, and anterior horns of the spinal cord.

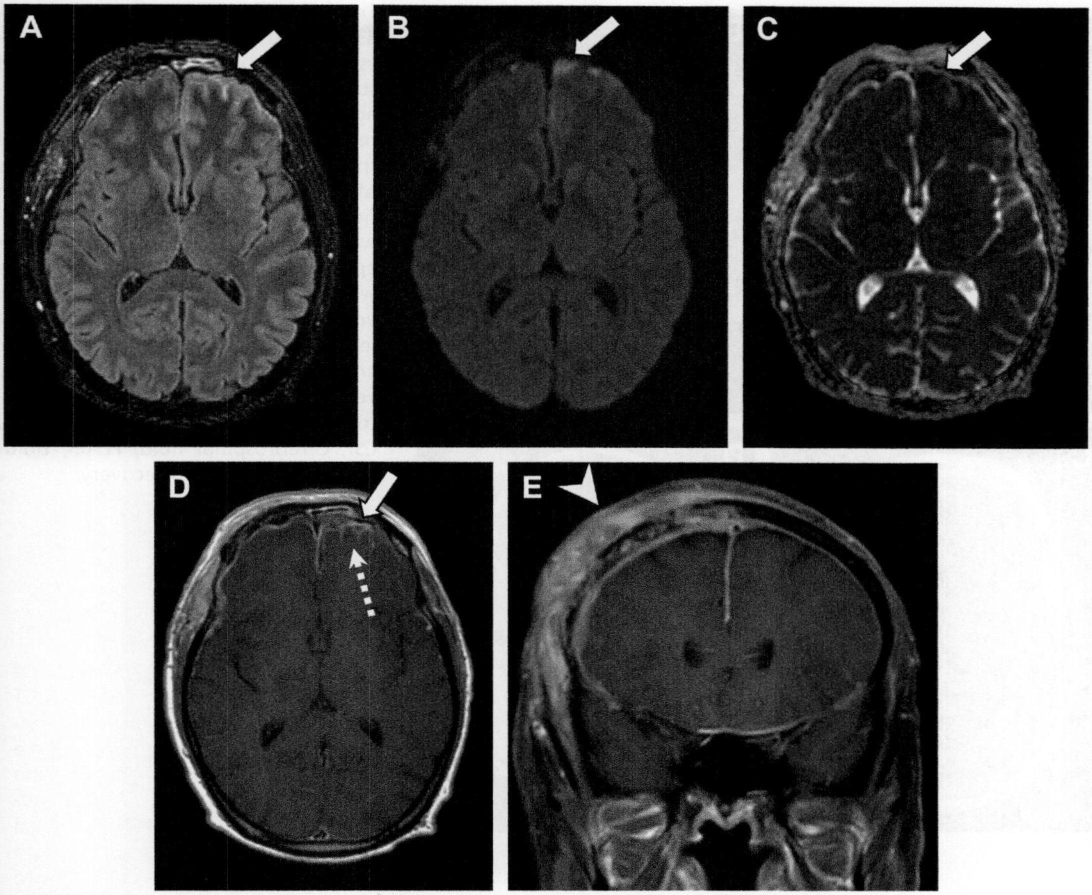

Fig. 7. A subdural empyema. A 67-year-old man with complicated frontal sinusitis presents with several months of headaches and unintended weight loss. Axial FLAIR (*A*), DWI (*B*), ADC map (*C*), axial (*D*), and coronal (*E*) post-contrast T1-weighted images show a thin rim-enhancing subdural collection with restricted diffusion along the left frontal convexity (*arrows* in figures *A–D*), consistent with subdural empyema. Note left frontal leptomeningeal enhancement (*dashed arrow* in figure *D*) and abnormal enhancement in the right frontal calvarium and overlying scalp soft tissue (*arrowhead* in figure *E*), consistent with meningitis and osteomyelitis, respectively. Following surgical evacuation, blood and pus cultures grew *Streptococcus milleri*. ADC, apparent diffusion coefficient; DWI, diffusion-weighted imaging; FLAIR, fluid-attenuated inversion recovery.

Human Herpes Viruses

HHVs are a large family of deoxyribonucleic acid viruses that are characterized by surface glycoproteins. Within this family, there are several notable viruses, including human simplex viruses (HSVs) type 1 (HSV-1) and type 2 (HSV-2), varicella-zoster virus (VZV), cytomegaloviruses, and Epstein-Barr virus. HHV can spread through the bloodstream or via neuronal axonal transport.[43] Following the primary infection, the virus enters a latent stage within neural tissue, where it remains dormant until reactivated by a stressor. The manifestations of HHV in the CNS depend on factors such as the viral strain, the patient's age, and their immune status, leading to various clinical and imaging presentations, including seizures, meningitis, ventriculitis, encephalitis, neuritis, and myelitis.[44] HHV infections, specifically HSV-1 and HSV-2, are typically contracted through direct contact with mucosal surfaces, conjunctiva, or disrupted skin exposed to infected bodily secretions. Among CNS manifestations, HSV encephalitis is the most common and can be fatal. Fortunately, despite the high prevalence of HSV infection, HSV encephalitis is relatively rare. Most cases of herpes encephalitis are associated with HSV-1, with only a small number attributed to HSV-2.[45] In adults and children over 3 months old, HSV encephalitis commonly affects the temporal lobe and limbic system. However, in infants under 3 months old, it has a more diffuse

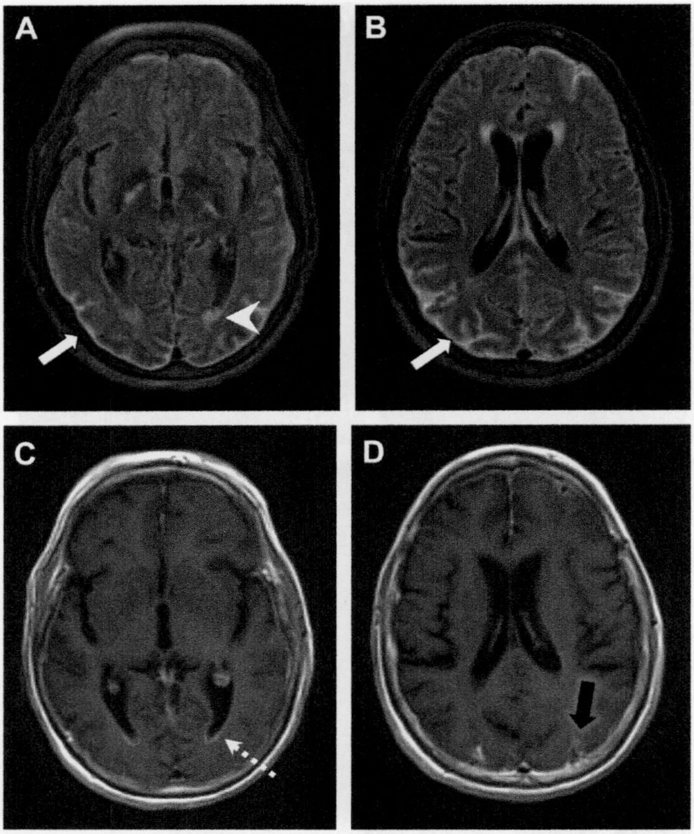

Fig. 8. Ventriculitis and meningitis. A 63-year-old man with a history of polysubstance abuse presents with mental status changes. Axial FLAIR (*A, B*) images show abnormal FLAIR hyperintense signal within the subarachnoid space (*arrows*) and the occipital horns of the lateral ventricles (*arrowhead* in figure *A*). Axial postcontrast T1-weighted (*C, D*) images show thin ependymal enhancement along the walls of the lateral ventricles (*dashed arrow* in figure *C*) as well as multifocal leptomeningeal enhancement (*black arrow* in figure *D*), characteristic of ventriculitis and meningitis. CSF culture grew *Streptococcus pneumoniae*. CSF, cerebrospinal fluid; FLAIR, fluid-attenuated inversion recovery.

presentation. Patients with HSV encephalitis typically present with altered mental status, fever, and headache. To diagnose this condition, CSF polymerase chain reaction viral analysis is considered the gold standard, with a sensitivity of 94% and specificity of 98%.[46] Treatment with acyclovir should begin immediately with any clinical suspicion of HSV encephalitis as the mortality rate approaches 70% without timely intervention, and with a high risk of neurologic morbidity in survivors.[47] With early administration of acyclovir, the mortality rate decreases to 20% to 30%.[48]

In HSV-1 encephalitis, CT findings typically show hypoattenuation within the temporal lobe and insula. On MR imaging, DWI, and T2 FLAIR sequences display restricted diffusion and increased T2 signal in the inferior frontal lobe, temporal lobe, and insula, while sparing the lentiform nuclei. Additionally, cortical and subcortical edema can be observed (**Fig. 13**A–H). Petechial hemorrhage may be present and appear as blooming on susceptibility-weighted imaging. It is important to note that isolated hippocampal involvement is uncommon, and if detected, other diagnostic possibilities should be considered.[49] In the early stages of the disease, the involvement is typically unilateral, but as the condition progresses, it may evolve into bilateral disease. Late findings include patchy or gyriform parenchymal enhancement, necrosis, and hemorrhage.

HSV-2 typically occurs in neonates with perinatal vertical transmission from maternal genital infection. In approximately 70% of infected neonates, CNS manifestations develop, with seizures being the most common.[50] The affected regions in the brain display T2 FLAIR hyperintense signal and/or restricted diffusion. Unlike HSV-1, HSV-2 does not show a preference for the temporal lobe; instead, it commonly involves the cortices, deep gray nuclei, and border zones. Regions with cytotoxic edema resulting from ischemic injury may progress to cortical laminar necrosis and encephalomalacia in later stages. DWI is the most sensitive sequence for identifying early disease and assessing the extent of involvement.[51]

VZV causes both chicken pox and shingles. Neurologic involvement commonly occurs in immunocompromised and elderly patients, resulting from the reactivation of latent virus. Patients present with cutaneous vesicular eruptions in a

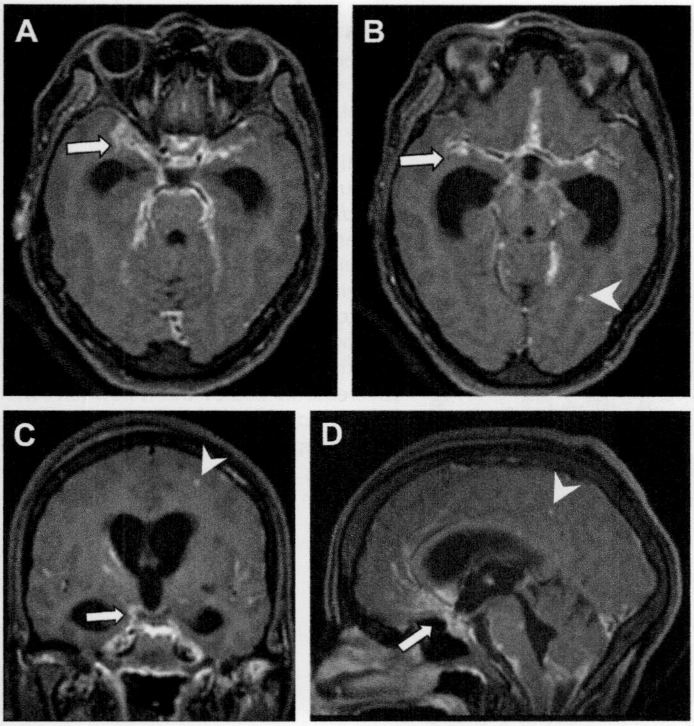

Fig. 9. Tuberculous meningitis. A 46-year-old woman with disseminated tuberculosis and CNS involvement presents with fever with acutely worsening mental status and bilateral lower extremity weakness. Initial chest CT scan showed left lower lobe pneumonia with diffuse miliary pulmonary nodules (not shown). QuantiFERON and sputum AFB tests were positive for tuberculosis. Axial (*A*, *B*), coronal (*C*), and sagittal (*D*) postcontrast T1-weighted images show diffuse, thick, nodular leptomeningeal enhancement greatest in the basal cisterns (*arrows*), characteristic of tuberculous meningitis. Additionally, there are several small foci of enhancement in the brain parenchyma (*arrowheads*), consistent with tuberculomas. Note hydrocephalus with dilatation of the lateral ventricles. ADC, apparent diffusion coefficient; AFB, acid-fast bacteria; CNS, central nervous system; CT, computed tomography.

dermatomal distribution. Neurologic manifestations of varicella can vary, encompassing conditions such as meningoencephalitis, cerebellitis, cranial and peripheral nerve palsies, vasculitis, and transverse myelitis. On MR imaging, increased T2 FLAIR hyperintense signal is typically observed, involving the brainstem, cerebellum, and, rarely, the parieto-temporal lobes. Reactivation of latent virus within the facial nerve geniculate ganglia can lead to Ramsay Hunt syndrome, which manifests as abnormal facial nerve enhancement on MR. Vasculitis may develop weeks to months after the cutaneous rash and is a significant factor in childhood ischemic stroke.[52] The virus directly infects the arterial adventitia and spreads toward the vessel lumen, causing focal stenosis, which can result in infarction. Myelitis is another uncommon complication of VZV infection that occurs weeks to months after the initial infection. It typically affects the same level as the cutaneous dermatomal distribution.

Human Immunodeficiency Virus

HIV is an RNA retrovirus that infects and compromises the functionality of the immune system. HIV can cross the blood-brain barrier and infect microglia, as well as a small population of astrocytes, which can serve as a reservoir for HIV.[53] Neurologic disease in HIV can arise from direct viral infection, opportunistic infections, HIV-related neoplasms, or as a side effect of antiretroviral therapy (ART). Since the advent of ART, the incidence of HIV-related CNS diseases, particularly opportunistic infections, has significantly declined. However, despite advances in therapy, approximately 50% of patients on ART still develop HIV-associated neurocognitive disorders (HAND).[54] HAND is further classified into 3 categories: (1) asymptomatic neurocognitive impairment (ANI), (2) mild neurocognitive impairment, and (3) HIV-associated dementia.[55] The use of ART has decreased the frequency of HIV-associated dementia but increased the occurrence of ANI and mild neurocognitive impairment. Diagnosis of HAND typically relies on neuropsychiatric testing and self-reported assessments of activities of daily living. However, MR imaging is useful in the diagnosis and management of HAND.[56] A common finding in HAND is diffuse cerebral atrophy and white matter injury manifest as symmetric confluent regions of hypoattenuation on CT or T2 FLAIR hyperintense signal abnormalities on MR imaging within the deep and periventricular white matter, with relative sparing of the subcortical U fibers and posterior fossa white matter (**Fig. 14**A–D). This pattern contrasts with progressive multifocal leukoencephalopathy, which

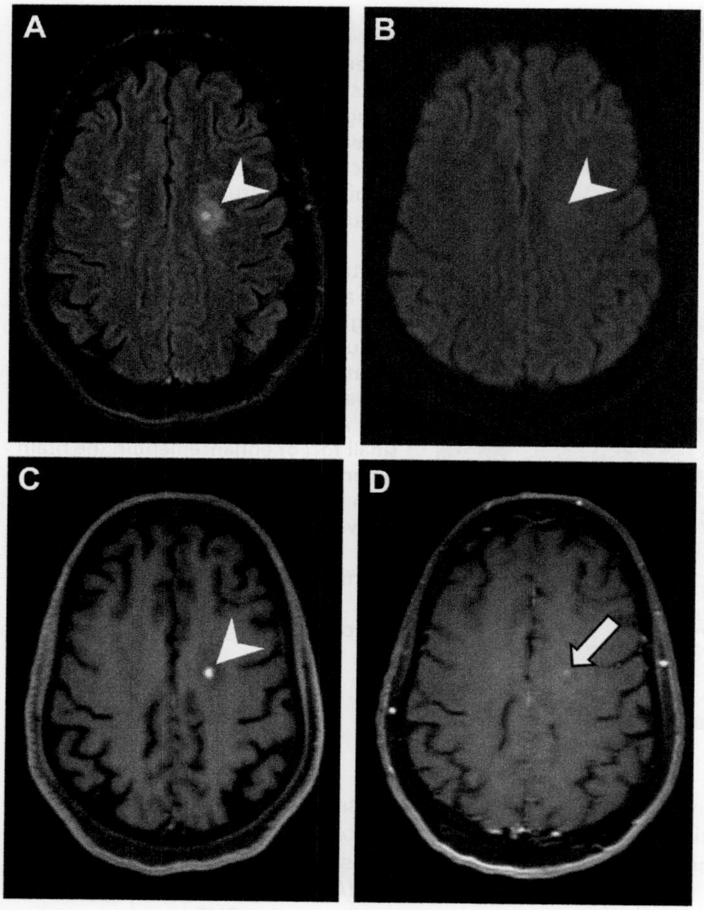

Fig. 10. A noncaseating tuberculoma. A 51-year-old woman with active disseminated tuberculosis. Sputum AFB was positive for mycobacterium. Axial FLAIR (*A*), DWI (*B*), and postcontrast T1-weighted (*C*) images show a small enhancing T2 FLAIR hyperintense nodule in the left frontal lobe (*arrowheads*), consistent with a noncaseating tuberculoma in the setting of known disseminated tuberculosis. There is no restricted diffusion. Follow-up axial postcontrast T1-weighted image (*D*) 4 months after treatment demonstrates treatment response with decrease in size of the lesion (*arrow*). AFB, acid-fast bacteria; CT, computed tomography; DWI, diffusion-weighted imaging; FLAIR, fluid-attenuated inversion recovery.

typically involves the U fibers, has a patchier and more asymmetric appearance. It is important to note that enhancement is not associated with HAND, and if present, it should raise suspicion for an alternative diagnosis.

MRS may be more sensitive than conventional MR imaging in detecting white matter changes in patients with ANI. MRS typically reveals reduced N-acetylaspartate and increased choline and myoinositol in the frontal cortices and basal ganglia, which is compatible with neuronal loss, inflammation, and gliosis. Some MRS research suggests that ART may be neuroprotective, as it has shown improvement in metabolites that serve as markers for glial injury.[57] However, conflicting MRS data exist, showing reduced N-acetylaspartate in the frontal white matter associated with ART, suggesting it may cause mitochondrial toxicity and neuronal impairment.[58] Volumetric MR imaging demonstrates significant cortical volume loss, with the degree of volume loss correlating with viral load and the extent of cognitive impairment.[59] DTI shows the degree of microstructural white matter injury, which is associated with duration of infection.[60] Additionally, DTI has shown elevated mean and radial diffusivity in the parietal white matter, which may reflect demyelination even in asymptomatic patients.[60] Blood-oxygen-level-dependent functional MR imaging has revealed impaired function of neuronal networks, correlating with the degree of neurocognitive impairment.[61] In the pre-ART era, fluorodeoxyglucose-PET imaging showed 2 unique metabolic signatures. Early infection showed hypermetabolic basal ganglia that switched to a hypometabolic state within the basal ganglia in chronic infection.[62] In the post-ART era, PET imaging has shown promise in complementing structural evaluation of HAND with investigational molecular studies evaluating glucose metabolism, neuroinflammation, amyloid deposition, and neurotransmitter function.[63] While there is no definitive cure for HAND, the current recommended therapy is CNS-penetrating combination

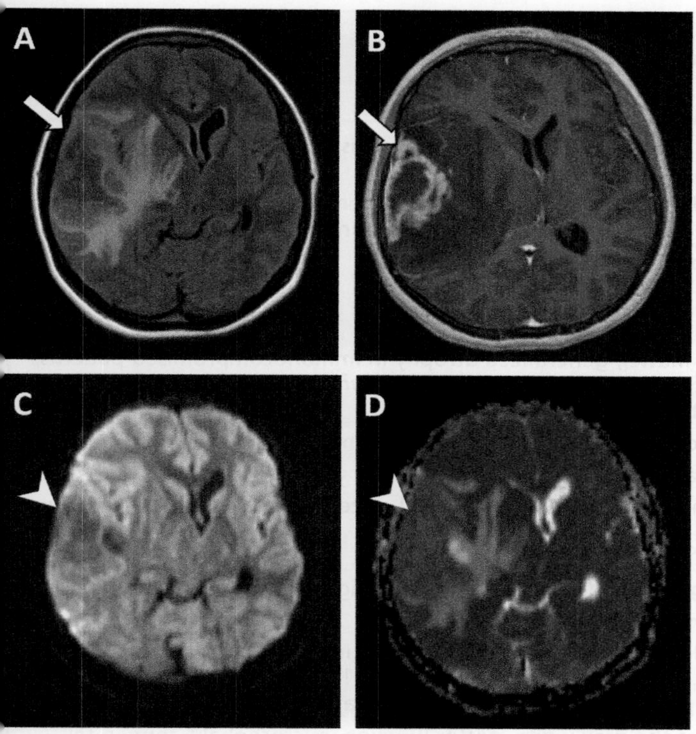

Fig. 11. A caseating tuberculoma. A 22-year-old woman presents with a new onset of headache, dizziness, and nausea. Axial FLAIR (*A*) and post-contrast T1-weighted (*B*) images show a large enhancing necrotic mass with surrounding edema in the right temporal lobe (*arrows*). The lesion demonstrates mild peripheral restricted diffusion (*arrowheads*) on DWI (*C*), confirmed on ADC map (*D*). Note mass effect with leftward midline shift. Due to concern for brain tumor, she underwent craniotomy with resection of the lesion, with final pathology showing necrotizing granulomatous inflammation. AFB of tissue was positive for mycobacterium. ADC, apparent diffusion coefficient; AFB, acid-fast bacteria; DWI, diffusion-weighted imaging; FLAIR, fluid-attenuated inversion recovery.

ART though there are still limited data available to fully support this recommendation.[64]

West Nile Virus

WNV is an RNA flavivirus belonging to the same family as the Japanese encephalitis virus. Transmission to humans typically occurs via mosquito bites, but rare cases of human-to-human transmission have been documented through transplacental, breastfeeding, organ transplantation, and blood transfusion routes. While WNV was initially identified in Uganda, it has since been found on all continents except Antarctica. Notably, approximately 80% of patients infected with WNV are asymptomatic.[65] However, adults over the age of 50 and immunocompromised patients are most likely to exhibit symptoms, which include fever, headache, myalgia, gastrointestinal symptoms, and a maculopapular rash. Muscle weakness is a common finding that may be useful in distinguishing WNV from other encephalitides.

Neurologic disease occurs in less than 1% of WNV cases, with variable clinical presentations, including meningitis, encephalitis, cranial neuropathies, movement disorders, and acute flaccid paralysis. The mortality rate for WNV infection ranges from 2% to 7%, with a higher mortality rate in patients who develop neuroinvasive disease.[66] The gold standard for diagnosis is serum and CSF serologic testing for mmunoglobulin M antibodies. CT findings are typically normal, and MR imaging findings can be transient and variable. In 20% to 70% of cases, MR imaging may show abnormalities.[67] The most common MR imaging abnormalities are increased DWI and T2 FLAIR signal abnormality within the deep gray matter (eg, bilateral basal ganglia, thalamus, and brainstem) and mesial temporal lobes (**Fig. 15**A–D).[68] Transient splenial lesions are occasionally observed, while leptomeningeal and periventricular enhancement is rare. Patients without MR imaging abnormalities tend to have a better prognosis.

CREUTZFELDT-JAKOB DISEASE

Prion diseases or transmissible spongiform encephalopathies are a heterogeneous group of incurable rapidly progressive neurodegenerative disorders caused by a prion. A prion is an abnormal protease-resistant protein that becomes misfolded and self-propagates misfolding via an autocatalytic process, resulting in aggregation of the abnormal protein leading to neuronal death. The incidence of prion diseases in the United States is approximately 1 per 1 million individuals.[69] One specific prion disease, Creutzfeldt-

Table 3
Summary of viral infections with characteristic imaging features.[76–78]

Viral Etiology	Characteristic Regions Affected and Imaging Patterns
Enterovirus	Posterior brain stem, substantia nigra, dentate nucleus, and anterior horns of the spinal cord
HSV 1	Unilateral or bilateral asymmetric involvement of anterior and medial temporal lobe, cingulate gyrus, and inferior frontal lobe with sparing of the basal ganglia
HSV2	Diffuse cortices, deep gray nuclei, and border zones
VZV	Cerebellum and brainstem, vasculopathy
EBV	Deep gray and subcortical white matter
CMV	Periventricular white matter, generalized atrophy in immunocompromised patients, periventricular calcifications and white matter, polymicrogyria, and anterior temporal lobes cysts in neonates
HIV	Symmetric periventricular and deep white matter with generalized atrophy
WNV	Deep gray matter, brain stem, mesial temporal lobes
Japanese encephalitis virus	Thalami, substantia nigra, basal ganglia, cerebral cortex, corpus striatum cerebellum
Rabies	Predilection for the gray matter, brainstem, basal ganglia, and thalamus
Dengue	Bilateral thalami, pons, medulla
Measles	ADEM pattern, measles inclusion body encephalitis in immunocompromised patients, nonspecific edema, atrophy, ventriculomegaly, and late manifestation subacute sclerosing panencephalitis shows decreased gray matter volume
Zika	Coarse calcifications at the grey-white matter junction, microcephaly, congenital anomalies
JC virus	Asymmetric subcortical U fiber white matter
Influenza	Diffuse edema, symmetric typically hemorrhagic involvement of thalami, brainstem, and cerebellum; ADEM pattern

Abbreviations: ADEM, acute disseminated encephalomyelitis; CMV, cytomegalovirus; EBV, Epstein-Barr virus; HIV, human immunodeficiency virus; HSV, herpes simplex virus; JC, human polyomavirus 2; VZV, varicella-zoster virus; WNV, West Nile virus.

Jakob disease (CJD), can be acquired through various means, such as ingesting infected beef or direct contact with infected neurologic tissue (eg, contaminated neurosurgical instruments, corneal transplants, or human pituitary hormones). CJD has different clinical and molecular subtypes, leading to diverse clinical and imaging features. These subtypes are classified as inherited (15%), idiopathic/sporadic (85%) (sCJD), or acquired/variant (1%) (vCJD).[70] This review will focus on sCJD, the most common subtype. Patients with sCJD typically present with rapidly progressive dementia along with at least 2 of the following symptoms: pyramidal/extrapyramidal symptoms, myoclonus, visual/cerebellar signs, or akinetic mutism. CSF analysis reveals increased 14-3-3 protein and electroencephalogram findings show periodic sharp wave complexes. The diagnostic criteria for sCJD are categorized into 3 levels: definite, probable, and possible sCJD.[68] Definite sCJD can be confirmed through brain biopsy or postmortem examination. Probable and possible sCJD cases rely on clinical features combined with positive paraclinical tests, including MR imaging.

MR imaging findings in sCJD can appear before clinical manifestations, making it a valuable tool for early diagnosis. In the early stage of sCJD, MR imaging may show focal or diffuse, symmetric, or asymmetric increased T2 FLAIR or DWI signal within the cerebral cortices and basal ganglia (**Fig. 16**A–F).[71] The most affected cortices are the insula, cingulate, and superior frontal gyrus followed by the precuneus and cuneus and paracentral lobule. The perirolandic cortices are usually spared, while cerebellar atrophy is common. In contrast to sCJD, the pulvinar and hockey stick signs are present in 90% of cases of vCJD and serve as accurate diagnostic signs for vCJD.[72] The pulvinar sign manifests as bilateral symmetric hyperintense T2 FLAIR signal within the pulvinar, and the hockey stick sign shows symmetric increased T2 FLAIR signal within the pulvinar and dorsomedial thalamus. If these signs are present

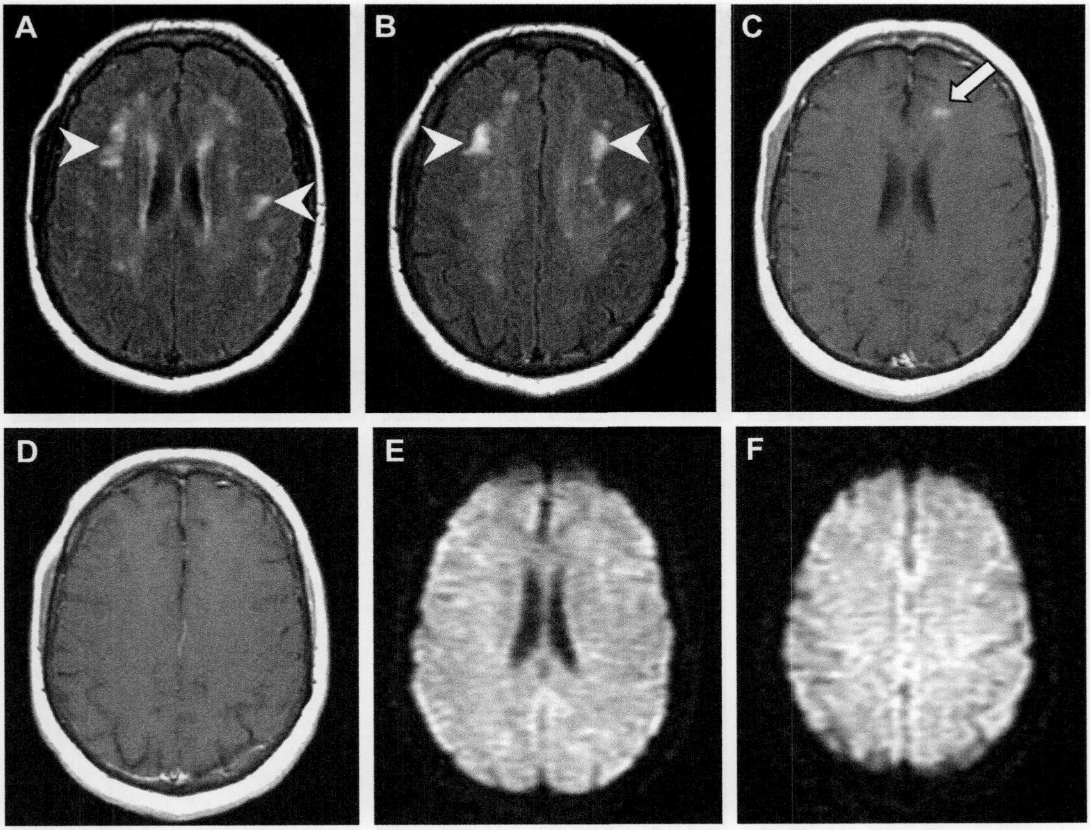

Fig. 12. Enterovirus encephalitis. A 60-year-old woman with a history of non-Hodgkin's lymphoma presents with intermittent fever, nausea, vomiting, and generalized weakness. CSF PCR for enterovirus was positive. Axial FLAIR (*A, B*) images show multiple focal and confluent areas of T2 FLAIR hyperintensity scattered in the cerebral white matter (*arrowheads*), most notable in subcortical region. Axial postcontrast T1-weighted images (*C, D*) show mild focal enhancement in the left frontal lobe (*arrow* in figure *C*). Axial DWI (*E, F*) demonstrates no restricted diffusion. CSF, cerebrospinal fluid; DWI, diffusion-weighted imaging; FLAIR, fluid-attenuated inversion recovery; PCR, polymerase chain reaction.

in sCJD, patients should also have increased T2 FLAIR signal within the caudate and putamen. Additionally, cortical T2 hyperintense signal is more common in sCJD than vCJD. T1-hyperintense signal abnormality in the globus pallidus is seen in patients with sCJD, which likely represents heavy deposition of prion proteins. Notably, there is no enhancement with CJD. Currently, the exact pathophysiology for the basis of reduced diffusion is not well understood and is believed to be related to vacuolar compartmentalization or prion protein deposition.[73] The degree and extent of signal intensity increase in the basal ganglia have been found to correlate with disease duration and may serve as a potential noninvasive biomarker.[74] In contrast, cortical signal intensity may fluctuate throughout the course of the disease. MRS shows decreased N-acetylaspartate and increased myoinositol, reflecting neuronal cell death and gliosis. MRS can detect abnormalities even in regions that appear normal on conventional MR imaging. While sCJD primarily affects gray matter, DTI has revealed microstructural abnormalities in white matter not observed with conventional MR imaging. DTI shows reduced fractional anisotropy within the corticospinal tracts, internal capsule, external capsule, fornix, and posterior thalamic radiation, suggesting a component of functional disconnection syndrome.[75] PET and single-photon emission computed tomography imaging can demonstrate decreased lobar metabolism and perfusion; however, these findings are nonspecific and not routinely used in evaluation. To avoid misdiagnosis, it is crucial to recognize the usual and unusual MR imaging findings of CJD within the appropriate clinical context, especially since many alternative diagnoses are treatable.

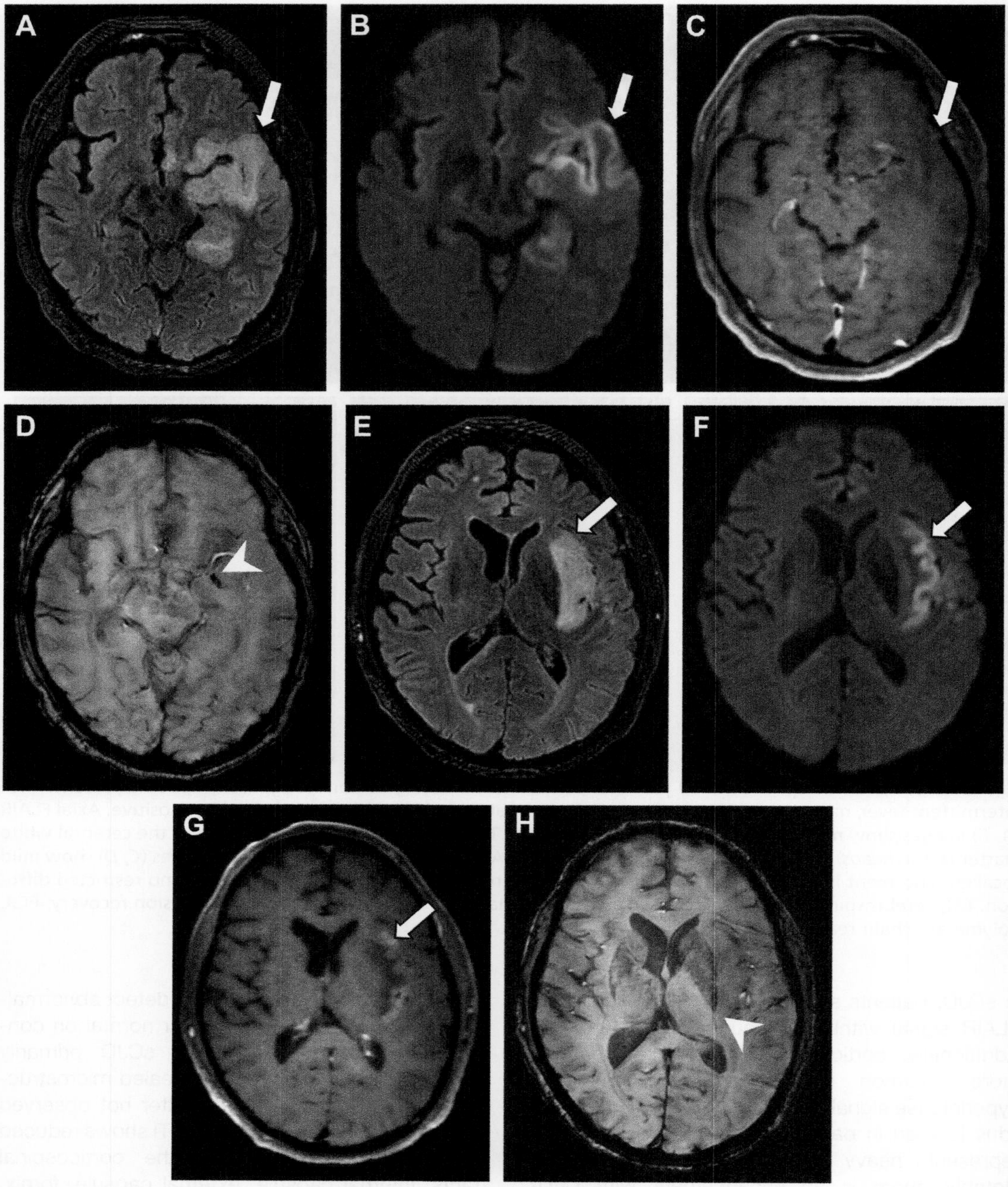

Fig. 13. HSV-1 encephalitis. A 76-year-old man with acute onset of fever, altered mental status, and expressive aphasia. Initial CSF analysis demonstrated lymphocyte-predominant pleocytosis and moderately elevated protein level. HSV-1 PCR in the CSF was positive. Axial FLAIR (*A*, *E*), DWI (*B*, *F*), and postcontrast T1-weighted images (*C*, *G*) show multifocal ill-defined areas of FLAIR hyperintense signal with restricted diffusion and gyriform enhancement within the left anterior temporal lobe, inferior frontal lobe, and insula (*arrows*), characteristic in distribution for HSV-1 encephalitis. Axial susceptibility-weighted images (*D*, *H*) demonstrate small areas of petechial hemorrhage in the affected regions (*arrowheads*). CSF, cerebrospinal fluid; DWI, diffusion-weighted imaging; FLAIR, fluid-attenuated inversion recovery; HSV-1, herpes simplex virus-1; PCR, polymerase chain reaction.

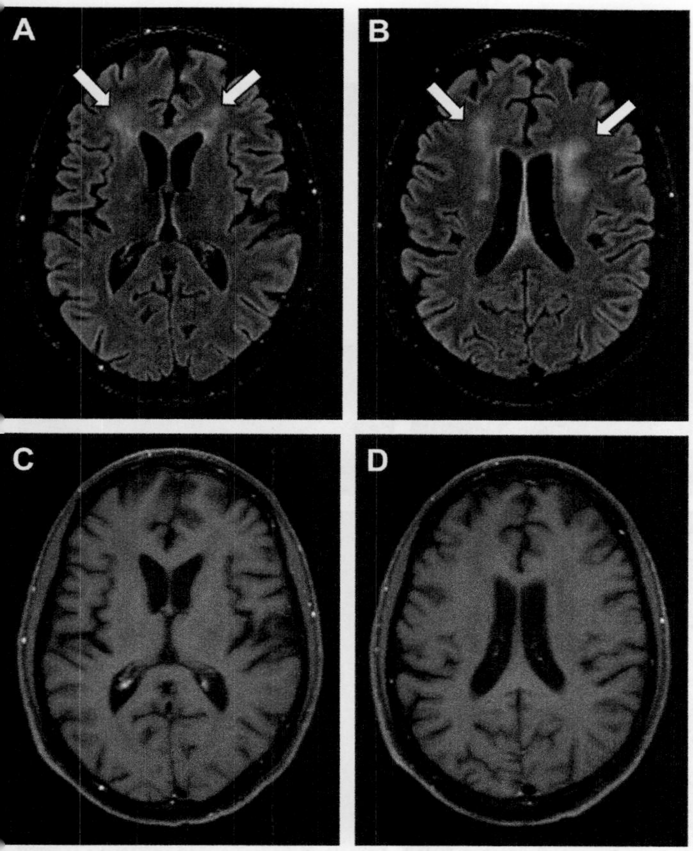

Fig. 14. HAND. A 40-year-old man with newly diagnosed HIV infection with low CD4 count and high viral load presents with confusion, hallucinations, and dyskinesia. Axial FLAIR (*A*, *B*) shows symmetric confluent areas of FLAR hyperintense signal in periventricular deep white matter with relative sparing of the subcortical U fibers (*arrows*). Axial post-contrast T1-weighted images (*C*, *D*) show no enhancement. Note diffuse cerebral parenchymal volume loss greater than expected for age. Extensive workup for opportunistic infections in the CSF was unrevealing. HAND was diagnosed based upon the clinical presentation and MR imaging findings. CSF, cerebrospinal fluid; DWI, diffusion-weighted imaging; FLAIR, fluid-attenuated inversion recovery; HIV, human immunodeficiency virus; HAND, human immunodeficiency virus–associated neurocognitive disorder.

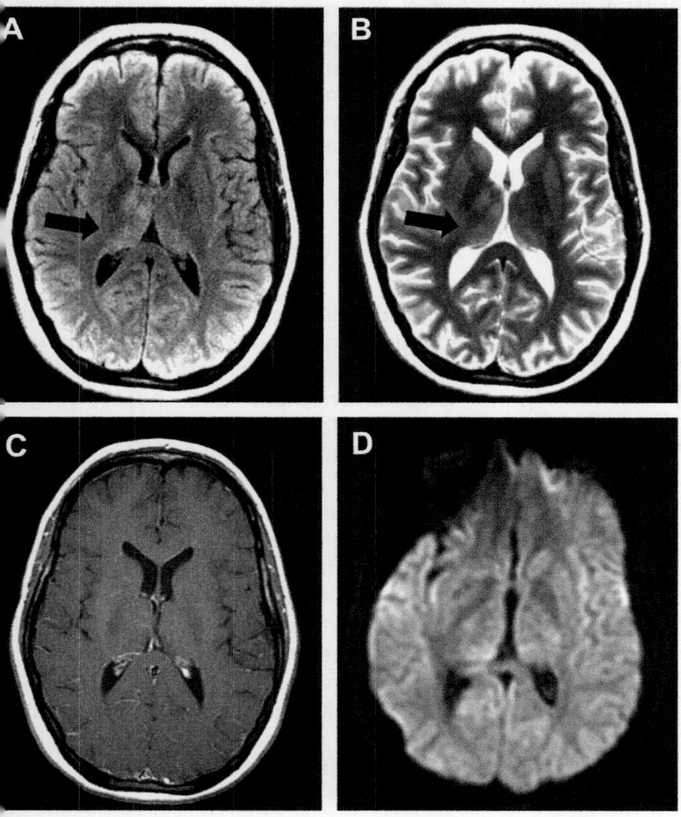

Fig. 15. WNV encephalitis. A 23-year-old woman with a history of juvenile rheumatoid arthritis presents with acute fever and mental status change. Molecular testing for WNV in CSF was positive. Axial FLAIR (*A*) and T2-weighted (*B*) images show abnormal T2 FLAIR hyperintense areas in the bilateral thalamus, more conspicuous on the right (*black arrows*). Axial post-contrast T1-weighted (*C*) and DWI (*D*) demonstrate no enhancement or restricted diffusion. CSF, cerebrospinal fluid; DWI, diffusion-weighted imaging; FLAIR, fluid-attenuated inversion recovery; WNV, West Nile virus.

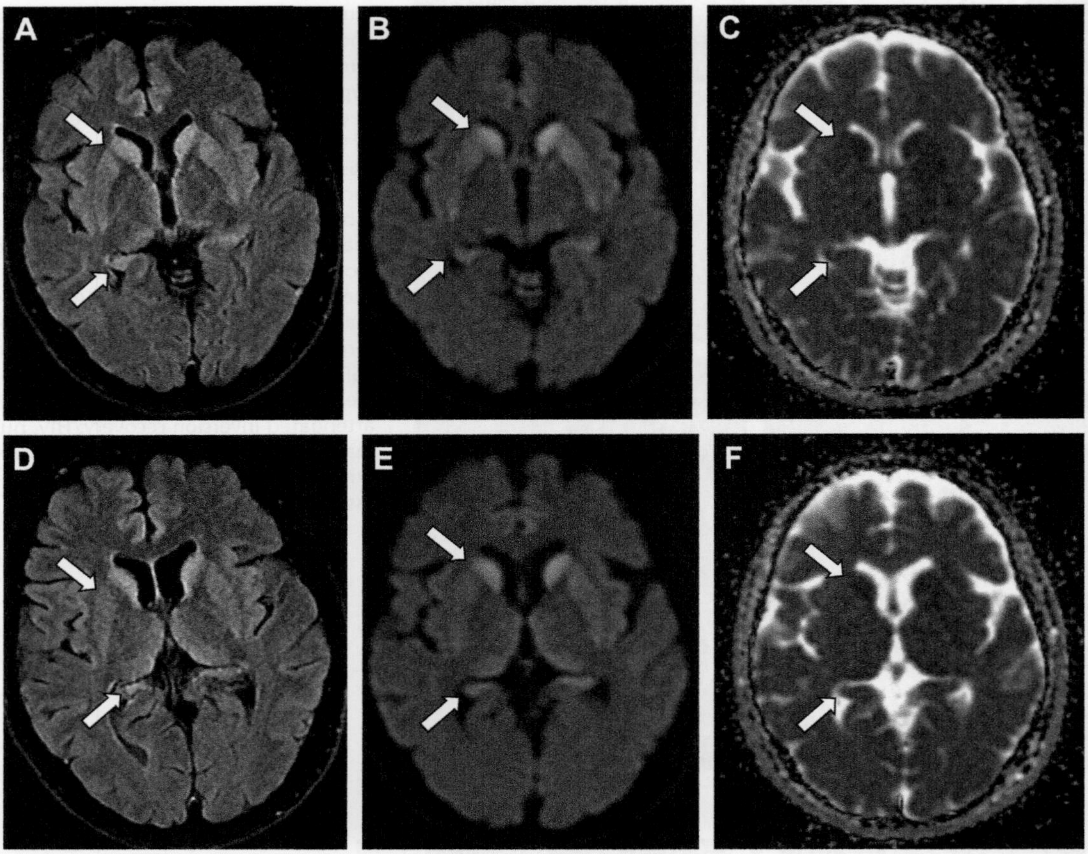

Fig. 16. Creutzfeldt-Jakob disease. A 60-year-old woman with a history of Sjogren's syndrome presents with rapidly progressive dementia. CSF analysis showed a markedly elevated level of 14-3-3 protein (124,692 AU/mL). Axial FLAIR (*A, D*), DWI (*B, E*), and ADC maps (*C, F*) demonstrate areas of FLAIR hyperintense signal and restricted diffusion symmetrically involving the bilateral caudate nuclei, putamina, medial thalami, and mesial temporal lobes (*arrows*). Note the characteristic involvement of the medial thalamus, also known as "hockey stick sign," an imaging feature frequently observed in cases of variant Creutzfeldt-Jakob disease. ADC, apparent diffusion coefficient; CSF, cerebrospinal fluid; DWI, diffusion-weighted imaging; FLAIR, fluid-attenuated inversion recovery.

SUMMARY

Bacterial and viral brain infections pose a significant global health burden. The imaging features of intracranial bacterial and viral infections vary based on the specific brain region affected. Imaging is essential for characterizing disease extent, assessing treatment response, and identifying complications. In tubercular meningitis, MR imaging typically shows thick nodular leptomeningeal enhancement in the basal cisterns, distinguishing it from bacterial and viral meningitis, which usually exhibit thin leptomeningeal enhancement. A ring-enhancing lesion with central restricted diffusion is classic but not pathognomonic of a brain abscess. Viral encephalitis is diagnosed based on the clinical scenario combined with imaging findings, CSF analysis, and serologic studies. Recognizing the characteristic pattern of herpes encephalitis with temporal lobe involvement and basal ganglia sparing is crucial for prompt and effective treatment. In the post-ART era, with increased life expectancy among HIV patients, understanding MR imaging presentations and potential mimics of HAND is essential for diagnosis and management. Early recognition of both typical and atypical MR imaging findings of CJD is vital for providing appropriate patient counseling. MR imaging is the preferred imaging modality for characterizing intracranial infections and when interpreted in conjunction with the clinical scenario, can lead to an accurate and timely diagnosis to optimize patient outcomes.

CLINICS CARE POINTS

- In the evaluation of meningitis, imaging should be interpreted in conjunction with the clinical presentation and CSF analysis to reach an accurate diagnosis because approximately 50% of patients may have negative imaging results.
- When HSV encephalitis is suspected clinically, prompt initiation of treatment with acyclovir is essential, without delay for imaging, as timely administration of antiviral therapy can substantially improve patient outcomes.
- With increased life expectancy in HIV patients in the post-ART era, the incidence of HAND is expected to rise; therefore, understanding the value of imaging in screening for HAND is essential for diagnosis and management.

DISCLOSURE

A.M. Condos: The views expressed in this presentation are those of the authors and do not necessarily reflect the official policy or position of the Department of the Navy, Department of Defense, or the US Government. The authors are military service members. This work was prepared as part of official duties. Title 17 U.S.C. 105 states that 'Copyright protection under this title is not available for any work of the United States Government.' The authors received no financial compensation for this presentation. Neither I nor my immediate family members have a financial relationship with any commercial organization that may have a direct or indirect interest in the content. P. Wangaryattawanich has no conflicts of interest to disclose and there were no financial incentives that would alter the contents of this article. T.J. Rath has no conflicts of interest to disclose and there were no financial incentives that would alter the contents of this article.

REFERENCES

1. Jessen NA, Munk AS, Lundgaard I, et al. The Glymphatic System: A Beginner's Guide. Neurochem Res 2015;40(12):2583–99.
2. Pauker SG, Kopelman RI. A rewarding pursuit of certainty. N Engl J Med 1993;329(15):1103–7. https://doi.org/10.1056/NEJM199310073291508.
3. Meningitis. Centers for Disease Control and Prevention website. http://www.cdc.gov/meningitis/index.html. Updated March 30, 2022.
4. Bender RG, Ikuta KS, Sharara F, et al. Global, regional, and national burden of meningitis and its aetiologies, 1990–2019: a systematic analysis for the Global Burden of Disease Study 2019. Lancet Neurol 2023;22(8):685–711.
5. Bacterial Meningitis. Centers for Disease Control and Prevention website. http://www.cdc.gov/meningitis/bacterial.html. Updated July 15, 2021.
6. van de Beek D, de Gans J, Spanjaard L, et al. Clinical features and prognostic factors in adults with bacterial meningitis. N Engl J Med 2004;351(18):1849–59.
7. Castillo M. Imaging of meningitis. Semin Roentgenol 2004;39(4):458–64.
8. Zunt JR, Kassebaum NJ, Blake N, et al. Global, regional, and national burden of meningitis, 1990–2016: a systematic analysis for the Global Burden of Disease Study 2016. Lancet Neurol 2018;17(12):1061–82.
9. Hasbun R, Abrahams J, Jekel J, et al. Computed tomography of the head before lumbar puncture in adults with suspected meningitis. N Engl J Med 2001;345(24):1727–33. https://doi.org/10.1056/NEJMoa010399.
10. Mohan S, Jain KK, Arabi M, et al. Imaging of meningitis and ventriculitis. Neuroimaging Clin N Am 2012;22(4):557–83.
11. Shih RY, Koeller KK. Bacterial, fungal, and parasitic infections of the central nervous system: radiologic-pathologic correlation and historical perspectives. Radiographics 2015;35(4):1141–69. https://doi.org/10.1148/rg.2015140317.
12. Wong J, Quint DJ. Imaging of central nervous system infections. Semin Roentgenol 1999;34(2):123–43.
13. Kremer S, Abu Eid M, Bierry G, et al. Accuracy of delayed post-contrast FLAIR MR imaging for the diagnosis of leptomeningeal infectious or tumoral diseases. J Neuroradiol 2006;33(5):285–91.
14. Osborn AG, GL Salzman KL. Osborn's brain: imaging pathology and anatomy. 2nd edition. Philadelphia PA: Elsevier; 2018.
15. Mathisen GE, Johnson JP. Brain abscess. Clin Infect Dis 1997 Oct;25(4):763–79. quiz 780-1.
16. Carpenter J, Stapleton S, Holliman R. Retrospective analysis of 49 cases of brain abscess and review of the literature. Eur J Clin Microbiol Infect Dis 2007;26(1):1–11.
17. Menon S, Bharadwaj R, Chowdhary A, et al. Current epidemiology of intracranial abscesses: a prospective 5-year study. J Med Microbiol 2008;57(Pt 10):1259–68.
18. Enzmann DR, Britt RH, Placone R. Staging of human brain abscess by computed tomography. Radiology 1983;146(3):703–8.
19. Tung GA, Rogg JM. Diffusion-weighted imaging of cerebritis. AJNR Am J Neuroradiol 2003 Jun-Jul;24(6):1110–3.
20. Toh CH, Wei KC, Chang CN, et al. Differentiation of pyogenic brain abscesses from necrotic glioblastomas with use of susceptibility-weighted imaging. AJNR Am J Neuroradiol 2012;33(8):1534–8.

21. Lai PH, Chang HC, Chuang TC, et al. Susceptibility-weighted imaging in patients with bacterial brain abscesses at 1.5T: characteristics of the abscess capsule. AJNR Am J Neuroradiol 2012; 33(5):910–4.
22. Rath TJ, Hughes M, Arabi M, et al. Imaging of cerebritis, encephalitis, and brain abscess. Neuroimaging Clin N Am 2012 Nov;22(4):585–607.
23. Hartmann M, Jansen O, Heiland S, et al. Restricted diffusion within ring enhancement is not pathognomonic for brain abscess. AJNR Am J Neuroradiol 2001 Oct;22(9):1738–42.
24. Tomar V, Yadav A, Rathore RK, et al. Apparent diffusion coefficient with higher b-value correlates better with viable cell count quantified from the cavity of brain abscess. AJNR. American journal of neuroradiology 2011;32(11):2120–5.
25. Nath K, Agarwal M, Ramola M, et al. Role of diffusion tensor imaging metrics and in vivo proton magnetic resonance spectroscopy in the differential diagnosis of cystic intracranial mass lesions. Magn Reson Imaging 2009;27(2):198–206.
26. Pal D, Bhattacharyya A, Husain M, et al. In vivo proton MR spectroscopy evaluation of bacterial brain abscesses: a report of 194 cases. AJNR Am J Neuroradiol 2010 Feb;31(2):360–6.
27. Hlavin ML, Kaminski HJ, Fenstermaker RA, et al. Intracranial suppuration: a modern decade of post-operative subdural empyema and epidural abscess. Neurosurgery 1994;34:974–80.
28. Wong AM, Zimmerman RA, Simon EM, et al. Diffusion-weighted MR imaging of subdural empyemas in children. AJNR Am J Neuroradiol 2004 Jun-Jul; 25(6):1016–21.
29. Tsuchiya K, Osawa A, Katase S, et al. Diffusion-weighted MRI of subdural and epidural empyemas. Neuroradiology 2003;45(4):220–3.
30. Karvouniaris M, Brotis A, Tsiakos K, et al. Current perspectives on the diagnosis and management of healthcare-associated ventriculitis and meningitis. Infect Drug Resist 2022;15:697–721.
31. Fukui MB, Williams RL, Mudigonda S. CT and MR imaging features of bacterial ventriculitis. AJNR Am J Neuroradiol 2001 Sep;22(8):1510–6.
32. Niederweis M, Danilchanka O, Huff J, et al. Mycobacterial outer membranes: in search of proteins. Trends Microbiol 2010;18(3):109–16.
33. Thwaites G, Chau TT, Mai NT, et al. Tuberculous meningitis [published correction appears in J Neurol Neurosurg Psychiatry 2000 Jun;68(6):802]. J Neurol Neurosurg Psychiatry 2000;68(3):289–99. https://doi.org/10.1136/jnnp.68.3.289.
34. Theron S, Andronikou S, Grobbelaar M, et al. Localized basal meningeal enhancement in tuberculous meningitis. Pediatr Radiol 2006;36(11):1182–5.
35. Vanjare HA, Gunasekaran K, Manesh A, et al. Evaluation of intracranial vasculitis in tuberculous meningitis using magnetic resonance vessel wall imaging technique. Int J Mycobacteriol 2021;10(3): 228–33.
36. Patkar D, Narang J, Yanamandala R, et al. Central nervous system tuberculosis: pathophysiology and imaging findings. Neuroimaging Clin N Am 2012; 22(4):677–705.
37. Gupta RK, Vatsal DK, Husain N, et al. Differentiation of tuberculous from bacterial brain abscesses with in vivo proton MR spectroscopy and magnetization transfer MR imaging. AJNR Am J Neuroradiol 2001 Sep;22(8):1503–9.
38. Koeller KK, Shih RY. Viral and Prion Infections of the Central Nervous System: Radiologic-Pathologic Correlation: From the Radiologic Pathology Archives. Radiographics 2017;37(1):199–233. https://doi.org/10.1148/rg.2017160149.
39. Zhang Y, Zhu Z, Yang W, et al. An emerging recombinant human enterovirus 71 responsible for the 2008 outbreak of hand foot and mouth disease in Fuyang city of China. Virol J 2010;7:94.
40. Chow FC, Glaser CA. Emerging and reemerging neurologic infections. Neurohospitalist 2014;4(4):173–84.
41. Chang PC, Chen SC, Chen KT. The current status of the disease caused by enterovirus 71 infections: epidemiology, pathogenesis, molecular epidemiology, and vaccine develop-ment. Int J Environ Res Public Health 2016;13(9):890.
42. Abdelgawad MS, El-Nekidy AE, Abouyoussef RAM, et al. MRI findings of enteroviral encephalomyelitis. Egypt J Radiol Nucl Med 2016;47(3):1031–6.
43. Kleinschmidt-DeMasters BK, Gilden DH. The expanding spectrum of herpesvirus infections of the nervous system. Brain Pathol 2001;11(4):440–51.
44. Meyding-Lamadé U, Strank C. Herpesvirus infections of the central nervous system in immunocompromised patients. Ther Adv Neurol Disord 2012; 5(5):279–96.
45. Whitley RJ. Herpes simplex encephalitis: adolescents and adults. Antiviral Res 2006;71(2–3): 141–8.
46. Lakeman FD, Whitley RJ. Diagnosis of herpes simplex encephalitis: application of polymerase chain reaction to cerebrospinal fluid from brain-biopsied patients and correlation with disease. National Institute of Allergy and Infectious Diseases Collaborative Antiviral Study Group. J Infect Dis 1995;171(4): 857–63. https://doi.org/10.1093/infdis/171.4.857.
47. Sabah M, Mulcahy J, Zeman A. Herpes simplex encephalitis. BMJ 2012;344:e3166.
48. Steiner I, Budka H, Chaudhuri A, et al. Viral meningoencephalitis: a review of diagnostic methods and guidelines for management. Eur J Neurol 2010;17(8):999. e57.
49. Soares BP, Provenzale JM. Imaging of Herpesvirus Infections of the CNS. AJR Am J Roentgenol 2016 Jan;206(1):39–48.

50. Berger JR, Houff S. Neurological complications of herpes simplex virus type 2 infection. Arch Neurol 2008;65(5):596–600. https://doi.org/10.1001/archneur.65.5.596.
51. Vossough A, Zimmerman RA, Bilaniuk LT, et al. Imaging findings of neonatal herpes simplex virus type 2 encephalitis. Neuroradiology 2008 Apr;50(4):355–66.
52. Amlie-Lefond C, Fullerton HJ. Rashes, sniffles, and stroke: a role for infection in ischemic stroke of childhood. Infect Disord: Drug Targets 2010 Apr;10(2):67–75.
53. Valdebenito S, Castellano P, Ajasin D, et al. Astrocytes are HIV reservoirs in the brain: A cell type with poor HIV infectivity and replication but efficient cell-to-cell viral transfer. J Neurochem 2021;158(2):429–43.
54. Heaton RK, Clifford DB, Franklin DR Jr, et al. HIV-associated neurocognitive disorders persist in the era of potent antiretroviral therapy: CHARTER Study. Neurology 2010;75(23):2087–96.
55. Antinori A, Arendt G, Becker JT, et al. Updated research nosology for HIV-associated neurocognitive disorders. Neurology 2007;69:1789–99.
56. Ances BM, Hammoud DA. Neuroimaging of HIV-associated neurocognitive disorders (HAND). Curr Opin HIV AIDS 2014;9(6):545–51. https://doi.org/10.1097/COH.0000000000000112.
57. Chang L, Ernst T, Leonido-Yee M, et al. Highly active antiretroviral therapy reverses brain metabolite abnormalities in mild HIV dementia. Neurology 1999;53(4):782–9.
58. Marra CM, Zhao Y, Clifford DB, et al. Impact of combination antiretroviral therapy on cerebrospinal fluid HIV RNA and neurocognitive performance. AIDS 2009;23:1359–66.
59. Patel SH, Kolson DL, Glosser G, et al. Correlation between percentage of brain parenchymal volume and neurocognitive performance in HIV-infected patients. AJNR Am J Neuroradiol 2002;23(4):543–9.
60. Zhu T, Zhong J, Hu R, et al. Patterns of white matter injury in HIV infection after partial immune reconstitution: a DTI tract-based spatial statistics study. J Neurovirol 2013;19(1):10–23.
61. Plessis SD, Vink M, Joska JA, et al. HIV infection and the fronto-striatal system: a systematic review and meta-analysis of fMRI studies. AIDS 2014;28(6):803–11.
62. von Giesen HJ, Antke C, Hefter H, et al. Potential time course of human immunodeficiency virus type 1-associated minor motor deficits: electrophysiologic and positron emission tomography findings. Arch Neurol 2000;57(11):1601–7.
63. Sinharay S, Hammoud DA. Brain PET Imaging: Value for Understanding the Pathophysiology of HIV-associated Neurocognitive Disorder (HAND). Curr HIV AIDS Rep 2019;16(1):66–75. https://doi.org/10.1007/s11904-019-00419-8.
64. Eggers C, Arendt G, Hahn K, et al. HIV-1-associated neurocognitive disorder: epidemiology, pathogenesis, diagnosis, and treatment. J Neurol 2017;264(8):1715–27. https://doi.org/10.1007/s00415-017-8503-2.
65. Debiasi RL, Tyler KL. West Nile virus meningoencephalitis. Nat Clin Pract Neurol 2006;2(5):264–75.
66. West Nile Virus. Centers for Disease Control and Prevention website. http://www.cdc.gov/westnile/index.html. Updated Jun 13, 2023.
67. Sejvar JJ. West Nile Virus Infection. Microbiol Spectr 2016;4(3). https://doi.org/10.1128/microbiolspec.EI10-0021-2016.
68. Ali M, Safriel Y, Sohi J, et al. West Nile virus infection: MR imaging findings in the nervous system. AJNR Am J Neuroradiol 2005;26(2):289–97.
69. Holman RC, Belay ED, Christensen KY, et al. Human prion diseases in the United States. PLoS One 2010;5(1):e8521.
70. Creutzfeldt-Jakob disease, classic (CJD). Centers for Disease Control and Prevention website. http://www.cdc.gov/prions/cjd/index.html. Updated October 18, 2021.
71. Tschampa HJ, Kallenberg K, Kretzschmar HA, et al. Pattern of cortical changes in sporadic Creutzfeldt-Jakob disease. AJNR Am J Neuroradiol 2007;28(6):1114–8.
72. Collie DA, Summers DM, Sellar RJ, et al. Diagnosing variant Creutzfeldt-Jakob disease with the pulvinar sign: MR imaging findings in 86 neuropathologically confirmed cases. AJNR Am J Neuroradiol 2003;24(8):1560–9.
73. Na DL, Suh CK, Choi SH, et al. Diffusion-weighted magnetic resonance imaging in probable Creutzfeldt-Jakob disease: a clinical-anatomic correlation. Arch Neurol 1999;56(8):951–7.
74. Eisenmenger L, Porter MC, Carswell CJ, et al. Evolution of diffusion-weighted magnetic resonance imaging signal abnormality in sporadic Creutzfeldt-Jakob disease, with his-topathological correlation. JAMA Neurol 2016;73(1):76–84.
75. Lee H, Cohen OS, Rosenmann H, et al. Cerebral white matter disruption in Creutzfeldt-Jakob disease. AJNR Am J Neuroradiol 2012;33(10):1945–50.
76. Jang S, Suh SI, Ha SM, et al. Enterovirus 71-related encephalomyelitis: usual and unusual magnetic resonance imaging findings. Neuroradiology 2012;54(3):239–45.
77. Takanashi J, Barkovich AJ, Yamaguchi K, et al. Influenza-associated encephalitis/encephalopathy with a reversible lesion in the splenium of the corpus callosum: a case report and literature review. AJNR Am J Neuroradiol 2004 May;25(5):798–802.
78. Buchanan R, Bonthius DJ. Measles Virus and Associated Central Nervous System Sequelae. Semin Pediatr Neurol 2012;19(3):107–14.

Bacterial and Viral Infectious Disease of the Spine

Pattana Wangaryattawanich, MD[a,*], Amy M. Condos, MD[b], Tanya J. Rath, MD[c]

KEYWORDS

• Spine • Bacterial infection • Viral infection • Spondylitis • Spondylodiscitis • Meningitis • Epidural abscess • Myelitis

KEY POINTS

- Bacterial infections affecting the spine encompass a broad range of conditions, including spondylitis, discitis, spondylodiscitis, paravertebral and intramuscular abscesses, septic arthritis of facet joints, epidural abscess, subdural abscess, leptomeningitis, myelitis, and intramedullary abscess.
- Viral infections in the spine can manifest as meningitis, myelitis, and radiculitis. In some cases, injury to the spinal cord and nerve roots may result from an immune-mediated inflammatory response triggered by a preceding viral infection or vaccination, such as acute disseminated encephalomyelitis and Guillain-Barré syndrome.
- MR imaging with contrast is the preferred imaging modality for evaluating spinal infections due to its superior soft tissue resolution, enabling a comprehensive assessment of the bony structures, intraspinal compartment, and surrounding soft tissues.

INTRODUCTION

Spinal infections are a diverse group of diseases affecting different compartments of the spine, resulting in variable clinical and imaging presentations. Diagnosis of spinal infections is based on a combination of clinical features, laboratory markers, and imaging studies. Diagnosing spinal infection can be challenging due to the often insidious and nonspecific clinical presentation.[1] Timely diagnosis is crucial for initiating appropriate treatment and preventing complications. Imaging plays a pivotal role in the diagnosis and management of spinal infections, characterizing the extent and severity of the disease, identifying complications, guiding biopsy or aspiration and monitoring treatment response.[2] In this article, the epidemiology, pathogenesis, clinical, and characteristic imaging manifestations of bacterial and viral spinal infections are discussed. Spinal infections from fungi, parasites, and other atypical organisms are discussed in another article within this issue.

AN OVERVIEW OF EPIDEMIOLOGY, PATHOGENESIS, AND CLINICAL MANIFESTATIONS OF SPINAL INFECTION

The incidence of spinal infections has increased in recent decades because of a combination of several predisposing factors.[3–5] Underlying medical comorbidities such as diabetes mellitus, cirrhosis, alcoholism, cancer, human immunodeficiency virus (HIV) infection, and chronic steroid usage impair the immune system and make individuals more susceptible to infections. Demographic changes, including an aging population,

[a] Department of Radiology, University of Washington School of Medicine, 1959 Northeast Pacific Street, Seattle, WA 98195-7115, USA; [b] Department of Radiology, University of Washington School of Medicine, 2545 Northeast 85th Street Seattle, WA 98115, USA; [c] Neuroradiology Section, Department of Radiology, Mayo Clinic Arizona, 5777 East Mayo Boulevard, Phoenix, AZ 85054, USA
* Corresponding author.
E-mail address: pattanaw@uw.edu

Magn Reson Imaging Clin N Am 32 (2024) 313–333
https://doi.org/10.1016/j.mric.2023.12.003

growing epidemic of intravenous drug abuse, and an increase in spinal surgical interventions, have also contributed to the increase of spinal infections.[4–8] The availability of diagnostic imaging tests including computed tomography (CT) and MR imaging has allowed for early detection of spinal infections.[9] Conditions that raise the risk of bacteremia, such as intravenous drug abuse and indwelling catheters, provide a pathway for bacteria to enter the bloodstream and potentially reach the spine.[8] Congenital spine anomalies, such as a congenital dermal sinus, can create openings in the skin that allow bacteria to enter the spinal area and increase the risk of infection.[10]

The main routes of spinal infections are as follows: (1) hematogenous spread, (2) direct inoculation, and (3) contiguous spread from nearby structures.[11] Hematogenous spread is the most common route of spread involving the arterial or venous systems. The anterolateral aspect of the vertebral endplate is typically the initial site of infection due to the presence of distal arteriolar arcades, which constitute a slow-flow arterial system, rendering this area more susceptible to infection. Retrograde venous spread to the spine through the valveless Batson's venous plexus originates from infections in the pelvic or intra-abdominal organs, such as urinary tract infections. Direct inoculation may occur due to earlier surgery, percutaneous interventions, or penetrating injuries, often affecting the posterior elements of the spine. Among spinal segments, the lumbar spine is the most frequently affected, followed by decreasing incidence in the thoracic and cervical spine.[1,8] In children, the small arterioles that supply the spine penetrate through narrow channels along the vertebral endplates and terminate near the intervertebral discs. Consequently, spinal infections in children may initiate in the intervertebral discs, a condition known as septic discitis. However, these small vessels become nonfunctional by the age of 30 years. Thus, in older children and adults, spinal infections typically develop in the vertebral endplates, as intervertebral discs become avascular structures.[12] Nonetheless, bacterial infections can still involve intervertebral discs due to the production of proteolytic enzymes by bacteria, which can digest the intervertebral disc substance.[8]

The clinical presentation of spinal infection often lacks specificity. Back pain is the most common symptom, affecting 80% to 90% of patients. Less common symptoms include fever, chills, malaise, radiculopathy, motor weakness, and bowel and bladder dysfunction.[1,13] Neurologic deficits, such as radiculopathy, motor weakness or paralysis, sensory loss, and urinary retention, are reported in approximately 34% of patients with pyogenic spondylodiscitis.[1] To evaluate clinically suspected spinal infection, laboratory tests such as white blood cell (WBC) count, erythrocyte sedimentation rate (ESR), C-reactive protein (CRP), and septic workup, including blood culture and urine culture, are typically performed.[2] It should be noted that the WBC count can be within the normal range in up to 40% of patients with pyogenic spondylodiscitis. Although ESR and CRP are sensitive inflammatory markers, they are not specific to spinal infection. Due to the nonspecific nature of the clinical presentation and laboratory findings, the diagnosis of spinal infection is often delayed by approximately 2 to 12 weeks after the onset of symptoms.[1]

IMAGING EVALUATION OF SPINAL INFECTION

Radiography, CT, MR imaging, and nuclear imaging studies are complementary imaging modalities for the diagnosis and evaluation of spinal infections. Radiography is often the initial modality used for assessing back or neck pain due to its widespread availability and low cost. However, it has limited sensitivity in detecting bone or soft tissue abnormalities and may be normal during the early course of disease.[9] Moreover, radiographic findings such as vertebral endplate erosion may lag behind the clinical course of spinal infection by at least 2 to 8 weeks (**Fig. 1**).[2,14] CT offers high-resolution thorough evaluation of bone integrity and nicely characterizes cortical erosion, which can occur in the setting of spondylodiscitis and septic arthritis of the facet joints. It is readily available and has a short acquisition time. CT is also useful for image-guided procedures such as spine biopsy or percutaneous drainage of fluid collections, serving both diagnostic and therapeutic purposes (**Fig. 2**). In addition, radiography and CT can assess spinal alignment, features of spinal instability, and the integrity of spinal instrumentation, if present.[9] However, CT has limited sensitivity in evaluating infections within the spinal canal.[15]

MR imaging is the preferred imaging modality for evaluating spinal infections due to its superior soft tissue resolution. It provides a comprehensive assessment of the intraspinal compartment and paraspinal soft tissues compared with CT.[9] MR imaging has a reported sensitivity, specificity, and accuracy of 96%, 92%, and 94%, respectively, in diagnosing spondylodiscitis.[16] A recent meta-analysis reported the sensitivity and specificity of MR imaging in diagnosing spondylodiscitis to be 90% and 72%, respectively.[17] Intravenous contrast is useful for assessing the disease extent and detecting abscesses. Following initiation of

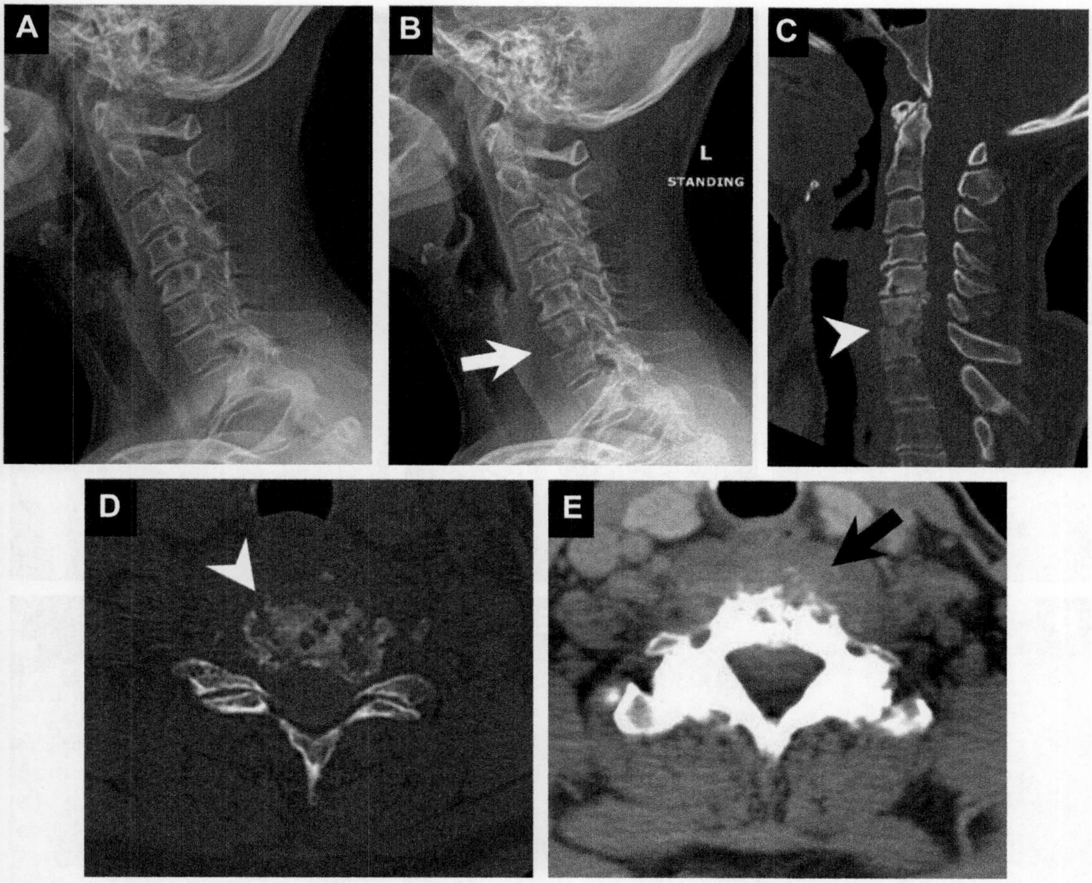

Fig. 1. Cervical spondylodiscitis. A 59-year-old woman presents with progressive neck pain for 3 weeks with no fever, chills, or other constitutional symptoms. Initial lateral cervical spine radiograph (*A*) shows mild degenerative changes with no bone erosion. Second cervical spine radiograph (*B*) performed 3 weeks after shows new subtle bone erosion of the C6 inferior vertebral endplate (*arrow*). Sagittal (*C*) and axial (*D*) CT in bone window shows erosive change of the C6-C7 vertebral endplates (*arrowheads*). Axial CT in soft tissue window (*E*) demonstrates surrounding paravertebral phlegmon (*black arrow*). Open spinal biopsy with tissue culture grows *Corynebacterium* species.

therapy, it is important to note that improvement in MR imaging abnormalities can lag behind clinical response to treatment or even seem worse despite clinical improvement.[2,18]

Nuclear imaging studies, including sequential bone scintigraphy with technetium 99m-methyldiphosphonate (Tc99 m MDP) or hydroxydiphosphonate, Gallium-67 scan, and ^{18}F-Fludeoxyglucose positron emission (F^{18} FDG) tomography/computed tomography (PET/CT) can serve as alternative imaging modalities for assessing spondylodiscitis when MR imaging is contraindicated or can be valuable problem-solving tools in equivocal cases.[2,9] Bone scintigraphy and Gallium-67 scan exhibit high sensitivity but low specificity. However, combining both modalities can increase the diagnostic accuracy to approximately 92%.[2,17] F^{18} FDG PET/CT has high sensitivity (93%–97%) and specificity (80%–91%) in diagnosing spondylodiscitis and may be helpful in equivocal cases.[9,17,19–21] In vitro labeled WBC scans have limited utility in spinal infections because they frequently depict nonspecific areas of decreased radiotracer uptake in the affected spine although the underlying mechanism of this phenomenon remains unknown.[8,22,23]

IMAGING MANIFESTATIONS OF BACTERIAL INFECTION IN THE SPINE

Bacterial infections affecting the spine encompass a broad range of conditions, including spondylitis, discitis, spondylodiscitis, paravertebral and intramuscular abscesses, septic arthritis of facet joints, epidural abscess, subdural abscess, leptomeningitis, myelitis, and intramedullary abscess. The most common pathogen is *Staphylococcus*

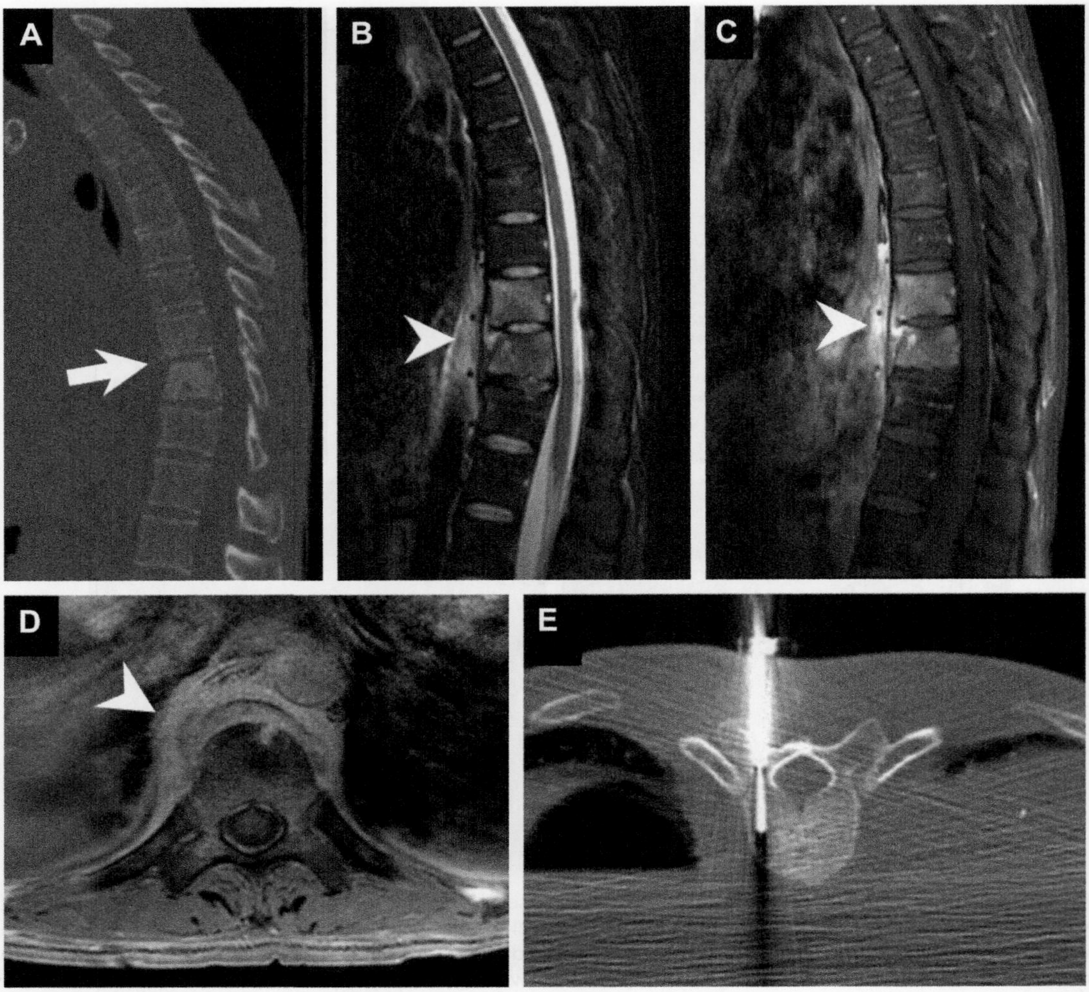

Fig. 2. Thoracic spondylodiscitis. A 46-year-old man with a history of diabetes and multiorgan transplant on chronic immunosuppression presents with worsening back pain for 1 month. Sagittal CT in bone window (*A*) shows erosive change of the T9-T10 vertebral endplates. Sagittal T2 STIR (*B*), sagittal (*C*), and axial (*D*) postcontrast fat suppressed T1-weighted images show marrow edema and enhancement of the affected endplates with phlegmon in the paravertebral soft tissues (*arrowheads*), characteristic of spondylodiscitis. CT-guided biopsy (*E*) with tissue culture grows *S aureus*.

aureus, responsible for approximately 60% of all pyogenic spinal infections.[1,8] Other causes include Streptococcal species, gram-negative bacilli, and anaerobic bacteria. The ensuing discussion will be based on the anatomic location of the disease.

SPONDYLITIS AND SPONDYLODISCITIS

Spondylitis, also known as vertebral osteomyelitis, and spondylodiscitis are inflammatory conditions that affect the vertebral bodies and intervertebral discs. These conditions are typically caused by bacterial infections that spread hematogenously, affecting the anteroinferior vertebral endplates. The infection can spread from the vertebral endplates to the adjacent intervertebral discs, vertebrae, paravertebral soft tissues, muscles, and even the intraspinal compartment, leading to the formation of phlegmon or abscess.[24] Initially, radiographic findings of spondylodiscitis are typically normal and become apparent approximately 2 to 4 weeks after the onset of the disease. Characteristic imaging findings include demineralization and loss of definition of the vertebral endplates, progressive narrowing of the intervertebral disc, and erosion of the vertebral bodies.[2,14,24]

CT is more sensitive than radiography and can detect subtle erosion of the vertebral endplates during the early stages of the disease (**Fig. 3**). CT

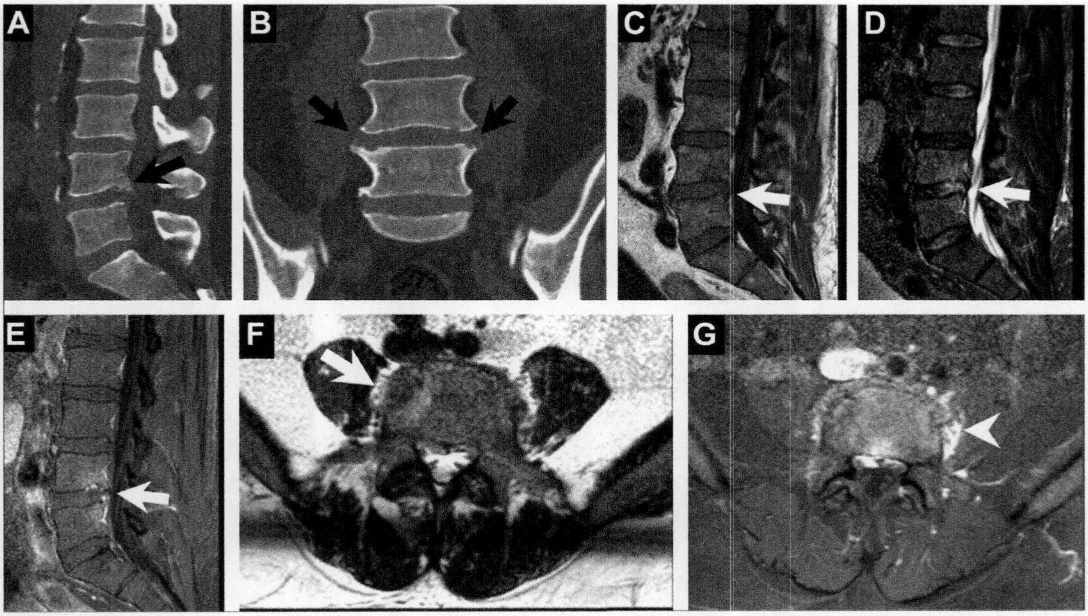

Fig. 3. Early spondylodiscitis. A 58-year-old man with a history of diabetes admitted due to *Streptococcus gordonii* sepsis and bacteremia with endocarditis and lumbar spondylodiscitis. Sagittal (*A*) and coronal (*B*) CT in bone window shows subtle bone erosion at the L4-L5 vertebral endplates (*black arrows*), an early imaging sign of spondylodiscitis. Sagittal T1-weighted image (*C*), T2 STIR (*D*), postcontrast fat suppressed T1-weighted image (*E*), axial T2-weighted image (*F*), and postcontrast fat suppressed T1-weighted image (*G*) show edematous change and enhancement of the corresponding vertebral endplate and adjacent intervertebral disc (*white arrows*). Note phlegmonous change with enhancement in the adjacent paravertebral soft tissue (*arrowhead* on *G*).

can also reveal soft tissue abnormalities such as loss of normal fat planes, gas, and fluid collection. Further evaluation with contrast-enhanced MR imaging is warranted to better characterize soft tissue abnormalities in the affected region. MR imaging findings include bone marrow edema with low T1 and high T2 signal and contrast enhancement in the subchondral bone and vertebral body (see **Fig. 2**) due to hyperemia with an inflammatory response.[8] Progressive destruction of the vertebral endplates and inflammation of the surrounding soft tissues and muscles may occur. Intervertebral discs typically show increased T2 signal and enhancement within the disc. In the early phase of the disease, there may be an increase in disc height followed by progressive disc height loss.[24] It is important to note that there are multiple noninfectious spinal disorders that may mimic spondylodiscitis on imaging, including Modic type I changes, spondyloarthropathy (eg, ankylosing spondylitis), pseudoarthrosis, crystal-induced arthropathy, and neuropathic spinal arthropathy (**Fig. 4**).[25] As such, imaging interpretation should always be integrated with clinical context. Diffusion-weighted imaging (DWI) can be useful in distinguishing between Modic type I changes and spondylodiscitis.[26–28] Modic type I changes on DWI demonstrate a characteristic "Claw sign," which appears as well-demarcated areas of high signal within the opposed vertebral endplates, localized at the interface between normal and abnormal marrow signal (**Fig. 5**).[26] The previously reported accuracy of the "Claw sign" for Modic type I changes was up to 97% to 100%.[26,27] As the disease progresses, it can lead to neurologic complications due to compression of the nerve roots or spinal cord, as well as fracture and collapse of the vertebral bodies, resulting in local instability and malalignment such as kyphosis or scoliosis (**Fig. 6**).[29] Long-term antibiotic therapy is the primary treatment of spondylodiscitis. Surgical intervention may be necessary for patients with epidural abscess, severe spinal destruction with mechanical instability, or when conservative treatment fails.[5] Reduction in soft tissue inflammation, reconstitution of normal bone marrow signal, and decreased enhancement in the affected spine and paraspinal soft tissues are imaging signs of healing although changes in the bones and intervertebral discs may persist after successful treatment.[11,18,30] These imaging signs are also correlated with normalization of inflammatory laboratory markers such as ESR and CRP, indicating response to treatment.[31]

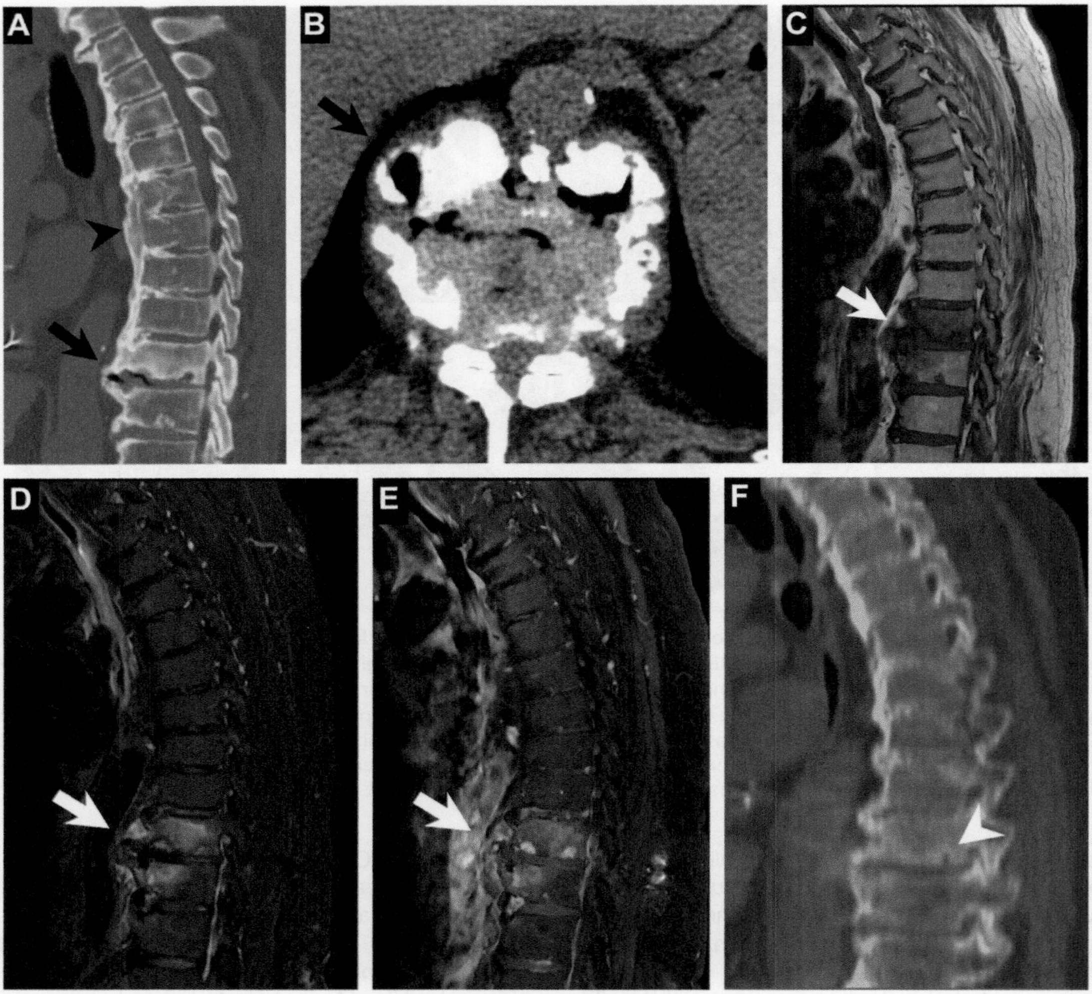

Fig. 4. Neuropathic spondyloarthropathy. Sagittal, bone window (*A*) and axial, soft tissue window (*B*) CT show diffuse endplate irregularity at T11-T12 level (*black arrows*), mimicking spondylodiscitis. Note foci of gas in the intervertebral disc of the same level, favoring vacuum phenomenon from degenerative process, and findings of diffuse idiopathic skeletal hyperostosis spanning the nearly the entire length of the thoracic spine (*black arrowhead*) cephalad to this level. Sagittal T1-weighted image (*C*), T2 STIR (*D*), and postcontrast fat suppressed T1-weighted image (*E*) show marrow edema and enhancement of the affected vertebrae and adjacent intervertebral disc (*white arrows*). Sagittal fused F^{18} FDG PET image (*F*) shows minimal FDG uptake along the T11 vertebral endplate around the Schmorl node (*arrowhead*).

EPIDURAL AND SUBDURAL ABSCESSES

Epidural abscess most commonly occurs in the lower thoracic and lumbar spine and is less frequent in the cervical and upper thoracic spine. It can be caused by hematogenous spread, direct extension from adjacent sites of infection such as spondylodiscitis or septic facet arthritis, or direct inoculation from previous spinal procedures.[32,33] The most common presenting symptom is back pain. Clinical manifestations of epidural abscess can be divided into 4 stages: Stage 1, characterized by back pain at the level of the disease; Stage 2, marked by radicular symptoms; Stage 3, involving motor or sensory deficits, bladder and bowel dysfunction; and Stage 4, the most serious stage, presenting with paralysis, which is a severe complication of epidural abscess.[33] Spinal cord injury resulting from epidural abscess is primarily caused by mechanical compression. The theory of spinal cord infarction from venous congestion or vasculitis remains controversial in animal models.[32] Cervical and thoracic epidural abscesses pose a higher risk of cord compression compared with those in the lumbar spine due to tighter intraspinal spaces.[32] Contrast-enhanced

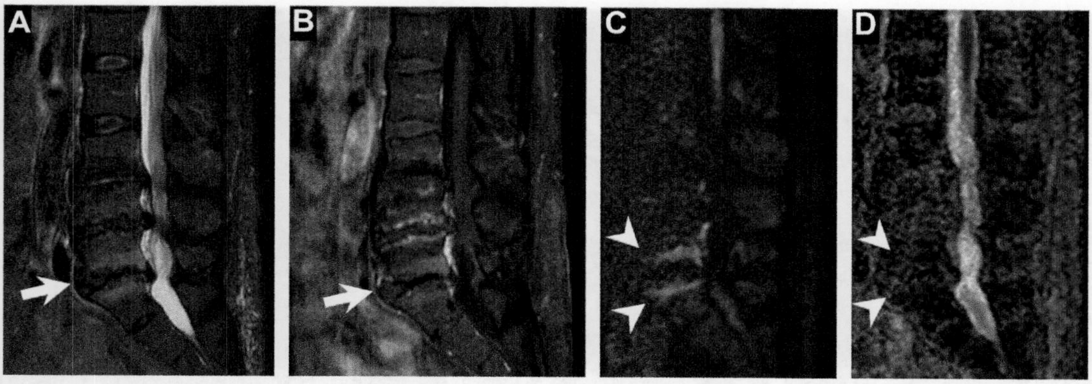

ig. 5. Claw sign on DWI. Sagittal T2 STIR (*A*), and postcontrast fat suppressed T1-weighted image (*B*) show Modic ype I endplate change with marrow edema and enhancement at the L5-S1 level (*arrows*). Sagittal DWI (*C*) and orresponding ADC map (*D*) show well-defined, paired band-like areas of diffusion restriction in the affected re- ions (*arrowheads*), known as the Claw sign, characteristic of Modic type I endplate change on DWI.

MR imaging is the preferred imaging modality for evaluating epidural abscess, revealing a rim-enhancing fluid collection centered in the epidural space. Thick, mucopurulent material within the abscess restricts diffusion on DWI (**Fig. 7**). Contiguous spinal infections, such as spondylodiscitis or septic arthritis of facet joints accompany epidural abscess in up to 80% of patients.[33] Treatment of epidural abscess includes antibiotics and surgical decompression, particularly in patients with neurologic deficits. Successful nonsurgical management of epidural abscess with antibiotic therapy has also been reported.[34]

Subdural abscess is a rare form of bacterial infection in the spine, with limited data available in the literature.[35–38] In a previous systematic review of spinal subdural abscesses in patients aged younger than 21 years, more than half of the patients (53%) were found to have congenital spinal anomalies such as spinal dysraphism.[35] The presenting symptoms are nonspecific and not distinguishable from other types of spinal infections. The key MR imaging feature is an enhancing fluid collection localized in the subdural space. However, differentiating between subdural and epidural collections on imaging can be challenging. Preservation of epidural fat is an important imaging clue indicating that the epicenter of the collection is in the subdural space (**Fig. 8**).[36] Prompt surgical drainage and antibiotic therapy are the mainstay treatments for spinal subdural abscess.[35,38,39]

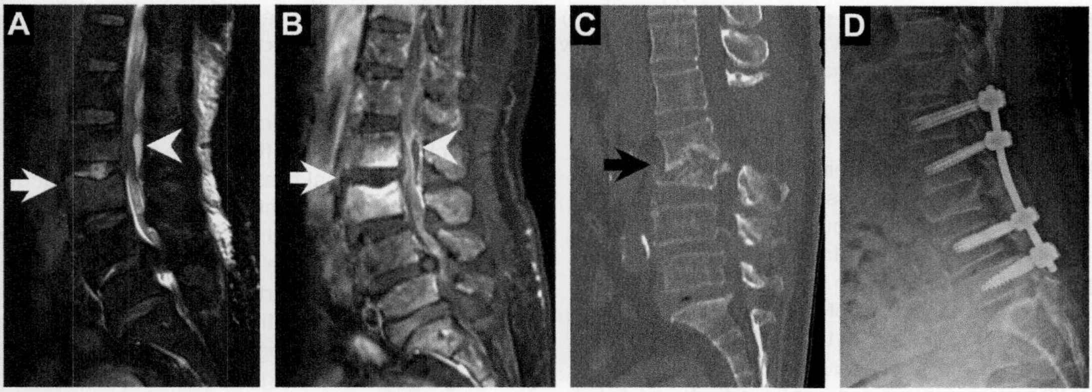

ig. 6. Spondylitis with vertebral body collapse. A 77-year-old woman with septic shock secondary to methicillin-sensitive *Staphyloccus aureus* (MSSA) bacteremia and lumbar spondylitis. Sagittal T2 STIR (*A*), and postcontrast at suppressed T1-weighted image (*B*) show marrow edema and enhancement at the L2-L3 vertebral endplates nd bodies (*white arrows*), consistent with spondylitis. Note dorsal epidural abscess in the spinal canal (*arrowheads*). Follow-up sagittal CT with bone window (*C*) after laminectomy with evacuation of dorsal epidural abscess hows severe collapse of the L3 vertebral body with mild kyphosis (*black arrow*). Surgical stabilization is required ue to local instability. Lateral lumbar spine radiograph (*D*) shows interval L1-L5 posterior spinal fusion, with mprovement of lumbar alignment.

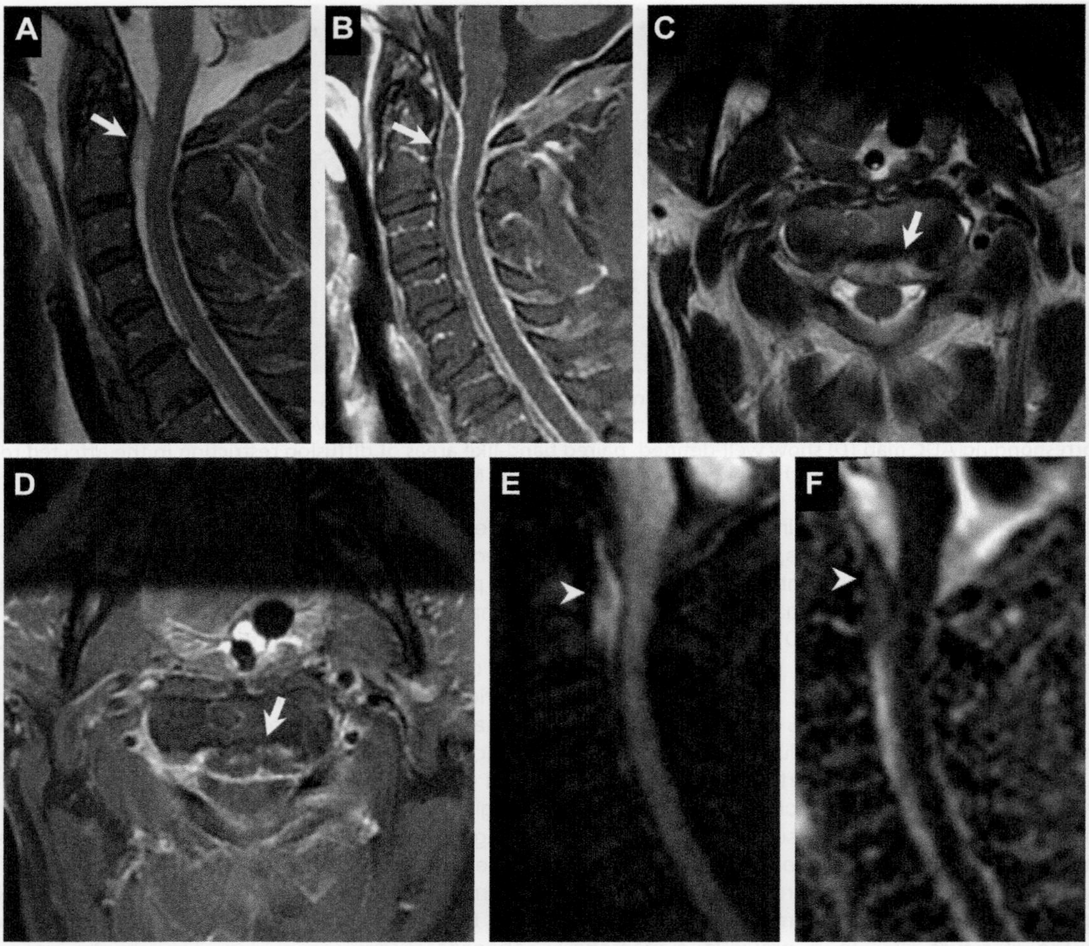

Fig. 7. Epidural abscess. A 65-year-old man with methicillin-susceptible *S aureus* (MSSA) bacteremia with cervical spinal epidural abscess. Sagittal T2 STIR (*A*), postcontrast fat suppressed T1-weighted image (*B*), and axial T2 (*C*) and postcontrast fat suppressed T1-weighted image (*D*) show large ventral epidural abscess (*arrows*) compressing the spinal cord. Sagittal DWI (*E*) and ADC map (*F*) show characteristic diffusion restriction within the abscess secondary to thick purulent material (*arrowheads*).

SEPTIC ARTHRITIS OF FACET JOINTS

Septic arthritis of facet joints is a well-recognized bacterial infection in the spine. The main route of infection is hematogenous spread, although it can also occur as an iatrogenic complication of spinal interventions such as facet joint injection, instrumentation, acupuncture, or epidural catheter placement.[40] *S aureus* is the most common pathogen, accounting for 60% to 70% of all cases.[41] Predisposing factors for septic arthritis of facet joints are similar to those of spondylodiscitis. The lumbar spine is the most frequently affected location.[41] Patients typically present with fever and acute severe back pain, often unilateral and worse with movement, becoming more constant as the disease progresses. Approximately half of the patients experience radicular symptoms radiating to the buttocks or extremities.[40,42] Clinical symptoms can be challenging to differentiate from spondylodiscitis, and atypical presentations such as acute abdominal pain or spontaneous bacterial peritonitis have been reported.[43,44]

Imaging plays a crucial role in the diagnosis and management of septic arthritis of facet joints. Plain radiography is not sensitive enough to detect joint changes, and initial radiographs are usually normal. Imaging evidence may lag behind clinical symptoms by approximately 6 to 12 weeks.[40,41] Plain radiographic findings may include erosion of the articular surfaces and widening or narrowing of the joint spaces. MR imaging is the preferred imaging modality and typically reveals joint effusion, abnormal marrow edema and enhancement, joint destruction, and surrounding soft tissue inflammation (**Fig. 9**).

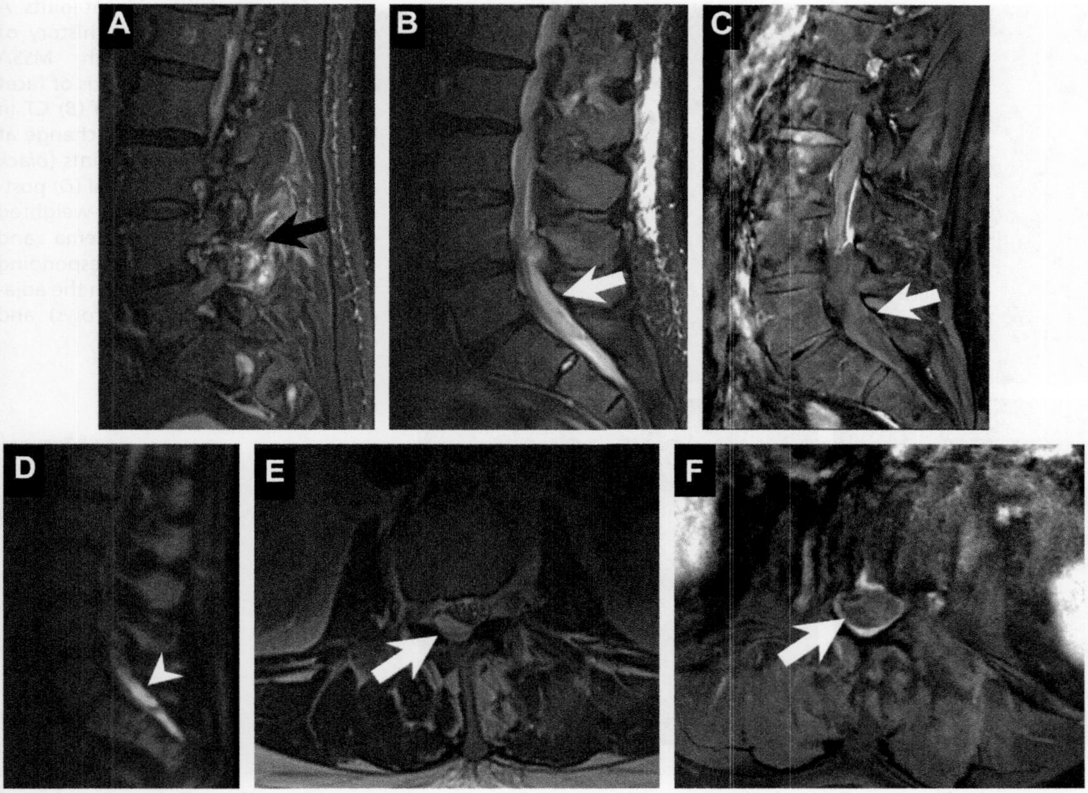

Fig. 8. Subdural abscess. A 54-year-old man with MSSA bacteremia and subdural abscess arising from septic arthritis of right L4-L5 facet joint. Sagittal T2 STIR (*A*) through the lateral aspect of the lumbar spine shows right L4-5 facet marrow edema with surrounding phlegmon consistent with septic arthritis. Sagittal T2 STIR (*B*), postcontrast fat suppressed T1-weighted image (*C*), DWI (*D*), and axial T2-weighted (*E*), and postcontrast fat suppressed T1-weighted image (*F*) show a crescentic fluid collection consistent with subdural abscess eccentric to the right (*arrows*) with diffusion restriction (*arrowhead* on *D*) reflecting the purulent content. Intraoperatively, the presence of a subdural abscess was confirmed.

Contiguous spread into the epidural space with epidural phlegmon or abscess occurs in up to 25% of patients with septic facet arthritis.[41] CT is typically used when MR imaging is contraindicated and demonstrates erosive changes of the affected facet joints and adjacent soft tissue inflammation. CT is particularly useful for imaging-guided diagnostic or therapeutic joint aspiration or bone biopsy. Nuclear medicine imaging with Tc-99m MDP and gallium-67 is highly sensitive in detecting abnormal radiotracer uptake in the affected joints, although the findings are nonspecific. Surgical intervention is indicated in patients with neurologic deficits, cord compression, or those who fail conservative management with ongoing symptoms or bacteremia.[11,40]

MENINGITIS, MYELITIS, AND INTRAMEDULLARY ABSCESS

Meningitis is a common bacterial infection characterized by inflammation of the leptomeninges in the brain and spine, most commonly caused by *Streptococcus pneumoniae* and *Neisseria meningitidis*.[45,46] The pathogenesis involves bacterial colonization, frequently in the upper respiratory tract, followed by invasion into the bloodstream and entry into the subarachnoid spaces. Neurologic damage results not only from the bacteria but also from the host immune response.[47] Symptoms can include fever, headaches, stiff neck, and altered mental status. However, the classic triad of fever, stiff neck, and altered mental status is observed in only 40% of patients with acute bacterial meningitis.[46] Cerebrospinal fluid (CSF) sampling is essential and should be promptly performed when suspected. Initial imaging may be normal but as the infection progresses, contrast-enhanced MR imaging reveals pathologic enhancement within the subarachnoid spaces and leptomeningeal membranes along the surface of the spinal cord and nerve roots. The enhancement patterns can be linear, nodular,

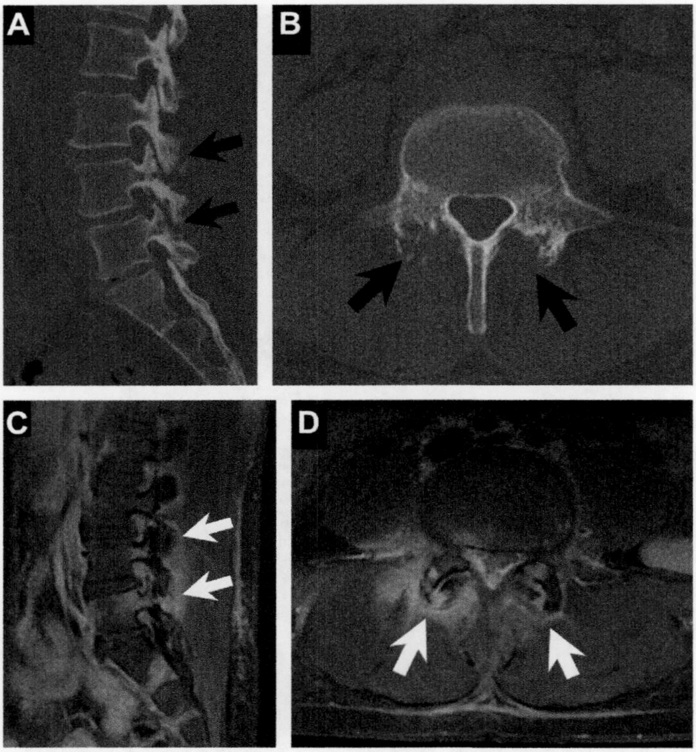

Fig. 9. Septic arthritis of facet joints. A 40-year-old woman with a history of polysubstance abuse with MSSA bacteremia and septic arthritis of facet joints. Sagittal (*A*) and axial (*B*) CT in bone window show erosive change at the L3-L4 and L4-L5 facet joints (*black arrows*). Sagittal (*C*) and axial (*D*) postcontrast fat suppressed T1-weighted images show marrow edema and enhancement of the corresponding facet joints with phlegmon in the adjacent soft tissue (*white arrows*) and epidural space.

or patchy, with clumping of the nerve roots (**Fig. 10**).[11] In chronic stages, adhesions and fluid loculations in the subarachnoid space can develop and cause syringohydromyelia due to CSF flow obstruction. The nerve roots may become abnormally thickened and adhered to the dural sac, resulting in the appearance of an empty sac.[48]

Myelitis and intramedullary abscess are rare manifestations of bacterial infection in the spine, with only around 250 cases reported.[49] They can occur through contiguous spread from nearby structures or systemic infection with hematogenous spread.[14,50] In some cases, the source of infection remains unidentified. Congenital dermal sinuses or epidermoid cysts are predisposing factors for developing intramedullary abscess in the pediatric population.[51] The most common causative bacteria are *S aureus* and *Escherichia coli*. It most frequently affects the thoracic cord.[49] Myelitis and intramedullary abscess represent a continuous disease process with variable MR imaging features according to the stage of the disease. Acute bacterial myelitis seems as an area of cord edema with T1 hypointensity, T2 hyperintensity, and minimal or no enhancement on postcontrast sequences (**Fig. 11**).[52] As myelitis

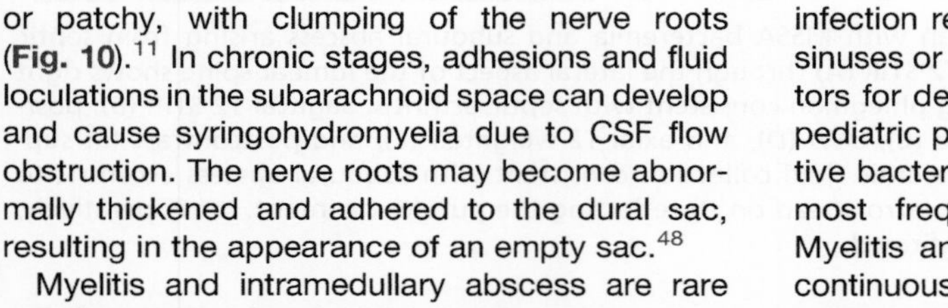

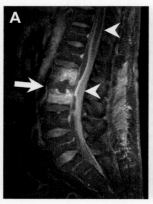

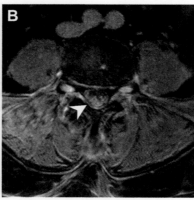

Fig. 10. Bacterial meningitis. A 74-year-old man with septic shock from *Enterococcus faecalis* bacteremia, with lumbar spondylodiscitis, and bacterial meningitis. Sagittal (*A*) and axial (*B*) postcontrast fat suppressed T1-weighted images show abnormal enhancement and destruction of the L3-L4 vertebral endplates and intervertebral disc (*arrow*) characteristic spondylodiscitis. There is extensive leptomeningeal enhancement along the surface of the spinal cord and cauda equina (*arrowheads*) consistent with associated leptomeningitis.

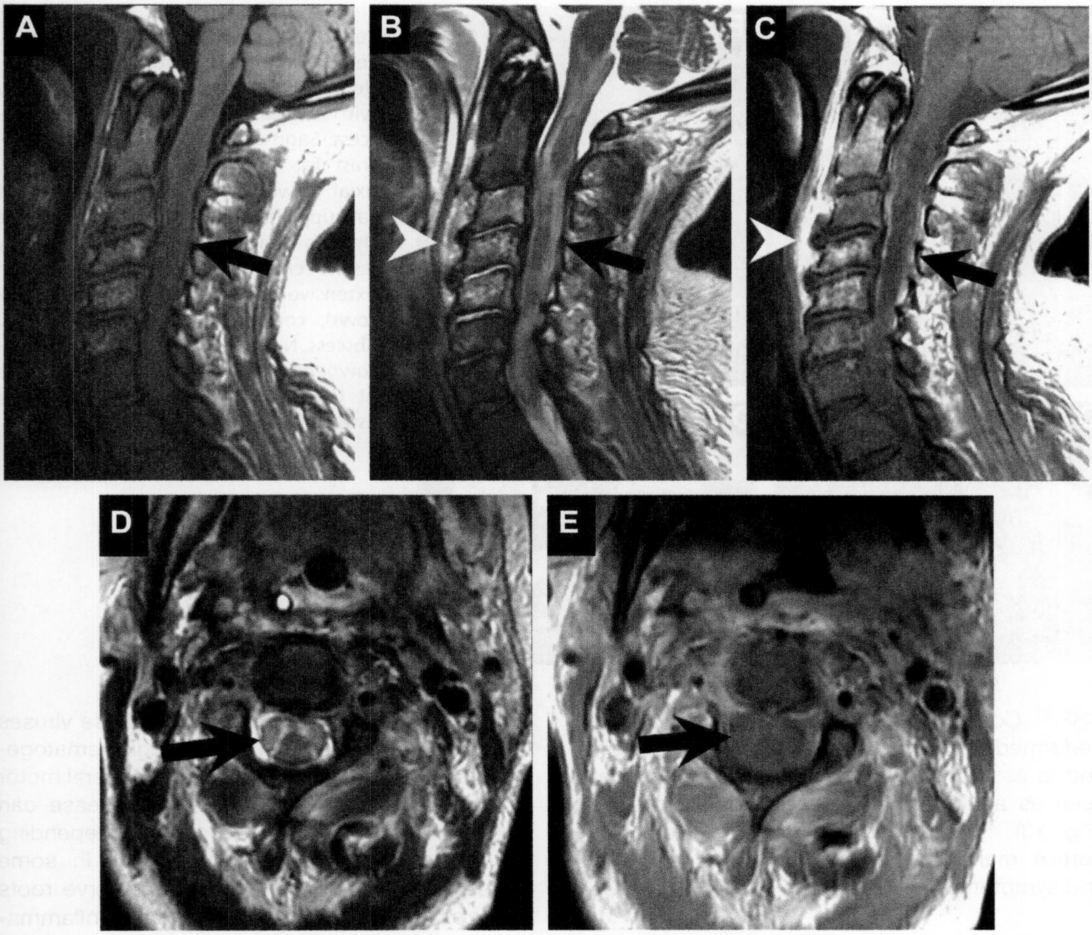

Fig. 11. Bacterial myelitis. A 56-year-old woman with septic shock from MSSA bacteremia, with cervical spondylitis, and myelitis. Sagittal T1-weighted (*A*), T2-weighted (*B*), and postcontrast T1-weighted (*C*) images, and axial T2-weighted (*D*), and postcontrast T1-weighted (*E*) images show diffuse cord expansion with abnormal intramedullary T2 hyperintensity, and heterogeneous enhancement (*black arrows*), suggestive of myelitis. Note spondylodiscitis at the C3-C5 level with phlegmon in the adjacent prevertebral soft tissue (*white arrowheads*).

progresses, intramedullary abscesses may form and seem as localized intramedullary fluid collections with enhancing walls and surrounding cord edema (**Fig. 12**).[14,52] DWI shows restricted diffusion in the central necrotic areas.[53,54] Abscesses may rupture and spread into the subarachnoid spaces.[55] The most common treatment of intramedullary abscess involves a combination of antibiotic therapy and surgical evacuation, although conservative management has been reported in select cases.[49,50]

IMAGING MANIFESTATIONS OF VIRAL INFECTION IN THE SPINE

Viral Meningitis

Viral meningitis, also known as aseptic meningitis, is a common manifestation of viral infection in the central nervous system (CNS), particularly in children. Human enteroviruses are the most common viral pathogen of viral meningitis, although other viruses such as herpesviruses and human influenza viruses can also be responsible.[56,57] Viruses typically enter the host through the respiratory or gastrointestinal tracts and subsequently infect the meninges. Symptoms of viral meningitis include fever, headache, stiff neck, sensitivity to light, nausea, and vomiting. In children and immunocompromised individuals, the manifestations may be severe, whereas in adults, they are typically mild and self-limiting.[57]

The diagnosis of viral meningitis is based on the clinical history, neurologic examination, and CSF analysis. The gold standard for confirming viral meningitis is the polymerase chain reaction (PCR) test, which detects viral DNA or RNA in the

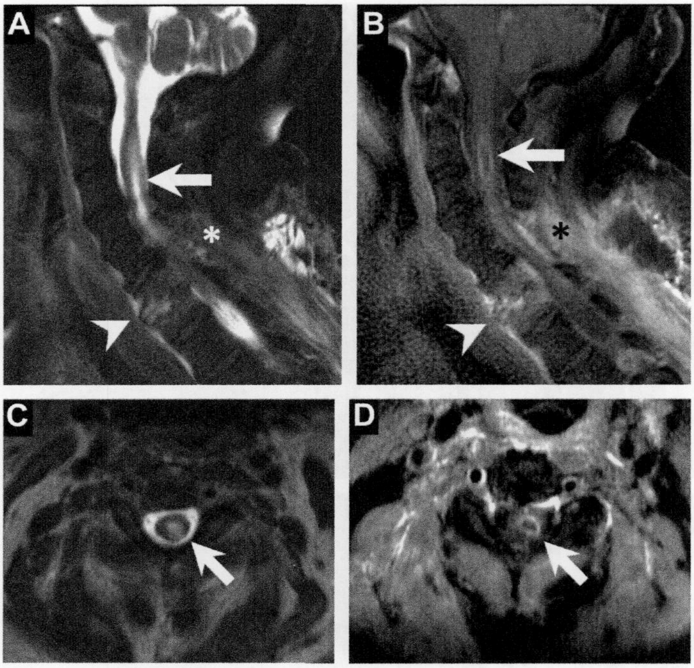

Fig. 12. Intramedullary abscess. A 66-year-old man with MSSA bacteremia, cervical spondylodiscitis, and intramedullary abscess status post laminectomy with surgical evacuation of epidural abscess. Sagittal T2 STIR (*A*) and postcontrast fat suppressed T1-weighted (*B*), axial T2-weighted (*C*) and postcontrast fat suppressed T1-weighted (*D*) images show a rim-enhancing intramedullary lesion centered at the C2-C3 level with extensive surrounding cord edema (*arrows*), consistent with intramedullary abscess. Note C6-C7 spondylodiscitis (*arrowheads*) and laminectomy changes at the C5-C6 level (*white* and *black asterisks*).

CSF.[57] Contrast-enhanced MR imaging may be performed to rule out other causes of symptoms and to assess for features of meningitis, typically seen as abnormal leptomeningeal enhancement (**Fig. 13**).[58] Treatment of viral meningitis is supportive management, including rest, hydration, and symptomatic relief.[57]

Viral Myelitis and Radiculitis

A wide range of viruses, including herpesviruses and enteroviruses, can lead to the inflammation of the spinal cord and nerve roots. These viruses can gain access to the CNS through hematogenous spread or dissemination via peripheral motor or sensory nerves.[56] The onset of disease can vary, ranging from acute to chronic, depending on the specific viruses involved.[59,60] In some cases, injury to the spinal cord and nerve roots may result from an immune-mediated inflammatory response triggered by a preceding viral infection or vaccination, such as acute disseminated encephalomyelitis (ADEM) and Guillain-Barré syndrome (GBS).[61] Contrast-enhanced MR imaging is

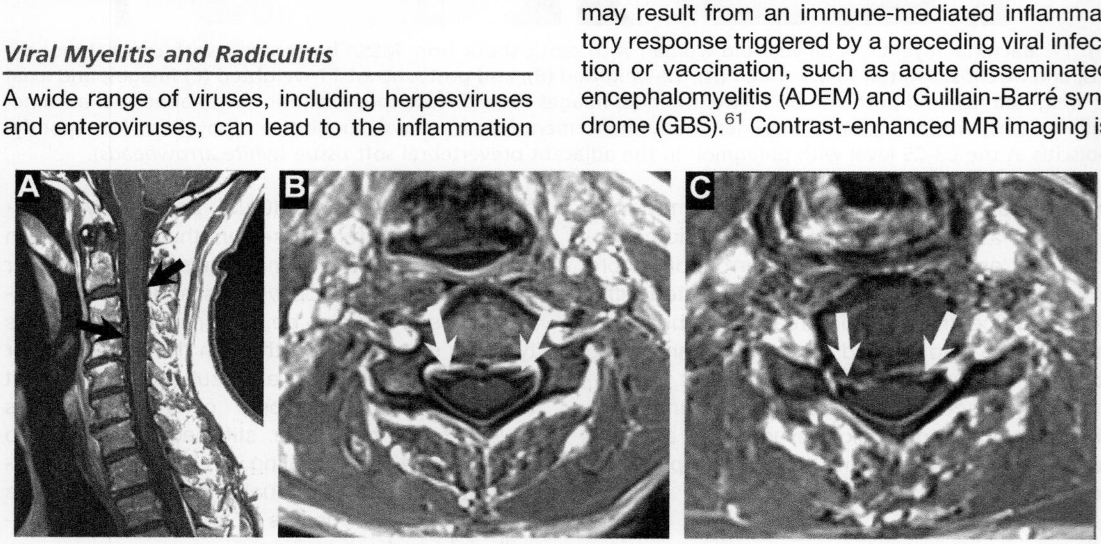

Fig. 13. West Nile virus meningitis and radiculitis. A 65-year-old man presented with progressive right arm weakness and bilateral shoulder pain in the context of recent febrile illness. Physical examination was notable for flaccid weakness of the right arm and left proximal arm and hyporeflexia of bilateral arms. West Nile virus IgG in serum and CSF was positive. Sagittal (*A*) axial (*B*, *C*) postcontrast T1-weighted images show mild leptomeningeal enhancement (*black arrows* on *A*) and enhancement along the bilateral cervical nerve roots (*arrows* on *B* and *C*), indicating leptomeningitis.

crucial for the diagnosis and clinical management of these conditions. In this section, we will explore the distinctive clinical and imaging features associated with various viral pathogens, as well as postinfectious inflammatory disorders of the spine.

Varicella Zoster Virus

Varicella zoster virus (VZV) is a highly neurotropic herpesvirus that commonly causes chickenpox and herpes zoster (shingles) in humans. Primary VZV infection typically occurs during childhood, followed by a latent infection in the trigeminal and peripheral dorsal root ganglia.[62] The virus remains dormant during this latent phase but can reactivate later in life, particularly in adults and the elderly. Myelitis, which is inflammation of the spinal cord, is a rare neurologic complication of VZV infection, with an incidence of 0.8% in the general population.[63] It often occurs during viral reactivation and can affect both immunocompromised and immunocompetent individuals.[62]

Neurologic deficits resulting from spinal cord dysfunction usually manifest within 2 to 3 weeks after the onset of the characteristic skin rash.[63] The mechanisms underlying spinal cord injury involve a combination of direct viral infection, immune-mediated inflammation, and viral-induced vasculitis, which can lead to spinal cord infarction.[63,64] MR imaging reveals longitudinal or multifocal intramedullary lesions that are hypointense on T1-weighted images, are hyperintense on T2-weighted images, and have variable enhancement (**Fig. 14**).[60,65,66] The spinal cord lesion location may correspond to the dermatome distribution of the associated skin rash.[66]

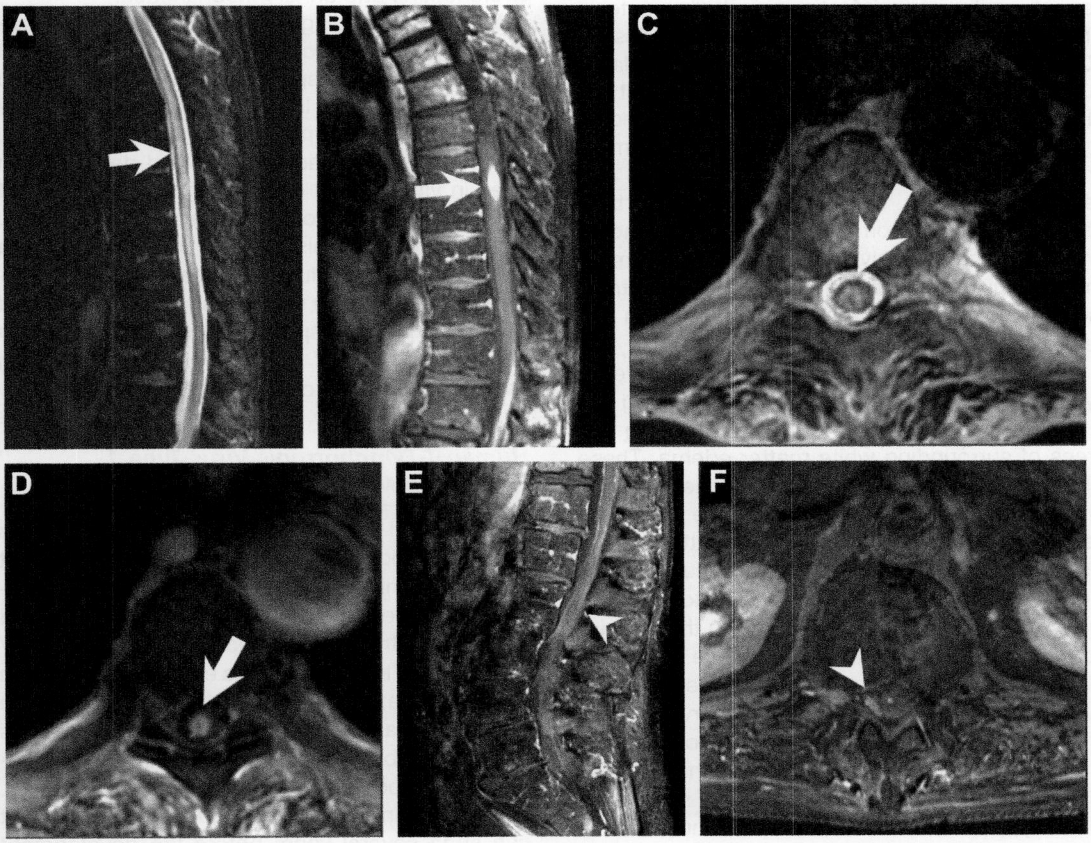

Fig. 14. VZV myelitis and radiculitis. A 71-year-old man with subacute onset of right hemiparesis. Vesicular lesions were also observed on the right side of his trunk, which were concerning for VZV reactivation. Skin swab with VZV index was positive, supporting the diagnosis. Sagittal T2 STIR (*A*), postcontrast fat suppressed T1-weighted (*B*), and axial T2-weighted (*C*) and postcontrast fat suppressed T1-weighted (*D*) images of the thoracic spine showed abnormal intramedullary T2 hyperintense signal with enhancement in the thoracic cord (*arrows*). Sagittal (*E*) and axial (*F*) postcontrast fat suppressed T1-weighted images of the lumbar spine show patchy enhancement of the cauda equina (*arrowheads*), consistent with myelitis and radiculitis secondary to disseminated VZV infection.

Additionally, radiculitis, characterized as abnormal enhancement of the nerve roots, may be present.[67] Treatment of VZV myelitis includes intravenous acyclovir along with corticosteroids to reduce inflammation. The prognosis and clinical outcomes of VZV myelitis vary depending on the individual's immune status.[68,69]

Poliovirus and Nonpolio Enterovirus

Poliovirus, enterovirus, and coxsackievirus belong to the family Picornaviridae and are commonly associated with acute flaccid myelitis (AFM).[59,70] Although poliovirus used to be the primary cause of AFM, global efforts to eradicate poliovirus have significantly reduced its incidence since 1988.[71] However, poliovirus remains endemic in certain regions, such as Afghanistan and Pakistan, where cases may be caused by oral vaccine-derived strains.[59,71] Conversely, the incidence of nonpolio enterovirus infections, including enterovirus D68, has decreased in recent decades. In 2014, the United States experienced a large outbreak of enterovirus D68.[70,72] The majority of AFM cases (85%) occur in children, with a median age of 6 years.[70] The primary sites of involvement are the anterior horn cells in the spinal cord and ventral nerve roots. Patients present with a brief period of viral prodromes, followed by the acute onset of flaccid paralysis affecting one or more limbs. Clinical examination reveals asymmetrical motor weakness, decreased deep tendon reflexes, and fasciculations.[70]

MR imaging reveals longitudinally extensive T2 hyperintense lesions predominantly affecting the gray matter of the spinal cord, with varying degrees of surrounding white matter edema. These lesions are minimally enhancing or nonenhancing. In the early acute phase, the lesions are typically ill defined and involve the entire gray matter. As the disease progresses into the subacute phase (approximately 1–4 weeks after symptom onset), the lesions become more localized to the anterior horn cells (**Fig. 15**). In some cases, the brainstem may also be affected, and there may be enhancement of the nerve roots or cranial nerves.[70,73,74] The treatment of AFM is supportive, focusing on managing symptoms and providing rehabilitation. Many patients experience incomplete neurologic recovery, with residual weakness and muscle atrophy, requiring long-term rehabilitation.[70]

Human Immunodeficiency Virus-associated Myelopathy

HIV-associated myelopathy, also known as vacuolar myelopathy (VM), is a slowly progressive condition that primarily affects individuals with advanced immunosuppression due to HIV infection. VM is characterized by the presence of vacuolization within the myelin sheath and macrophage infiltration in the spinal white matter, particularly in the dorsal and lateral columns of the thoracic cord.[75–77] Autopsy study has shown that VM is present in approximately 40% to 50% of patients with acquired immunodeficiency syndrome, although only 27% of those with pathologically confirmed VM experience symptomatic manifestations.[78] The exact underlying mechanisms of VM are not fully understood but several hypotheses have been proposed. These include macrophage infiltration, secretion of neurotoxic cytokines, and impaired metabolism of vitamin B12. Clinical symptoms of VM include painless progressive spastic paraparesis (weakening of the lower limbs with increased muscle tone), sensory ataxia (loss of coordination due to sensory dysfunction), and urinary incontinence.[76,77]

MR imaging findings in VM reveal spinal cord atrophy and nonspecific T2 hyperintense signal changes within the spinal cord, without a specific distribution pattern. In some cases, there may be preferential involvement of the dorsal columns, resembling the subacute combined degeneration seen in vitamin B12 deficiency.[60] Diagnosing VM involves excluding other causes of myelopathy, including opportunistic infections, through a comprehensive evaluation. Treatment of VM focuses on supportive measures, including physical therapy to manage spasticity, medications to alleviate symptoms of spasticity, and addressing neurogenic bladder dysfunction.[77]

Human T-Lymphotropic Virus Type 1-Associated Myelopathy

Human T-cell lymphotropic virus type 1 (HTLV-1) is a highly oncogenic retrovirus known to cause adult T-cell leukemia/lymphoma and various inflammatory disorders, including HTLV-1-associated myelopathy/tropical spastic paraparesis (HAM/TSP).[79,80] HTLV-1 infection is endemic in Southern Japan, Africa, central and southern America, the Caribbean, and central Australia. The virus is transmitted between individuals through breastfeeding, blood transfusions, and sexual contact. After infection, there is a long latency period that can span several years before the development of hematologic malignancies and inflammatory disorders.

HAM/TSP is a chronic progressive myelopathy that affects 1% to 2% of individuals with HTLV-1 infection.[59,80] The presence of a high HTLV-1 proviral load is a strong predictor for the development of HAM/TSP. Inflammatory changes can occur in

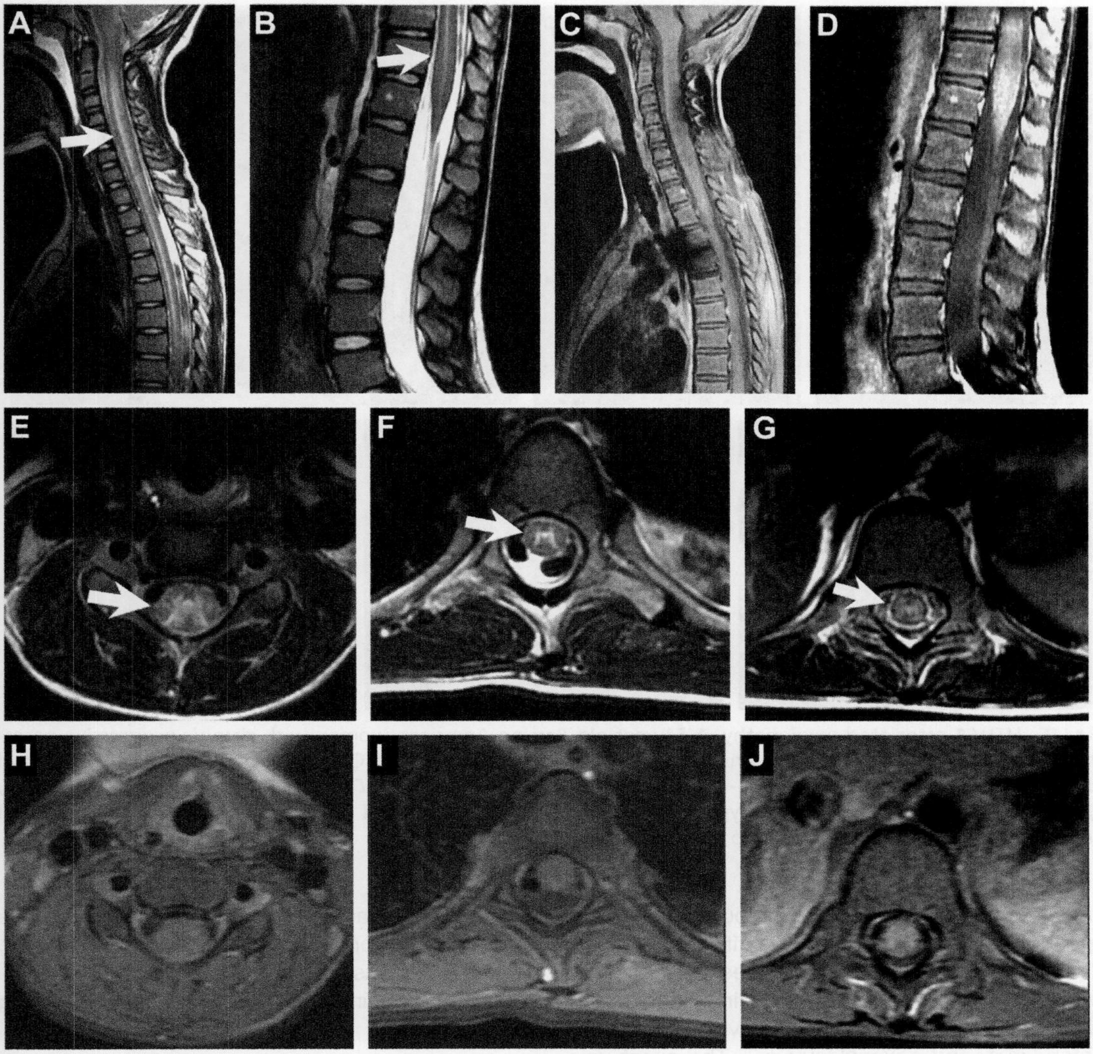

Fig. 15. Acute flaccid myelitis. An 8-year-old girl with acute febrile illness, diffuse weakness, and acute respiratory failure secondary to acute flaccid myelitis, presumably from enterovirus infection. Sagittal T2-weighted (*A, B*) and postcontrast fat suppressed T1-weighted (*C, D*), and axial T2-weighted (*E–G*) and postcontrast fat suppressed T1-weighted (*H–J*) images show longitudinally extensive intramedullary T2 hyperintensity throughout the spinal cord, conforming to the gray matter (*arrows*). There is no enhancement on postcontrast sequences.

various parts of the CNS but the upper thoracic spinal cord is most commonly affected. Clinical features of HAM/TSP include subacute or chronic progressive spastic paraparesis, lower back pain, distal paresthesia in the hands and feet, and urinary and anal sphincter dysfunction.[80] Laboratory assessment for HAM/TSP includes the detection of HTLV-1 antibodies or HTLV-1 DNA using PCR in the blood and CSF, which can provide a definitive diagnosis. MR imaging findings in HAM/TSP are generally nonspecific, and the primary purpose of MR imaging is to exclude other diseases. The appearance of the spinal cord on MR imaging can vary and may show normal findings, cord edema, or atrophy, depending on the stage of the disease (**Fig. 16**).[60,80,81] There is currently no specific antiviral therapy available for HAM/TSP, and supportive treatment aims to alleviate pain, manage spasticity, and address other associated complications.[80]

POSTINFECTIOUS MYELOPATHY AND POLYRADICULOPATHY

Acute Disseminated Encephalomyelitis

ADEM is an immune-mediated demyelinating disorder that primarily affects children between the ages of 3 and 7 years.[82,83] It often occurs following

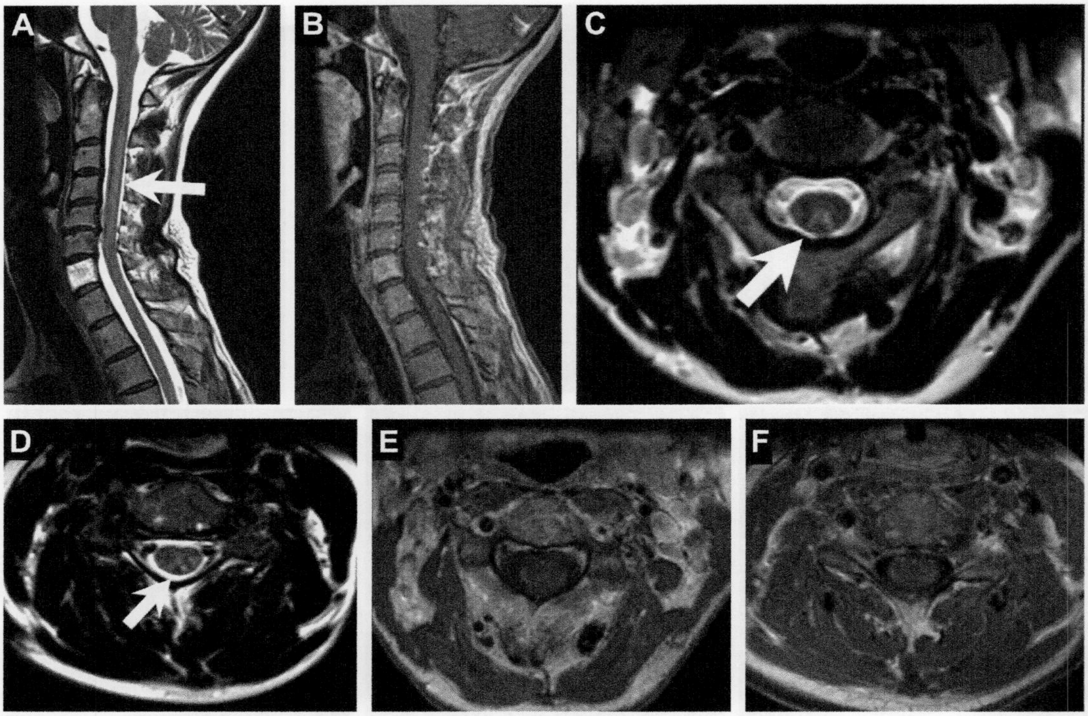

Fig. 16. HTLV-1 associated myelopathy. A 51-year-old Persian American woman with chronic progressive paresthesia and spasticity of the upper and lower extremities. HTLV-1 PCR of CSF and blood was positive. Sagittal T2-weighted (*A*) and postcontrast T1-weighted (*B*), axial T2-weighted (*C, D*), and postcontrast T1-weighted (*E, F*) images show intramedullary T2 hyperintensity within the cervical cord predominantly involving the dorsal and lateral columns (*arrows*), with no contrast enhancement.

an infection or vaccination, although it can be spontaneous without an identifiable trigger. Various microorganisms have been associated with the development of ADEM, including measles, rubella, VZV, herpes simplex virus, influenza, enterovirus, and coxsackievirus.[82] The exact underlying mechanism of ADEM remains unclear but it is thought to involve an abnormal immune response to pathogens or environmental factors in genetically susceptible individuals.[82] Symptoms of ADEM usually emerge within 2 to 4 weeks after an infection and rapidly progress to maximum severity within 2 to 7 days.[82,83] Patients with ADEM typically present with altered mental state and multifocal neurologic deficits, such as ataxia, visual changes, or weakness.[82] Approximately 30% of patients with ADEM develop spinal cord lesions.[84,85] MR imaging reveals intramedullary T2 hyperintense signal within the spinal cord usually without enhancement.[85] The length of cord lesions can vary, with some extending across 2 to 3 vertebral segments and others spanning the entire length of the spinal cord (**Fig. 17**). ADEM is primarily diagnosed based on clinical presentation with no specific laboratory markers for the condition. Treatment of active ADEM includes high-dose intravenous corticosteroids, plasma exchange, and intravenous immunoglobulin, aimed at suppressing the immune response and reducing inflammation.[82]

Guillain-Barré Syndrome

GBS is an acute immune-mediated polyradiculopathy that can develop following an infection, and less commonly, after vaccination. Approximately 70% to 80% of patients with GBS have a preceding infection usually within 4 weeks before the onset of neurologic symptoms.[61] Various microorganisms have been associated with the occurrence of GBS, including *Campylobacter jejuni*, *Mycoplasma pneumoniae*, influenza, cytomegalovirus, and the severe acute respiratory syndrome coronavirus 2.[61] The pathophysiology of GBS involves the production of antibodies against specific glycolipids or proteins in the nerves or myelin. GBS can be classified into 2 main phenotypes: acute inflammatory demyelinating polyradiculopathy (AIDP) and acute motor axonal neuropathy (AMAN), depending on the primary

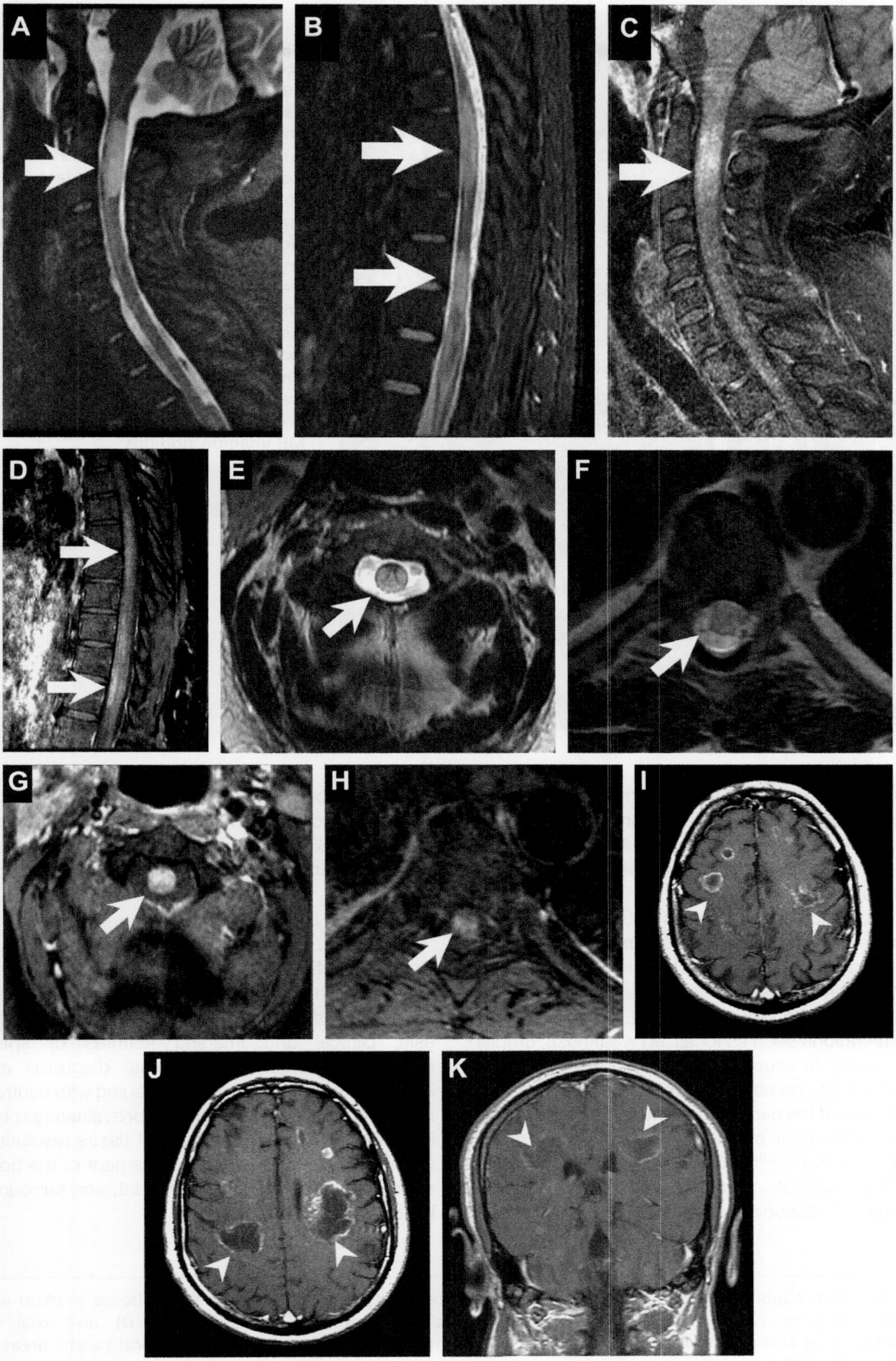

Fig. 17. Acute disseminated encephalomyelitis. A 43-year-old man with rapidly progressive paresthesia, quadriplegia, and urinary retention following a recent episode of viral infection. CSF analysis showed elevated protein,

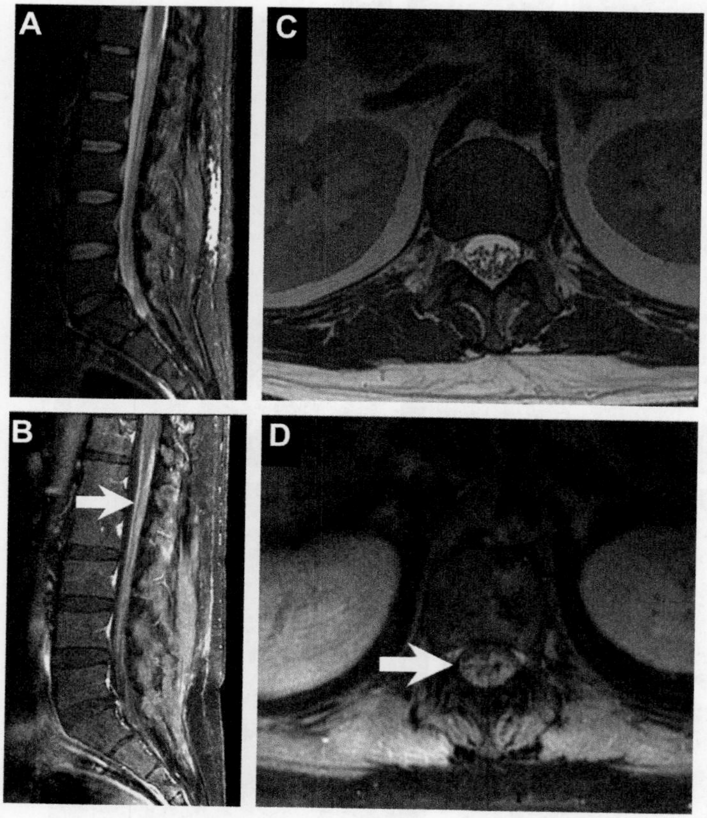

Fig. 18. Guillain-Barré syndrome. A 32-year-old man with a history of alcohol use disorder and hypertension presents with diffuse severe weakness. Physical examination was notable for areflexia, flaccid tone, and paralysis except for movement of face, neck, and shoulders, suggestive of polyneuropathy. CSF protein was markedly elevated. Sagittal T2-weighted (*A*) and postcontrast fat suppressed T1-weighted (*B*), axial T2-weighted (*C*), and postcontrast fat suppressed T1-weighted (*D*) images show smooth extensive diffuse enhancement of the cauda equina (*white arrows*). GBS was diagnosed based on the clinical presentation, electromyography, and MR imaging findings.

sites of antigens. In AIDP, inflammatory demyelination and destruction of the myelin sheaths are the primary features, whereas in AMAN, axonal injury without significant demyelination leads to abnormal nerve conduction.[61]

The classic clinical features of GBS include progressive ascending weakness starting in the lower limbs, along with associated hyporeflexia on clinical examination. However, some patients may present with variants of GBS, exhibiting different clinical manifestations such as localized weakness, cranial neuropathy, or acute bulbar palsy.[61] MR imaging in GBS typically reveals abnormal enhancement and thickening of the nerve roots, with differential or uniform involvement of the ventral and dorsal nerve roots (**Fig. 18**).[60,86,87] Diagnosis of GBS is based on the clinical presentation, CSF albumin-cytological dissociation (elevated protein levels without a corresponding increase in WBCs), and electrodiagnostic studies. The mainstay of treatment of GBS during the acute phase is plasma exchange and intravenous immunoglobulin therapy.[61]

SUMMARY

Spinal infections encompass a wide range of diseases with diverse clinical and imaging presentations. Understanding the epidemiology, pathogenesis, clinical and imaging features of spinal infections is crucial for accurate diagnosis and appropriate management. MR imaging with contrast is the preferred imaging modality for evaluating spinal infections due to its superior soft tissue resolution, enabling a comprehensive assessment of the bony structures, intraspinal compartment, and surrounding soft tissues.

with negative oligoclonal bands and aquaporin-4 antibody testing. Extensive infectious disease workup was negative. Sagittal T2-weighted (*A, B*) and postcontrast fat suppressed T1-weighted (*C, D*), and axial T2-weighted (*E, F*) and postcontrast fat suppressed T1-weighted (*G, H*) images showed multifocal patchy areas of intramedullary T2 hyperintensity and contrast enhancement throughout the spinal cord (*white arrows*). Simultaneous axial (*I, J*) and coronal (*K*) postcontrast T1-weighted images of the brain showed multiple rim enhancing lesions in the bilateral cerebral white matter (*arrowheads*).

CLINICS CARE POINTS

- Radiography has limited sensitivity in detecting bone or soft tissue abnormalities and may be normal during the early course of spinal infection. Radiographic findings such as vertebral endplate erosion may lag behind the clinical course of spinal infection by at least 2 to 8 weeks.
- In vitro labeled WBC scan has limited utility in spinal infections due to nonspecific areas of decreased radiotracer uptake in the affected spine, for which the mechanism remains unknown.
- Multiple noninfectious spinal disorders that mimic spondylodiscitis can often be differentiated by careful assessment of accompanying imaging features interpreted in the context of the clinical history.

DISCLOSURE

P. Wangaryattawanich and T.J. Rath have no conflicts of interest to disclose, and there were no financial incentives that would alter the contents of this article. A.M. Condos: The views expressed in this presentation are those of the authors and do not necessarily reflect the official policy or position of the Department of the Navy, Department of Defense, or the United States Government. The authors are military service members. This study was prepared as part of official duties. Title 17 U.S C. 105 provides that "Copyright protection under this title is not available for any work of the United States Government." The authors received no financial compensation for this presentation. Neither I nor my immediate family members have a financial relationship with a commercial organization that may have a direct or indirect interest in the content.

REFERENCES

1. Mylona E, Samarkos M, Kakalou E, et al. Pyogenic vertebral osteomyelitis: a systematic review of clinical characteristics. Semin Arthritis Rheum 2009; 39(1):10–7.
2. Lazzeri E, Bozzao A, Cataldo MA, et al. Joint EANM/ESNR and ESCMID-endorsed consensus document for the diagnosis of spine infection (spondylodiscitis) in adults. Eur J Nucl Med Mol Imaging 2019; 46(12):2464–87.
3. Issa K, Diebo BG, Faloon M, et al. The epidemiology of vertebral osteomyelitis in the United States From 1998 to 2013. Clin Spine Surg 2018;31(2):E102–8.
4. Nagashima H, Yamane K, Nishi T, et al. Recent trends in spinal infections: retrospective analysis of patients treated during the past 50 years. Int Orthop 2010;34(3):395–9.
5. Waheed G, Soliman MAR, Ali AM, et al. Spontaneous spondylodiscitis: review, incidence, management, and clinical outcome in 44 patients. Neurosurg Focus 2019;46(1):E10.
6. Zhou J, Wang R, Huo X, et al. Incidence of surgical site infection after spine surgery: a systematic review and meta-analysis. Spine (Phila Pa 1976) 2020;45(3):208–16.
7. DiGiorgio AM, Stein R, Morrow KD, et al. The increasing frequency of intravenous drug abuse-associated spinal epidural abscesses: a case series. Neurosurg Focus 2019;46(1):E4.
8. Raghavan M, Palestro CJ. Imaging of spondylodiscitis: an update. Semin Nucl Med 2023;53(2):152–66.
9. Expert Panel on Neurological I, Ortiz AO, Levitt A, et al. ACR Appropriateness Criteria(R) Suspected Spine Infection. J Am Coll Radiol 2021;18(11S): S488–501.
10. Prasad GL, Hegde A, Divya S. Spinal intramedullary abscess secondary to dermal sinus in children. Eur J Pediatr Surg 2019;29(3):229–38.
11. Tali ET, Oner AY, Koc AM. Pyogenic spinal infections. Neuroimaging Clin 2015;25(2):193–208.
12. Offiah AC. Acute osteomyelitis, septic arthritis and discitis: differences between neonates and older children. Eur J Radiol 2006;60(2):221–32.
13. Hetem SF, Schils JP. Imaging of infections and inflammatory conditions of the spine. Semin Muscoskel Radiol 2000;4(3):329–47.
14. DeSanto J, Ross JS. Spine infection/inflammation. Radiol Clin North Am 2011;49(1):105–27.
15. Shroyer S, Boys G, April MD, et al. Imaging characteristics and CT sensitivity for pyogenic spinal infections. Am J Emerg Med 2022;58:148–53.
16. Modic MT, Feiglin DH, Piraino DW, et al. Vertebral osteomyelitis: assessment using MR. Radiology 1985;157(1):157–66.
17. Maamari J, Grach SL, Passerini M, et al. The use of MRI, PET/CT, and nuclear scintigraphy in the imaging of pyogenic native vertebral osteomyelitis: a systematic review and meta-analysis. Spine J 2023; 23(6):868–76.
18. Gillams AR, Chaddha B, Carter AP. MR appearances of the temporal evolution and resolution of infectious spondylitis. AJR Am J Roentgenol 1996; 166(4):903–7.
19. Treglia G, Pascale M, Lazzeri E, et al. Diagnostic performance of (18)F-FDG PET/CT in patients with spinal infection: a systematic review and a bivariate meta-analysis. Eur J Nucl Med Mol Imaging 2020; 47(5):1287–301.
20. Smids C, Kouijzer IJ, Vos FJ, et al. A comparison of the diagnostic value of MRI and (18)F-FDG-PET/CT

in suspected spondylodiscitis. Infection 2017;45(1): 41–9.
21. Prodromou ML, Ziakas PD, Poulou LS, et al. FDG PET is a robust tool for the diagnosis of spondylodiscitis: a meta-analysis of diagnostic data. Clin Nucl Med 2014;39(4):330–5.
22. Gemmel F, Dumarey N, Palestro CJ. Radionuclide imaging of spinal infections. Eur J Nucl Med Mol Imaging 2006;33(10):1226–37.
23. Love C, Palestro CJ. Nuclear medicine imaging of bone infections. Clin Radiol 2016;71(7):632–46.
24. Prodi E, Grassi R, Iacobellis F, et al. Imaging in spondylodiskitis. Magn Reson Imaging Clin N Am 2016;24(3):581–600.
25. Boudabbous S, Paulin EN, Delattre BMA, et al. Spinal disorders mimicking infection. Insights Imaging 2021;12(1):176.
26. Patel KB, Poplawski MM, Pawha PS, et al. Diffusion-weighted MRI "claw sign" improves differentiation of infectious from degenerative modic type 1 signal changes of the spine. AJNR Am J Neuroradiol 2014;35(8):1647–52.
27. Daghighi MH, Poureisa M, Safarpour M, et al. Diffusion-weighted magnetic resonance imaging in differentiating acute infectious spondylitis from degenerative Modic type 1 change; the role of b-value, apparent diffusion coefficient, claw sign and amorphous increased signal. Br J Radiol 2016;89(1066):20150152.
28. Dumont RA, Keen NN, Bloomer CW, et al. Clinical utility of diffusion-weighted imaging in spinal infections. Clin Neuroradiol 2019;29(3):515–22.
29. Huyskens J, Van Goethem J, Faure M, et al. Overview of the complications and sequelae in spinal infections. Neuroimaging Clin 2015;25(2):309–21.
30. Mavrogenis AF, Megaloikonomos PD, Igoumenou VG, et al. Spondylodiscitis revisited. EFORT Open Rev 2017;2(11):447–61.
31. Ahn KS, Kang CH, Hong SJ, et al. The correlation between follow-up MRI findings and laboratory results in pyogenic spondylodiscitis. BMC Musculoskelet Disord 2020;21(1):428.
32. Babic M, Simpfendorfer CS, Berbari EF. Update on spinal epidural abscess. Curr Opin Infect Dis 2019;32(3):265–71.
33. Darouiche RO. Spinal epidural abscess. N Engl J Med 2006;355(19):2012–20.
34. Suppiah S, Meng Y, Fehlings MG, et al. How best to manage the spinal epidural abscess? a current systematic review. World Neurosurg 2016;93:20–8.
35. Sandler AL, Thompson D, Goodrich JT, et al. Infections of the spinal subdural space in children: a series of 11 contemporary cases and review of all published reports. a multinational collaborative effort. Childs Nerv Syst 2013;29(1):105–17.
36. Khalil JG, Nassr A, Diehn FE, et al. Thoracolumbosacral spinal subdural abscess: magnetic resonance imaging appearance and limited surgical management. Spine (Phila Pa 1976) 2013;38(13): E844–7.
37. McCabe JJ, Murphy RP. Spinal subdural abscess. JAMA Neurol 2013;70(2):266–7.
38. Lenga P, Fedorko S, Gulec G, et al. Intradural extramedullary pyogenic abscess: incidence, management, and clinical outcomes in 45 patients with a mean follow up of 2 years. Global Spine J 2023. 21925682231151640.
39. Martin RJ, Yuan HA. Neurosurgical care of spinal epidural, subdural, and intramedullary abscesses and arachnoiditis. Orthop Clin North Am 1996; 27(1):125–36.
40. Babic M, Simpfendorfer CS. Infections of the spine. Infect Dis Clin North Am 2017;31(2):279–97.
41. Anaya JEC, Coelho SRN, Taneja AK, et al. Differential diagnosis of facet joint disorders. Radiographics 2021;41(2):543–58.
42. Cabet S, Perge K, Ouziel A, et al. Septic arthritis of facet joint in children: a systematic review and a 10-year consecutive case series. Pediatr Infect Dis J 2021;40(5):411–7.
43. Rajeev A, Choudhry N, Shaikh M, et al. Lumbar facet joint septic arthritis presenting atypically as acute abdomen - A case report and review of the literature. Int J Surg Case Rep 2016;25:243–5.
44. Lopes Correia B, Diniz SE, Lopes da Silva E, et al. Septic arthritis of the lumbar facet joint presenting as spontaneous bacterial peritonitis: a rare case requiring surgical intervention. Eur J Orthop Surg Traumatol 2020;30(1):175–8.
45. Oordt-Speets AM, Bolijn R, van Hoorn RC, et al. Global etiology of bacterial meningitis: A systematic review and meta-analysis. PLoS One 2018;13(6): e0198772.
46. Hasbun R. Progress and challenges in bacterial meningitis: a review. JAMA 2022;328(21):2147–54.
47. McGill F, Heyderman RS, Panagiotou S, et al. Acute bacterial meningitis in adults. Lancet 2016; 388(10063):3036–47.
48. Wright MH, Denney LC. A comprehensive review of spinal arachnoiditis. Orthop Nurs 2003;22(3):215–9. quiz 220-211.
49. Satyadev N, Moore C, Khunkhun SK, et al. Intramedullary spinal cord abscess management: case series, operative video, and systematic review. World Neurosurg 2023;174:205–12. e6.
50. Cerecedo-Lopez CD, Bernstock JD, Dmytriw AA, et al. Spontaneous intramedullary abscesses caused by Streptococcus anginosus: two case reports and review of the literature. BMC Infect Dis 2022;22(1):141.
51. Szmyd B, Jabbar R, Lusa W, et al. What is currently known about intramedullary spinal cord abscess among children? a concise review. J Clin Med 2022; 11(15).

52. Murphy KJ, Brunberg JA, Quint DJ, et al. Spinal cord infection: myelitis and abscess formation. AJNR Am J Neuroradiol 1998;19(2):341–8.
53. Dorflinger-Hejlek E, Kirsch EC, Reiter H, et al. Diffusion-weighted MR imaging of intramedullary spinal cord abscess. AJNR Am J Neuroradiol 2010;31(9):1651–2.
54. Roh JE, Lee SY, Cha SH, et al. Sequential magnetic resonance imaging finding of intramedullary spinal cord abscess including diffusion weighted image: a case report. Korean J Radiol 2011;12(2):241–6.
55. Akimoto T, Hirose S, Mizoguchi T, et al. Ruptured long intramedullary spinal cord abscess successfully treated with antibiotic treatment. J Clin Neurosci 2020;82(Pt B):249–51.
56. Swanson PA 2nd, McGavern DB. Viral diseases of the central nervous system. Curr Opin Virol 2015; 11:44–54.
57. Kohil A, Jemmieh S, Smatti MK, et al. Viral meningitis: an overview. Arch Virol 2021;166(2):335–45.
58. Handique SK. Viral infections of the central nervous system. Neuroimaging Clin 2011;21(4):777–94.
59. Asundi A, Cervantes-Arslanian AM, Lin NH, et al. Infectious myelitis. Semin Neurol 2019;39(4):472–81.
60. Yokota H, Yamada K. Viral infection of the spinal cord and roots. Neuroimaging Clin 2015;25(2):247–58.
61. Shahrizaila N, Lehmann HC, Kuwabara S. Guillain-barre syndrome. Lancet 2021;397(10280):1214–28.
62. Steiner I, Kennedy PG, Pachner AR. The neurotropic herpes viruses: herpes simplex and varicella-zoster. Lancet Neurol 2007;6(11):1015–28.
63. Devinsky O, Cho ES, Petito CK, et al. Herpes zoster myelitis. Brain 1991;114(Pt 3):1181–96.
64. Gilden D, Cohrs RJ, Mahalingam R, et al. Varicella zoster virus vasculopathies: diverse clinical manifestations, laboratory features, pathogenesis, and treatment. Lancet Neurol 2009;8(8):731–40.
65. Friedman DP. Herpes zoster myelitis: MR appearance. AJNR Am J Neuroradiol 1992;13(5):1404–6.
66. Hirai T, Korogi Y, Hamatake S, et al. Case report: varicella-zoster virus myelitis–serial MR findings. Br J Radiol 1996;69(828):1187–90.
67. Oak P, Modi T, Patkar D. Zoster neuritis of lumbar nerves: A clinical, magnetic resonance imaging, and electrodiagnostic evaluation. J Postgrad Med 2022;68(1):48–50.
68. Wang X, Zhang X, Yu Z, et al. Long-term outcomes of varicella zoster virus infection-related myelitis in 10 immunocompetent patients. J Neuroimmunol 2018;321:36–40.
69. Hung CH, Chang KH, Kuo HC, et al. Features of varicella zoster virus myelitis and dependence on immune status. J Neurol Sci 2012;318(1–2):19–24.
70. Murphy OC, Messacar K, Benson L, et al. Acute flaccid myelitis: cause, diagnosis, and management. Lancet 2021;397(10271):334–46.
71. Stehling-Ariza T, Wilkinson AL, Diop OM, et al. Surveillance To Track Progress Toward Poliomyelitis Eradication - Worldwide, 2021-2022. MMWR Morb Mortal Wkly Rep 2023;72(23):613–20.
72. Sooksawasdi Na Ayudhya S, Laksono BM, van Riel D. The pathogenesis and virulence of enterovirus-D68 infection. Virulence 2021;12(1):2060–72.
73. Okumura A, Mori H, Fee Chong P, et al. Serial MRI findings of acute flaccid myelitis during an outbreak of enterovirus D68 infection in Japan. Brain Dev 2019;41(5):443–51.
74. Maloney JA, Mirsky DM, Messacar K, et al. MRI findings in children with acute flaccid paralysis and cranial nerve dysfunction occurring during the 2014 enterovirus D68 outbreak. AJNR Am J Neuroradiol 2015;36(2):245–50.
75. Levin SN, Lyons JL. HIV and spinal cord disease. Handb Clin Neurol 2018;152:213–27.
76. Paruk HF, Bhigjee AI. Review of the neurological aspects of HIV infection. J Neurol Sci 2021;425: 117453.
77. McArthur JC, Brew BJ, Nath A. Neurological complications of HIV infection. Lancet Neurol 2005;4(9): 543–55.
78. Dal Pan GJ, Glass JD, McArthur JC. Clinicopathologic correlations of HIV-1-associated vacuolar myelopathy: an autopsy-based case-control study. Neurology 1994;44(11):2159–64.
79. Mohanty S, Harhaj EW. Mechanisms of innate immune sensing of HTLV-1 and viral immune evasion. Pathogens 2023;12(5).
80. Bangham CR, Araujo A, Yamano Y, et al. HTLV-1-associated myelopathy/tropical spastic paraparesis. Nat Rev Dis Prim 2015;1:15012.
81. Shakudo M, Inoue Y, Tsutada T. HTLV-I-associated myelopathy: acute progression and atypical MR findings. AJNR Am J Neuroradiol 1999;20(8): 1417–21.
82. Wang CX. Assessment and management of acute disseminated encephalomyelitis (adem) in the pediatric patient. Paediatr Drugs 2021;23(3): 213–21.
83. Pohl D, Alper G, Van Haren K, et al. Acute disseminated encephalomyelitis: Updates on an inflammatory CNS syndrome. Neurology 2016;87(9 Suppl 2):S38–45.
84. Wendebourg MJ, Nagy S, Derfuss T, et al. Magnetic resonance imaging in immune-mediated myelopathies. J Neurol 2020;267(5):1233–44.
85. Rossi A. Imaging of acute disseminated encephalomyelitis. Neuroimaging Clin 2008;18(1):149–61, ix.
86. Althubaiti F, Guiomard C, Rivier F, et al. Prognostic value of contrast-enhanced MRI in Guillain-Barre syndrome in children. Arch Pediatr 2022;29(3): 230–5.
87. Byun WM, Park WK, Park BH, et al. Guillain-Barre syndrome: MR imaging findings of the spine in eight patients. Radiology 1998;208(1):137–41.

Infectious Diseases of the Brain and Spine
Fungal Diseases

Dhairya A. Lakhani, MD, Francis Deng, MD, Doris D.M. Lin, MD, PhD*

KEYWORDS

• Atypical central nervous system infections • Fungal central nervous system infections
• Transmissible central nervous system infections

KEY POINTS

- Fungal infection in the central nervous system can be life-threatening and most frequently affects people who are immunocompromised.
- Leptomeningitis is the most common manifestation of yeast (*Candida* and *Cryptococcus*) infection; however, microabscesses are characteristic of neurocandidiasis and gelatinous pseudocysts are unique in cryptococcal infection.
- Invasive rhinosinusitis due to molds (*Aspergillus* and *Mucor*) is characterized by angioinvasion resulting in mucosal necrosis, aggressive soft-tissue infiltration, orbital and cerebral involvement with cerebritis, abscess, or infarction.
- Persons with normal immune system can be infected with dimorphic fungi (*Coccidioides, Histoplasma, and Blastomyces*) in endemic regions including the Southwestern and Midwestern United States.

INTRODUCTION

Infectious diseases remain a significant burden in certain regions of the world and have only recently begun to recede.[1] Because of the ease of global travel and immigration, radiologists will encounter infections that are not endemic in their region. Furthermore, the incidence of atypical infections has increased as patients are living longer under treatment for autoimmune diseases, acquired immunodeficiency syndrome (AIDS), and organ transplantation.[2–4] Unusual infections can rarely affect even persons with normal immune status.[5] Hence, familiarity with a wide range of infectious agents that can afflict the brain and spinal cord remains an important part of diagnostic neuroradiology. In this review, using case examples, the authors provide an in-depth review of fungal diseases of the central nervous system (CNS).

Fungi are eukaryotic organisms that derive nutrition from decomposition of organic matter. More than a hundred thousand fungal species are recognized, but only a few hundred cause clinically important infection in humans. Out of these, only 10% to 15% of pathologic fungi are known to produce systemic or CNS manifestations.[6–9] Fungi generally have low pathogenicity and rarely infect normal subjects. However, opportunistic CNS fungal infections in immunocompromised hosts have increased in recent decades, due to improved survival, long-term immunosuppressant use, and the increased use of CNS devices.

Opportunistic fungi with ubiquitous distribution include *Aspergillus* spp, *Candida* spp, and *Cryptococcus* spp. These provide no long-term immunity to previously infected patients.[9] Commonly encountered, endemic pathogenic fungi include

Funding: None.
Division of Neuroradiology, Russell H. Morgan Department of Radiology and Radiological Science, Johns Hopkins University School of Medicine, 600 N. Wolfe Street, Phipps B-100 Baltimore, MD 21287, USA
* Corresponding author.
E-mail address: ddmlin@jhmi.edu

Magn Reson Imaging Clin N Am 32 (2024) 335–346
https://doi.org/10.1016/j.mric.2024.02.001
1064-9689/24/

mri.theclinics.com

Coccidioides spp, and *Histoplasma* spp. They have a restricted geographic distribution and produce acute clinical syndrome in immunocompetent hosts, which once resolved, provides lifelong immunity. Fungal pathogens can be subclassified into 3 morphologic categories: yeast, mold, and dimorphic fungus. These forms have distinct patterns of growth and neuroimaging patterns.[5,10]

YEASTS

Microbiology, Epidemiology, and Pathogenesis

Yeasts are unicellular fungi. The main yeasts causing CNS infections are *Cryptococcus* spp and *Candida* spp. These yeasts can disseminate in the bloodstream and traverse the blood-brain barrier by penetrating microvascular endothelial cells, resulting in meningitis or meningoencephalitis. These infections are usually opportunistic, occurring in immunocompromised hosts, especially those with impaired cell-mediated immunity.[11,12]

Within the genus *Cryptococcus*, *Cryptococcus neoformans* is the main pathogenic species, while *C. gatti* infection occurs less commonly overall but more often affects immunocompetent patients.[13,14] *Cryptococcus* spp are found in soil around the world. The mode of transmission is typically environmental inhalation. In the lungs, the organism can cause pneumonia and gain access to the bloodstream. It disseminates with a tropism for the CNS, which is believed to be related to the presence of essential nutrients and the absence of complement pathway factors in the cerebrospinal fluid (CSF).[15] The most common risk factor associated with cryptococcal meningoencephalitis is AIDS. Cryptococcal meningoencephalitis is the most common fungal disease of the CNS worldwide and still accounts for a fifth of AIDS-related deaths annually.[16]

Within the genus *Candida*, by far the most common pathogenic species is *C. albicans*, but CNS infections can occur with several other species: *C. parapsilosis*, *C. tropicalis*, *C. glabrata,* and *C. krusei. Candida* spp are part of normal skin, gut and vaginal flora.[17] *Candida* can gain access to the bloodstream by translocating across the mucosa that it colonizes or via indwelling vascular catheters. Risk factors for candidemia, and by extension neurocandidiasis, include critical illness requiring intensive care, immunocompromise such as neutropenia, injection drug use, and prematurity in neonates. In addition to hematogenous spread, *Candida* can enter the CNS as a neurosurgical contaminant on devices such as ventricular shunts. Candida produces biofilms on synthetic materials, which facilitates adhesion of fungi to the devices and renders them relatively refractory to medical therapy.[18]

Cryptococcal and candida meningitis/meningoencephalitis typically present on a subacute-to-chronic course, but an acute presentation mimicking bacterial meningitis is also possible.

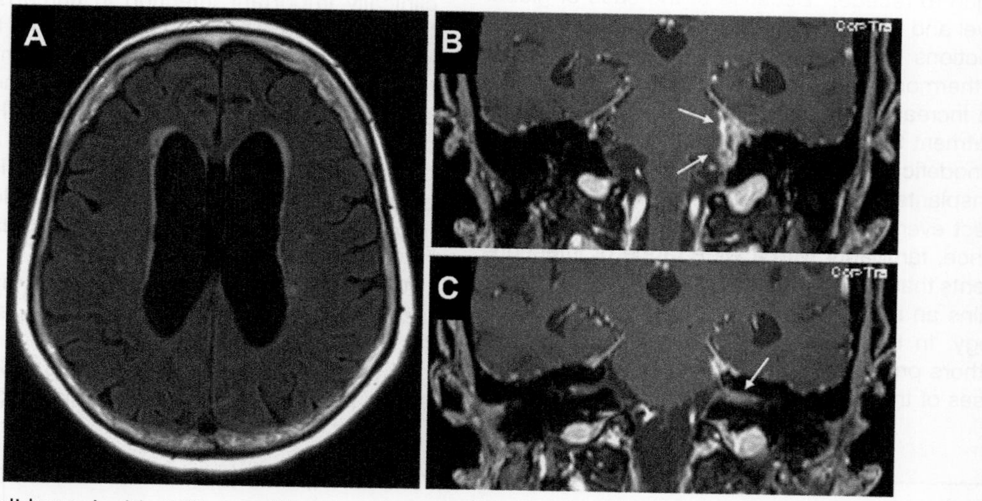

Fig. 1. Candida meningitis. A 77-year-old woman with previous planum sphenoidale meningioma resection 2 and a half months ago presents with new-onset headaches. Axial FLAIR (*A*) and coronal T1 fat-suppressed postcontrast (*B, C*) images show moderate hydrocephalus and irregular, thick dural enhancement in the left cerebellopontine angle cistern and internal auditory canal (*B* and *C, arrows*). *Candida albicans* was confirmed on next-generation metagenomic sequencing on CSF analysis. Localized, thick dural enhancement is nonspecific but can be seen in atypical infectious meningitis. CSF, cerebrospinal fluid; FLAIR, fluid-attenuated inversion recovery.

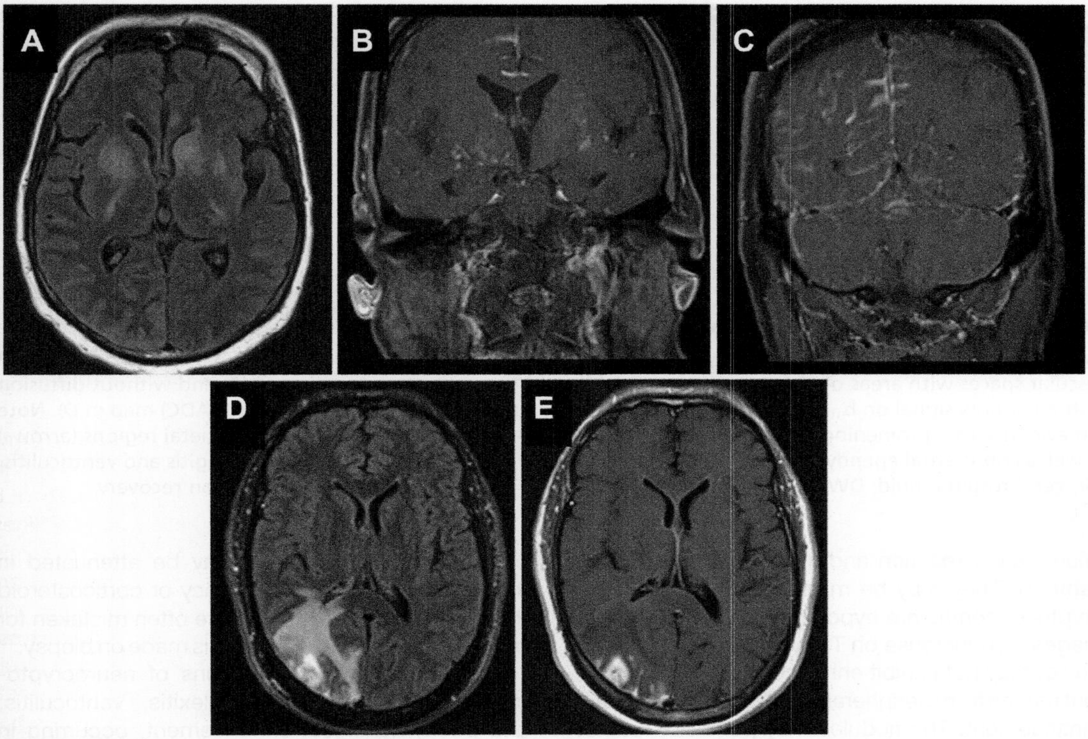

Fig. 2. Cryptococcal meningitis in 2 different patients. In patient 1, (*A*) axial FLAIR image shows hyperintense signal abnormality in the bilateral striatocapsular regions, common areas of cryptococcal involvement, as well as a lack of CSF suppression in the right more than left parietal-occipital sulci. Coronal postcontrast T1-weighted fat-saturated images (*B*, *C*) show punctate and patchy enhancement in the bilateral basal ganglia, involving frontal sulci and more extensive leptomeningeal enhancement of bilateral parieto-occipital regions (right greater than left) and cerebellum. In patient 2, (*D*) axial FLAIR shows localized right parieto-occipital vasogenic edema and (*E*) thickened, masslike focal leptomeningeal enhancement. CSF, cerebrospinal fluid; FLAIR, fluid-attenuated inversion recovery.

Imaging Presentation

The most common imaging findings in both cryptococcal and candida infection are those of leptomeningitis (**Figs. 1** and **2**). On MRI, postcontrast T1-weighted images show contrast enhancement along the leptomeningeal surfaces of the brain, especially along the basal cisterns but often also within the cerebellar fissures and cerebral sulci. Postcontrast 3-dimensional fluid-attenuated inversion recovery (FLAIR) images can provide additional accuracy for leptomeningeal enhancement.[19] Accompanying features may include foci of restricted diffusion in the subarachnoid spaces and communicating hydrocephalus. These findings indicate meningitis but are not specific for fungal etiology. In fungal meningitis, enhancement is often thicker and more nodular than that seen in bacterial and viral meningitis and may mimic carcinomatous meningitis (leptomeningeal metastatic disease).[20] The clinical history and CSF analysis can help distinguish, as can the presence of additional imaging features that are described in the following sections.

Cryptococcosis

Dilatation of the perivascular spaces is a characteristic finding of neurocryptococcosis, wherein the budding yeast produces gelatinous pseudocysts,[21] most commonly in the basal ganglia (**Fig. 3**). On MRI, these spaces have a round or oval "soap bubble appearance," with a low-to-intermediate signal on T1-weighted images, and high signal on T2-weighted images that variably suppresses on T2-FLAIR. Spaces can coalesce and have mild mass effect. Typically, these spaces do not demonstrate surrounding edema or significant enhancement[22] (**Table 1**).

Cyptococcomas (cryptococcal granulomas) may develop (**Fig. 4**), most commonly in immunocompetent hosts.[23,24] Cryptococcomas are intraparenchymal masses of fungi that are hematogenously seeded the brain and generate a granulomatous

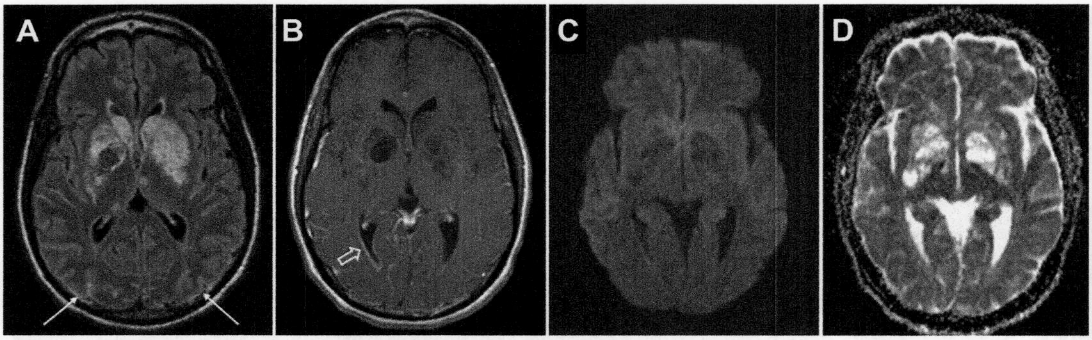

Fig. 3. Cryptococcal gelatinous pseudocysts. Soap bubble appearance of mucoid material within the dilated perivascular spaces with areas of FLAIR hyperintensity (*A*), without contrast enhancement (*B*) and without diffusion restriction (low signal on b_{1000} DWI in *C* and high signal on apparent diffusion coefficient (ADC) map in *D*). Note the evidence of leptomeningeal enhancement and CSF non-suppression in the bilateral parietal regions (*arrows*) as well as right atrial ependymal enhancement (block *arrow*) indicating concomitant meningitis and ventriculitis. CSF, cerebrospinal fluid; DWI, diffusion-weighted imaging; FLAIR, fluid-attenuated inversion recovery.

inflammatory reaction and mucoid material[25] (see **Table 1**). They may be miliary (<3 mm) or larger. Cryptococcomas are hypointense on T1-weighted images, hyperintense on T2-weighted images, and may or may not exhibit enhancement, which if present ranges from peripheral nodular to homogenous enhancement. The nodules may permit or restrict diffusion and may have surrounding vasogenic edema.[23,24,26,27] As is the case with any infection, edema and enhancement may be attenuated in the context of immunodeficiency or corticosteroid therapy.[28] Cryptococcomas are often mistaken for brain tumors and the diagnosis is made on biopsy.[29]

Less common manifestations of neurocryptococcosis include choroid plexitis, ventriculitis, and pachymeningeal enhancement, occurring in isolation or concomitantly with other MRI findings.[24] Choroid plexitis appears as multilobulated

Table 1
Imaging features characteristic of certain infectious etiologies

Fungal Infections	Finding	MRI Appearance
Cryptococcosis	Gelatinous pseudocysts (dilated perivascular spaces containing yeast and mucoid material)	Round or oval "soap bubble appearance," with low to intermediate T1-signal, and high T2-signal that variably suppress on T2 FLAIR
Candidiasis	Cerebral microabscesses (<3 mm)	Like other brain abscesses, including hyperintensity on DWI and nodular contrast enhancement
Angioinvasive mold infection (aspergillosis and mucormycosis)	Invasive rhinosinusitis, bone erosion, soft-tissue infiltration, extension into the periantral fat, orbit, and intracranial compartment	Non-enhancing nasal mucosa, "black turbinate" sign. Cerebral infarcts (restricted diffusion), cerebritis (restricted diffusion and vasogenic edema with no or little enhancement), and abscess. Hypointensity on SWI due to fungal hyphae or microhemorrhage
Endemic mycoses (coccidioidomycosis and histoplasmosis)	Basilar meningitis, vasculitis, and intraparenchymal granuloma (more so for *Histoplasma*)	Nodular leptomeningeal enhancement in the basal cisterns, deep cerebral infarcts, and small nodular enhancing lesions

Abbreviations: DWI, diffusion-weighted imaging; FLAIR, fluid-attenuated inversion recovery; SWI, susceptibility-weighted imaging.

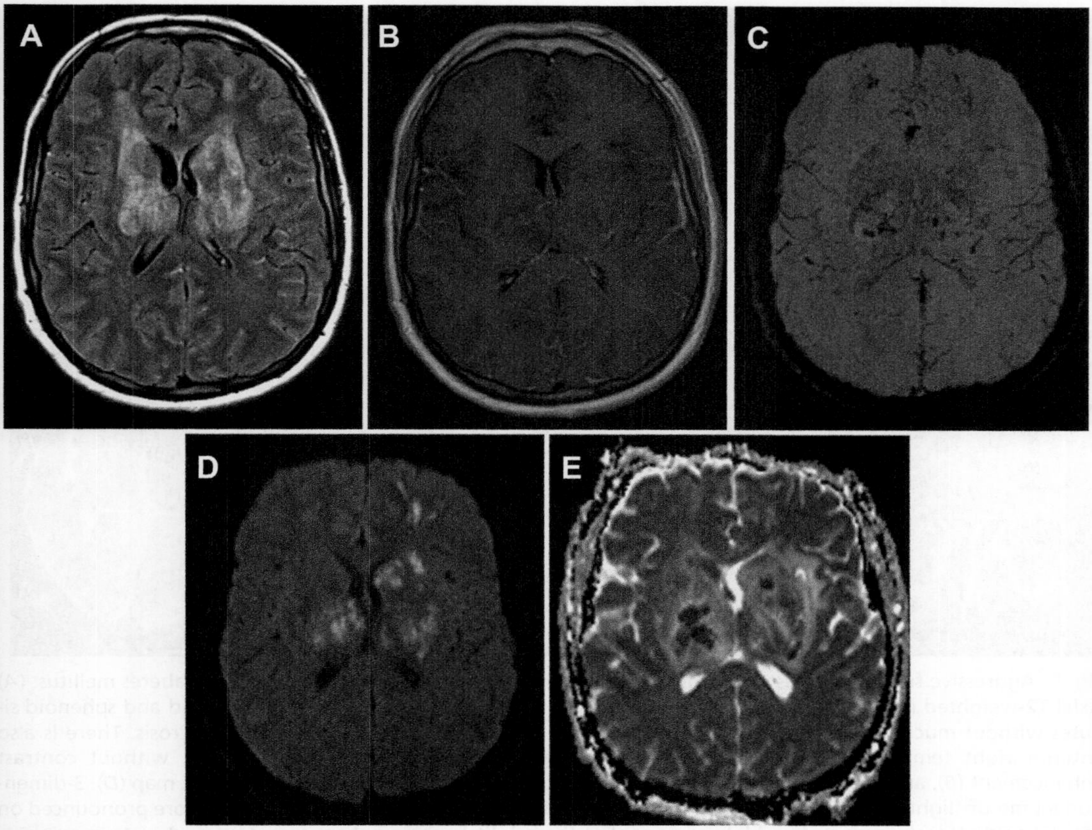

ig. 4. Disseminated cryptococcomas and meningitis in a 27-year-old with rheumatoid arthritis on immunosup-
ression. (*A*) Heterogeneous FLAIR hyperintense lesions centered in the bilateral deep gray nuclei and scattered n the frontal white matter. (*B*) Postcontrast axial T1-weighted image shows faint peripheral contrast enhance-ment in some of the deep gray lesions. (*C*) Axial susceptibility-weighted imaging (SWI) demonstrates multiple oci of dark signal consistent with microhemorrhages scattered in the frontal regions, basal ganglia, and thalami ilaterally. (*D*) DWI and (*E*) ADC show larger areas of multifocal restricted mixed with facilitated diffusion in the rontal and deep gray nuclei. These findings suggest a combination of meningoencephalitis-induced infarction nd hemorrhage. ADC, apparent diffusion coefficient; DWI, diffusion-weighted imaging; FLAIR, fluid-ttenuated inversion recovery.

ystic appearance of choroid plexus, with bnormal T2-FLAIR hyperintense signal and avid contrast enhancement.[24,30] Ventriculitis appears as linear ependymal enhancement, periventricular edema, and debris with restricted diffusion within he ventricles.[31]

Candidiasis

Cerebral microabscesses are a characteristic inding of neurocandidiasis that occurs by hema-ogenous seeding of brain parenchyma. These microabscesses are less than 3 mm, multiple, and diffusely distributed at the cerebral gray-white matter junction, basal ganglia, and cerebellum.[32] Magnetic resonance signal characteristics are similar to that of other brain abscesses, including hyperintensity on diffusion-weighted imaging.[32,33]

It is important to note that computed tomography (CT) and lumbar punctures do not usually contribute to diagnosis, as the size of the abscesses is below the resolution of CT and CSF culture is usually sterile. In rare cases, macroabscesses have been reported both in immunocompromised and immunocompetent hosts.[32] Other less common imaging findings include angioinvasion with thrombosis and mycotic aneurysms, resulting in ischemic and hemorrhagic stroke[32] (see **Table 1**).

Candida vertebral osteomyelitis can be acquired via a hematogenous route or by direct inoculation; however, hematogenous spread to vertebral bodies is more common.[34] Similar to bacterial osteomyelitis/discitis, the infection usually centers around the intervertebral disc, leading to disc height loss and erosion of the vertebral

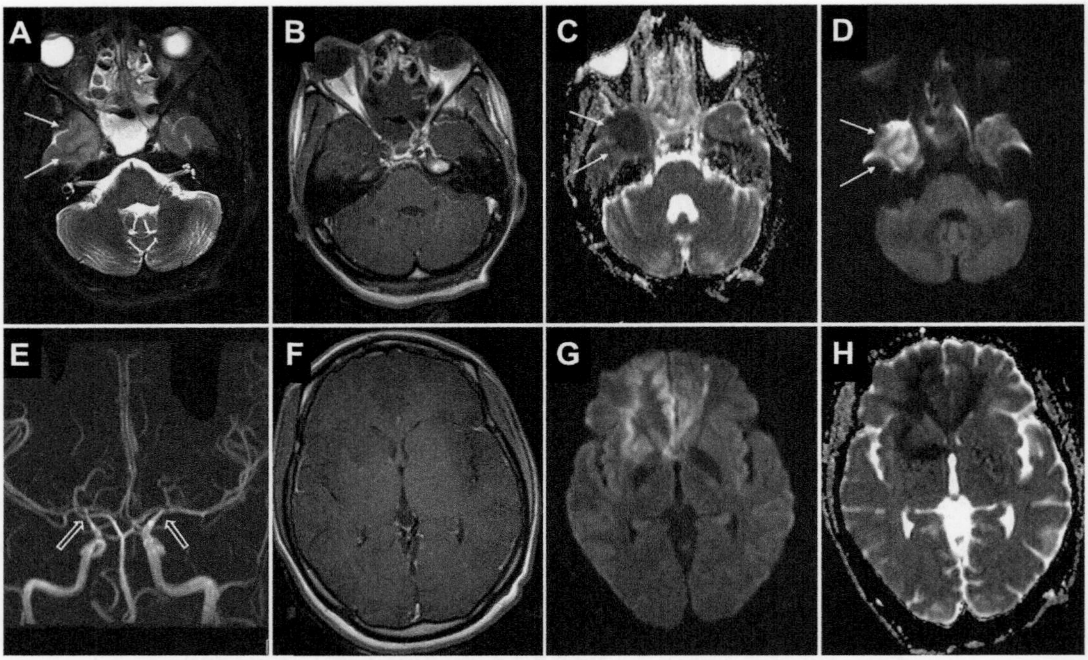

Fig. 5. Aggressive fungal sinusitis due to mucormycosis in a 29-year-old female with type 1 diabetes mellitus. (*A*) Axial T2-weighted images show extensive hyperintense mucosal inflammation in the ethmoid and sphenoid sinuses without mucosal enhancement on postcontrast T1-weighted images (*B*) reflecting necrosis. There is also anterior right temporal lobe gyral edema demonstrating T2 hyperintensity (*A, arrows*), without contrast enhancement (*B*), and with restricted diffusion (*arrows*) on axial DWI trace image (*C*) and ADC map (*D*). 3-dimensional time-of-flight MRA (*E*) shows stenosis of the distal internal carotid arteries bilaterally, more pronounced on the right side (*block arrows*). At a higher image slice there is little or no enhancement on postcontrast axial T1-weighted image (*F*), but with mixed regions of restricted diffusion (*G, H*) in bilateral frontal lobes, right greater than left, suggesting cerebritis and ischemic infarction from angioinvasion. Angioinvasive fungal sinusitis, potentially with skullbase, orbit, and cerebral invasion, can be seen in both mucormycosis and aspergillosis. ADC, apparent diffusion coefficient; DWI, diffusion-weighted imaging; MRA, magnetic resonance angiography.

endplates. MRI signal changes would be similar as well, with T1-hypointense and T2-hyperintense signal characteristics, with the exception that T2 changes would be less pronounced compared to bacterial discitis/osteomyelitis. Less pronounced T2 signal may be attributed to the relatively blunted immune response in affected patients.[35,36]

MOLDS

Microbiology, Epidemiology, and Pathogenesis

Unlike yeasts, molds grow as multicellular filaments (hyphae), which can transform into macroscopic networks (mycelia).[6] The most common pathogenic molds are *Aspergillus* spp and those in the order Mucorales. Aspergillosis refers to infection by the genus *Aspergillus*, the most common pathogenic species of which is *A. fumigatus*, followed by *A. flavus*, *A. niger*, and *A. terreus*. The fungal division Mucoromycota (formerly Zygomycota) contains the order Mucorales. Related infections, known as mucormycosis (formerly zygomycosis), are most commonly due to the genera *Mucor*, *Rhizopus*, and *Rhizomucor*. Rarely, dematiaceous fungi cause an infection known as phaeohyphomycosis, so-named for their dark melaninlike pigmentation on histology. The most common of the agents of phaeohyphomycosis is *Cladophialophora bantiana*.

These molds are ubiquitous in the soil and spores can be inhaled into the respiratory tract. They may then enter the CNS either hematogenously or directly from the paranasal sinuses.[37,38] *Aspergillus* spp and the agents of mucormycosis often cause symptomatic pulmonary and sinonasal infection, but dematiaceous fungi do not. Aspergillosis and mucormycosis carry a propensity for vascular invasion, facilitated by production of elastase. Unlike yeast, the multicellular hyphae are too large for the meningeal microcirculation and instead are more likely to cause invasive

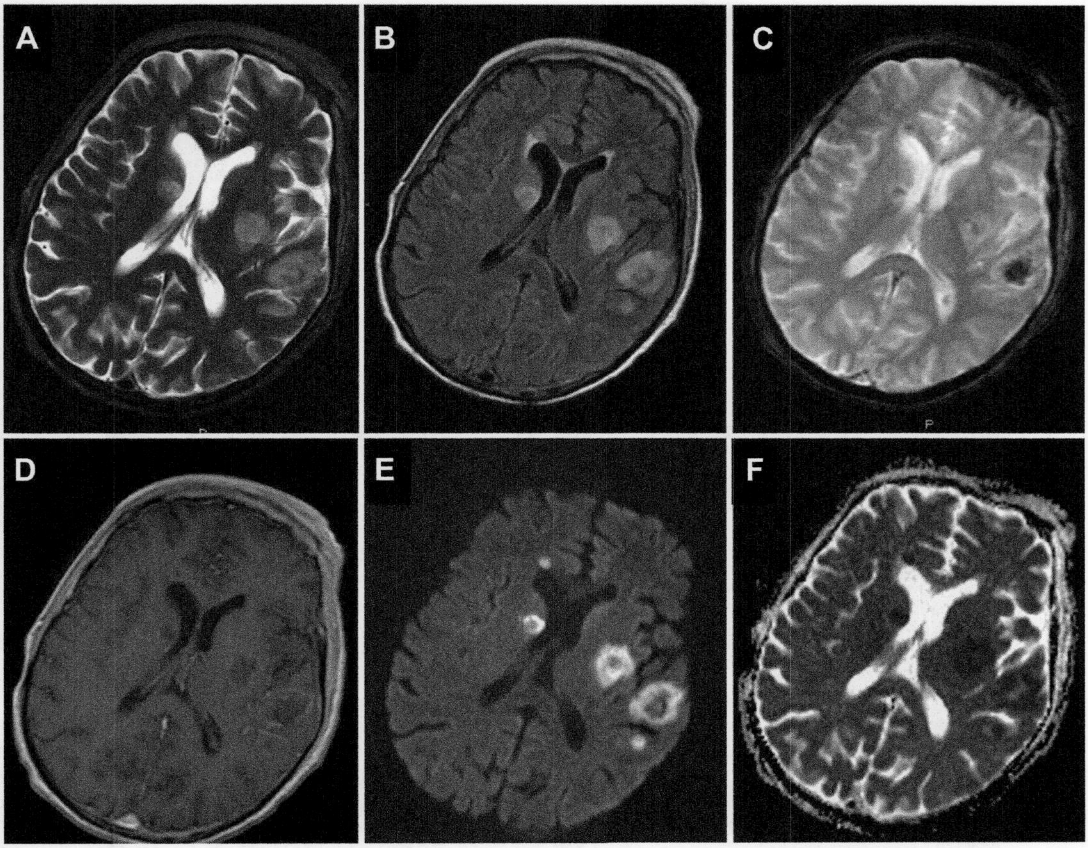

Fig. 6. Aspergillus cerebral abscesses. A 48-year-old man with type 3 glycogen storage disease, hepatocellular carcinoma, and liver transplant, presenting with marked decline in mental status. (*A*) Axial T2 and (*B*) FLAIR images show multiple hyperintense parenchymal masses with central areas of susceptibility artifact on T2*-weighted gradient recalled echo sequence (*C*) that may reflect minerals associated with fungal hyphae or microhemorrhages. (*D*) Axial postcontrast T1-weighted image shows mild peripheral enhancement. (*E*) DWI trace image and (*F*) ADC map show thick peripheral restricted diffusion but central facilitated diffusion. ADC, apparent diffusion coefficient; DWI, diffusion-weighted imaging; FLAIR, fluid-attenuated inversion recovery.

parenchymal disease (cerebritis, brain abscess, and infarction) than meningitis.

These infections are opportunistic, especially affecting immunocompromised patients such as those with neutropenia due to hematologic malignancy and bone marrow transplantation.[39] Additional risk factors include the use of steroids and other immunosuppressants, AIDS, and the recent coronavirus disease 2019 infection. Mucormycosis commonly also affects patients with diabetes mellitus, especially during episodes of diabetic ketoacidosis. Cerebral mucormycosis without rhinosinusitis has also been repeatedly described with people who inject intravenous drugs.[40] Intracranial involvement by mucormycosis or aspergillosis has a fulminant course associated with a high mortality rate of more than 90%.[38,39,41]

Imaging Presentation

Because brain infection may result from local extension from the paranasal sinuses, brief mention is warranted of the imaging findings of invasive fungal rhinosinusitis due to aspergillosis and mucormycosis (**Fig. 5**). CT findings include sinonasal mucosal thickening and opacification, stranding in the periantral fat, pterygopalatine fossa, nasolacrimal duct, lacrimal sac, and orbit; bone erosion and dehiscence; and nasal septal ulceration.[42] As the hallmark of angioinvasive fungal infection is necrosis rather than purulent inflammation, the degree of sinonasal mucosal thickening and opacification may be minimal compared to that of bacterial or viral sinusitis. MRI is more sensitive in detecting angioinvasive disease, as early in the disease course, sinonasal mucosal infarction results in

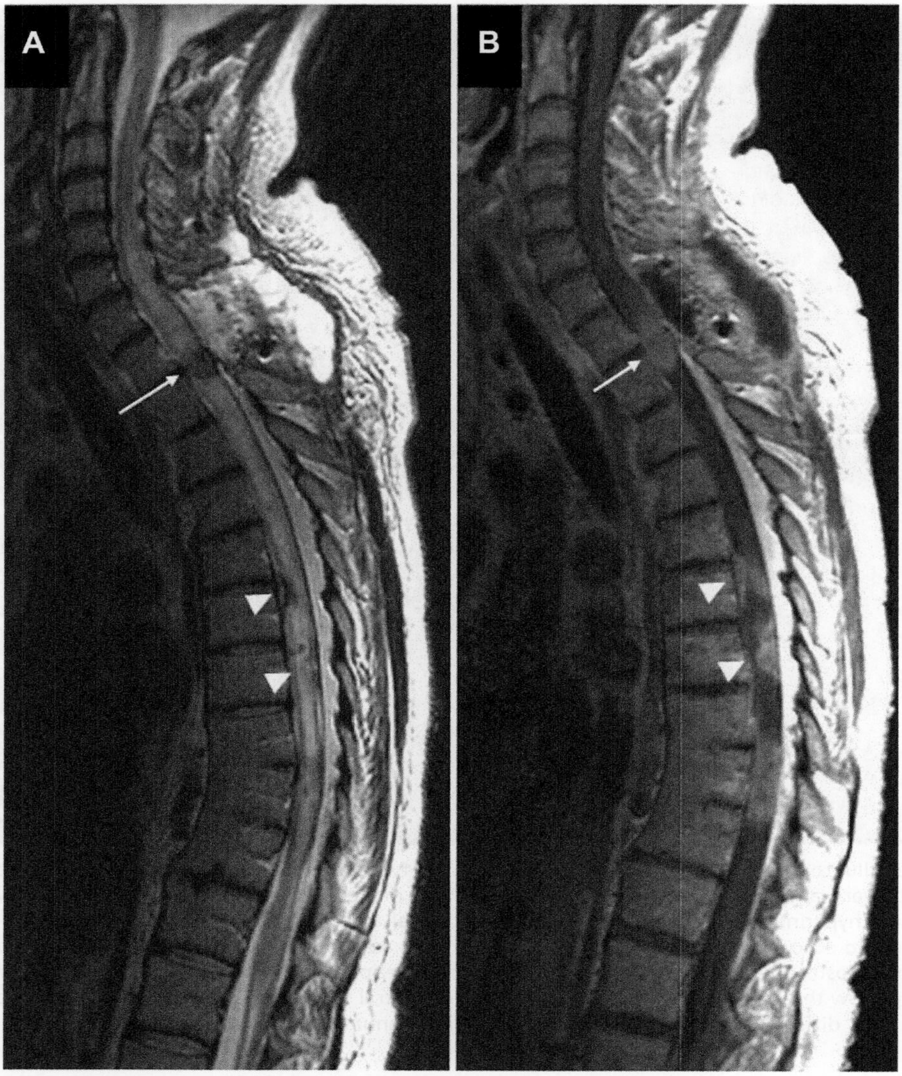

Fig. 7. Spinal aspergillosis. Sagittal T2-weighted (*A*) and postcontrast T1-weighted (*B*) images in a 40-year-old woman with a history of airway disease and asthma show extensive expansile T2-hyperintensity reflecting edema throughout the spinal cord, with multiple intramedullary (*arrows*) and intradural extramedullary (*arrowheads*) T2-hypointense masses that demonstrate larger enhancement with irregular and fluffy margins.

lack of contrast enhancement giving a characteristic "black turbinate" sign[43] (see **Table 1**). On CT, bone erosion and subtle stranding of the periantral fat can be the first imaging finding of invasion, but MRI is generally more sensitive for detection of extra-sinus soft-tissue involvement including orbital and intracranial extension.[42] Intracranial extension of invasive fungal rhinosinusitis initially appears as pachymeningeal thickening and enhancement on postcontrast T1-weighted images.[39]

When involving the brain, the angioinvasive mold infections lead initially to acute infarction and later extend into surrounding tissue as infectious cerebritis or abscess (see **Fig. 5**). MRI reveals restricted diffusion and relatively larger areas of vasogenic edema. Mycotic aneurysms and intracerebral hemorrhage can also occur. This mechanism has a predilection for the frontal and temporal lobes when the source is local extension of rhinosinusitis and for the basal ganglia when the source is hematogenous, which are uncommonly affected by other infectious organisms or metastasis.[44,45]

Fungal abscesses exhibit different imaging characteristics compared to bacterial abscesses (**Figs. 6** and **7**). First, the walls show irregular ring or heterogenous or faint enhancement. Subtle

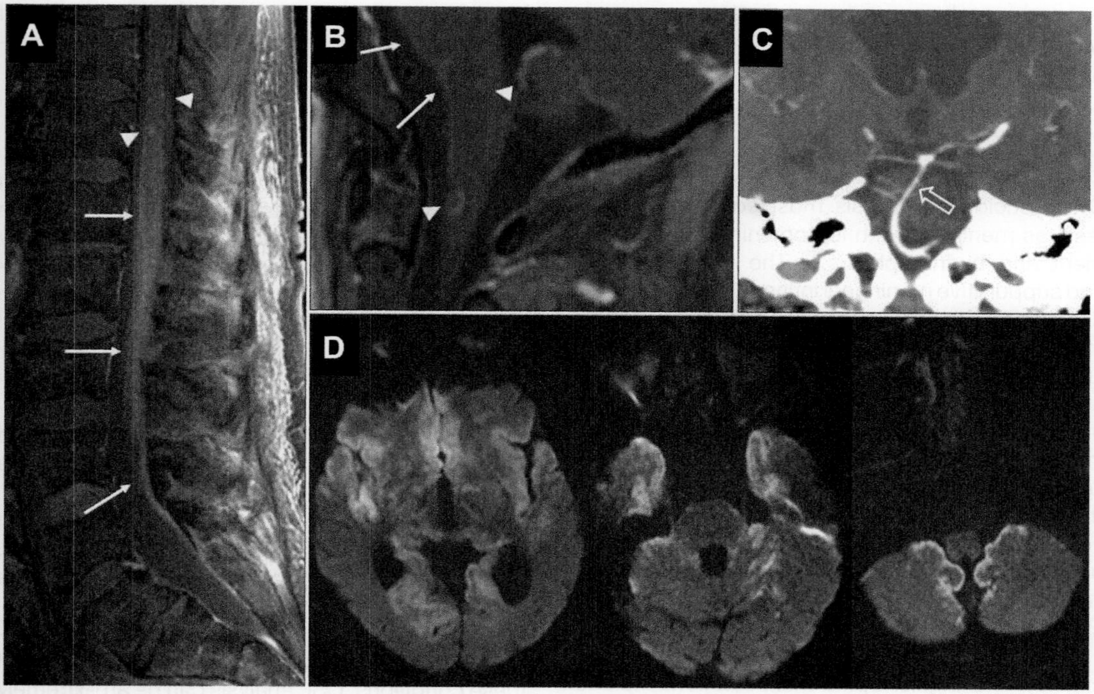

ig. 8. CNS histoplasmosis in a 77-year-old man who spent summer vacation in his farm in Missouri, presenting vith a month of imbalance, falls, headache, and weight loss. (*A*) Sagittal postcontrast fat-saturated T1-weighted mage shows diffuse pial enhancement of the cauda equina nerve roots and surface of the lower spinal cord (*ar-ows*), as well as a few punctate cord parenchymal enhancement foci (*arrowheads*). (*B*) Additional enhancement long the surface of the visualized brainstem (*arrows*) and a few small intraparenchymal enhancing foci in the nedulla, and upper cervical cord (*arrowheads*). (*C*) Coronal head CTA shows mild narrowing of the mid to distal egments of the basilar artery (block *arrow*). (*D*) Axial b_{1000} DWI trace images show multifocal diffusion restriction n a distribution concentrated along the surface of the lower parts of the brain. CNS, central nervous system; CTA, omputed tomography angiography; DWI, diffusion-weighted imaging.

eripheral enhancement is seen much more ommonly than well-defined ring enhancement.[10] Second, the peripheral enhancing component re-tricts diffusion, while the central contents permit liffusion.[37] Proliferating hyphae may be depicted s intracavitary T2-hypointense projections that estrict diffusion.[46]

IMORPHIC FUNGI

Aicrobiology, Epidemiology, and athogenesis

Dimorphic fungi are unicellular at body tempera-ure and multicellular mycelia (mold) at room tem-erature. The mold form resides in the soil and elease conidia (spores) into the air. Dimorphic ungi transition into spherules (not yeast) when in ost and then reproduce by rupturing and eleasing endospores (instead of budding). Geographic locations where a wet season (allow-ng robust growth of mold) is followed by a dry sea-on (allowing spore dispersal in dust) had higher ncidence of infection by dimorphic fungi.[47]

Dimorphic fungi cause endemic mycoses. *Coccidioides immitis* and *Coccidioides posadasii*, which cause coccidioidomycosis, are endemic to areas of the Southwestern United States as well as Northern Mexico, and parts of Central and South America.[48] *Histoplasma capsulatum*, which causes histoplasmosis, is endemic in the Midwestern United States, Canada, Mexico, Central and South America, and less commonly in other continents.[49] *Blastomyces dermatitidis*, which causes blastomycosis, is endemic in the Midwestern and Southeastern United States as well as part of Central Canada.[50,51]

Spore inhalation manifests as primary pulmonary disease in 40% of patients, chronic pulmonary disease in 5% to 10%, and disseminated disease affecting the skin, bones, and meninges in 1%.[47,52] Disseminated infection is more likely in immunocompromised patients. These dimorphic fungi can cause both meningitis and focal brain lesions.[5] Overall, about 5% to 10% of progressive disseminated histoplasmosis will have CNS involvement.[49,53] The disease course is more indolent compared to bacterial meningitis or abscess, so the presentation can mimic a neoplastic process.[54,55]

Imaging Presentation

Coccidioidomycosis

CNS coccidioidomycosis most commonly manifests as meningitis with leptomeningeal enhancement and hydrocephalus.[56] The granulomatous and suppurative meningeal inflammation has a predilection for the basal cisterns. Additionally, inflammation can occur within the outer layers of small arteries and arterioles, which can lead to ischemia and exudates.[48,57–59] Up to 40% of cases exhibit this infectious vasculitis, resulting in deep brain infarcts.[60] Granulomatous inflammation of large vessels can rarely result in subarachnoid hemorrhage.[61] In addition to meningitis and vasculitis, cerebritis may develop (especially in immunocompromised patients) due to fungal extension along vessel walls or in perivascular spaces.[62] Parenchymal abscesses are less common.

Spinal involvement occurs in most cases of coccidioidal meningitis. Spine manifestations include leptomeningeal enhancement, nerve root clumping and thickening (adhesive arachnoiditis), and, less commonly, intramedullary spinal cord edema or syrinx formation.[56,63] Focal intradural extramedullary lesions can occur, representing adhesive inflammatory exudate or abscess just as in the basal cisterns of the head. Myelograms can reveal CSF blocks due to these lesions.

Histoplasmosis

The most frequent manifestation of CNS histoplasmosis is intra-axial ring-enhancing lesions (histoplasmomas), which are typically small (<2 cm) and multifocal. These lesions have been described in the subcortical gray matter structures, the gray-white junction, the cerebellum, the brain stem, and the spinal cord.[50] Slightly less commonly, CNS histoplasmosis manifests as subacute or chronic meningitis, which appears as leptomeningeal enhancement and hydrocephalus.[53] Like coccidioidal and tuberculous meningitis, histoplasma meningitis has a basal predominance. Rare findings included diffuse white matter changes representing encephalitis, infarcts due to vasculitis, and spinal cord involvement in about 5% of cases (**Fig. 8**). When the spinal cord was involved, the most common presentation was the presence of enhancing lesions and non-mass cord lesions.[53]

Blastomycosis

CNS blastomycosis is rare. The few available case reports and series showed enhancing intra-axial mass lesions with central diffusion restriction compatible with abscess, leptomeningeal enhancement indicative of meningitis, or a combination of these 2.[50,64]

SUMMARY

There is a significant amount of overlap in imaging findings when it comes to various fungal infections affecting the CNS. These findings frequently resemble those seen in atypical bacterial infections, noninfectious inflammatory and neoplastic conditions. For example, subacute or chronic basal meningitis invites a differential of the yeast or dimorphic fungal meningitides, in addition to tuberculosis, sarcoidosis, and carcinomatosis. Nonetheless, particular imaging characteristics can aid in distinguishing certain unusual infectious causes (see **Table 1**).

It is of utmost importance to differentiate between infectious and noninfectious inflammatory causes, as the use of steroids could exacerbate infectious diseases. Similarly, distinguishing between infectious and neoplastic causes could help minimize unnecessary invasive procedures. In the majority of these conditions, CSF analysis can be an extremely valuable tool for narrowing down the potential causes, often leading to a definitive diagnosis.

CLINICS CARE POINTS

- Imaging characteristics of a fungal abscess differ from that of bacterial abscesses. Fungal abscess will have subtle peripheral enhancement, the enhancing component restricts diffusion, while the central contents permit diffusion and proliferating hyphae may be depicted as intracavitary T2-hypointense projections that restrict diffusion.
- Most common imaging finding in neurocryptococcosis, neurocandidasis, and neurococcidioidomycosis is of posterior predominant leptomeningitis.
- A unique finding of neurocryptococcosis is dilatation of the perivascular spaces.
- A characteristic finding of neurocandidiasis is cerebral microabscesses.
- Most common imaging finding in CNS histoplasmosis is of multifocal small (<2 cm) intra-axial ring-enhancing lesions.

DISCLOSURE

None.

REFERENCES

1. Murray CJ, Ortblad KF, Guinovart C, et al. Global, regional, and national incidence and mortality for HIV, tuberculosis, and malaria during 1990-2013: a systematic analysis for the Global Burden of Disease Study 2013. Lancet 2014;384(9947):1005–70.
2. Stenehjem E, Armstrong WS. Central nervous system device infections. Infect Dis Clin North Am 2012;26(1):89–110.
3. Hasbun R. Central Nervous System Device Infections. Curr Infect Dis Rep 2016;18(11):34.
4. Martin RM, Zimmermann LL, Huynh M, et al. Diagnostic Approach to Health Care- and Device-Associated Central Nervous System Infections. J Clin Microbiol 2018;56(11).
5. Shih RY, Koeller KK. Bacterial, Fungal, and Parasitic Infections of the Central Nervous System: Radiologic-Pathologic Correlation and Historical Perspectives. Radiographics 2015;35(4):1141–69.
6. Mathur M, Johnson CE, Sze G. Fungal infections of the central nervous system. Neuroimaging Clin N Am 2012;22(4):609–32.
7. Sun S, Hoy MJ, Heitman J. Fungal pathogens. Curr Biol 2020;30(19):R1163–9.
8. Kurtzman CP. Molecular taxonomy of the yeasts. Yeast 1994;10(13):1727–40.
9. Raman Sharma R. Fungal infections of the nervous system: current perspective and controversies in management. Int J Surg 2010;8(8):591–601.
10. Ashdown BC, Tien RD, Felsberg GJ. Aspergillosis of the brain and paranasal sinuses in immunocompromised patients: CT and MR imaging findings. AJR Am J Roentgenol 1994;162(1):155–9.
11. Rathore SS, Sathiyamoorthy J, Lalitha C, et al. A holistic review on Cryptococcus neoformans. Microb Pathog 2022;166:105521.
12. Chang YC, Stins MF, McCaffery MJ, et al. Cryptococcal yeast cells invade the central nervous system via transcellular penetration of the blood-brain barrier. Infect Immun 2004;72(9):4985–95.
13. Harris JR, Lockhart SR, Debess E, et al. Cryptococcus gattii in the United States: clinical aspects of infection with an emerging pathogen. Clin Infect Dis 2011;53(12):1188–95.
14. Suchitha S, Sheeladevi CS, Sunila R, et al. Disseminated cryptococcosis in an immunocompetent patient: a case report. Case Rep Pathol 2012;2012:652351.
15. Igel HJ, Bolande RP. Humoral defense mechanisms in cryptococcosis: substances in normal human serum, saliva, and cerebrospinal fluid affecting the growth of Cryptococcus neoformans. J Infect Dis 1966;116(1):75–83.
16. Zhao Y, Ye L, Zhao F, et al. Cryptococcus neoformans, a global threat to human health. Infect Dis Poverty 2023;12(1):20.
17. Cohen R, Roth FJ, Delgado E, et al. Fungal flora of the normal human small and large intestine. N Engl J Med 1969;280(12):638–41.
18. Kojic EM, Darouiche RO. Candida infections of medical devices. Clin Microbiol Rev 2004;17(2):255–67.
19. Fukuoka H, Hirai T, Okuda T, et al. Comparison of the added value of contrast-enhanced 3D fluid-attenuated inversion recovery and magnetization-prepared rapid acquisition of gradient echo sequences in relation to conventional postcontrast T1-weighted images for the evaluation of leptomeningeal diseases at 3T. AJNR Am J Neuroradiol 2010; 31(5):868–73.
20. Rohde S. Inflammatory Diseases of the Meninges, Inflammatory Diseases of the Brain, 21 (2012), 127–137.
21. Berkefeld J, Enzensberger W, Lanfermann H. Cryptococcus meningoencephalitis in AIDS: parenchymal and meningeal forms. Neuroradiology. Feb 1999;41(2):129–33.
22. Lakhani DA, Joseph J. Giant Tumefactive Perivascular Spaces. Radiology 2023;307(4):e222559.
23. Anjum SH, Bennett JE, Dean O, et al. Neuroimaging of Cryptococcal Meningitis in Patients without Human Immunodeficiency Virus: Data from a Multi-Center Cohort Study. J Fungi (Basel) 2023;9(5).
24. Duarte SBL, Oshima MM, Mesquita JVDA, et al. Magnetic resonance imaging findings in central nervous system cryptococcosis: comparison between immunocompetent and immunocompromised patients. Radiol Bras 2017;50(6):359–65.
25. Cheng YC, Ling JF, Chang FC, et al. Radiological manifestations of cryptococcal infection in central nervous system. J Chin Med Assoc 2003;66(1):19–26.
26. Kamezawa T, Shimozuru T, Niiro M, et al. MRI of a cerebral cryptococcal granuloma. Neuroradiology 2000;42(6):441–3.
27. Ho TL, Lee HJ, Lee KW, et al. Diffusion-weighted and conventional magnetic resonance imaging in cerebral cryptococcoma. Acta Radiol 2005;46(4):411–4.
28. Saigal G, Post MJ, Lolayekar S, et al. Unusual presentation of central nervous system cryptococcal infection in an immunocompetent patient. AJNR Am J Neuroradiol 2005;26(10):2522–6.
29. Chastain DB, Rao A, Yaseyyedi A, et al. Cerebral Cryptococcomas: A Systematic Scoping Review of Available Evidence to Facilitate Diagnosis and Treatment. Pathogens 2022;11(2).
30. Kumari R, Raval M, Dhun A. Cryptococcal choroid plexitis: rare imaging findings of central nervous system cryptococcal infection in an immunocompetent individual. Br J Radiol 2010;83(985):e14–7.
31. Mohan S, Jain KK, Arabi M, et al. Imaging of meningitis and ventriculitis. Neuroimaging Clin N Am 2012; 22(4):557–83.
32. Sánchez-Portocarrero J, Pérez-Cecilia E, Corral O, et al. The central nervous system and infection by

Candida species. Diagn Microbiol Infect Dis 2000; 37(3):169–79.
33. Mao J, Li J, Chen D, et al. MRI-DWI improves the early diagnosis of brain abscess induced by Candida albicans in preterm infants. Transl Pediatr 2012;1(2):76–84.
34. Slenker AK, Keith SW, Horn DL. Two hundred and eleven cases of Candida osteomyelitis: 17 case reports and a review of the literature. Diagn Microbiol Infect Dis 2012;73(1):89–93.
35. Williams RL, Fukui MB, Meltzer CC, et al. Fungal spinal osteomyelitis in the immunocompromised patient: MR findings in three cases. AJNR Am J Neuroradiol 1999;20(3):381–5.
36. Stäbler A, Reiser MF. Imaging of spinal infection. Radiol Clin North Am 2001;39(1):115–35.
37. Gabelmann A, Klein S, Kern W, et al. Relevant imaging findings of cerebral aspergillosis on MRI: a retrospective case-based study in immunocompromised patients. Eur J Neurol 2007;14(5):548–55.
38. Nussbaum ES, Hall WA. Rhinocerebral mucormycosis: changing patterns of disease. Surg Neurol 1994; 41(2):152–6.
39. Herrera DA, Dublin AB, Ormsby EL, et al. Imaging findings of rhinocerebral mucormycosis. Skull Base 2009;19(2):117–25.
40. Terry AR, Kahle KT, Larvie M, et al. Case records of the massachusetts general hospital. case 5-2016. A 43-year-old man with Altered Mental Status and a History of Alcohol Use. N Engl J Med 2016;374(7): 671–80.
41. Schwartz S, Thiel E. Update on the treatment of cerebral aspergillosis. Ann Hematol 2004;83(Suppl 1): S42–4.
42. Kamalian S, Avery L, Lev MH, et al. Nontraumatic Head and Neck Emergencies. Radiographics 2019;39(6):1808–23.
43. Safder S, Carpenter JS, Roberts TD, et al. The "Black Turbinate" sign: An early MR imaging finding of nasal mucormycosis. AJNR Am J Neuroradiol 2010;31(4):771–4.
44. Tempkin AD, Sobonya RE, Seeger JF, et al. Cerebral aspergillosis: radiologic and pathologic findings. Radiographics 2006;26(4):1239–42.
45. Yamada K, Shrier DA, Rubio A, et al. Imaging findings in intracranial aspergillosis. Acad Radiol 2002; 9(2):163–71.
46. Luthra G, Parihar A, Nath K, et al. Comparative evaluation of fungal, tubercular, and pyogenic brain abscesses with conventional and diffusion MR imaging and proton MR spectroscopy. AJNR Am J Neuroradiol 2007;28(7):1332–8.
47. Hirschmann JV. The early history of coccidioidomycosis: 1892-1945. Clin Infect Dis 2007;44(9):1202–7.
48. Jackson NR, Blair JE, Ampel NM. Central Nervous System Infections Due to Coccidioidomycosis. J Fungi (Basel) 2019;5(3).
49. Riddell J, Wheat LJ. Central Nervous System Infection with. J Fungi (Basel). 2019;5(3).
50. Starkey J, Moritani T, Kirby P. MRI of CNS fungal infections: review of aspergillosis to histoplasmosis and everything in between. Clin Neuroradiol 2014; 24(3):217–30.
51. Fang W, Washington L, Kumar N. Imaging manifestations of blastomycosis: a pulmonary infection with potential dissemination. Radiographics 2007;27(3): 641–55.
52. Galgiani JN, Ampel NM, Blair JE, et al. Coccidioidomycosis. Clin Infect Dis 2005;41(9):1217–23.
53. Wheat J, Myint T, Guo Y, et al. Central nervous system histoplasmosis: Multicenter retrospective study on clinical features, diagnostic approach and outcome of treatment. Medicine (Baltimore) 2018; 97(13):e0245.
54. Paphitou NI, Barnett BJ. Solitary parietal lobe histoplasmoma mimicking a brain tumor. Scand J Infect Dis 2002;34(3):229–32.
55. Khalaf SA, Patel P, Caruso CR, et al. CNS Histoplasmosis as a Gliosarcoma mimicker: The diagnostic dilemma of solitary brain lesions. IDCases 2022;27: e01364.
56. Lammering JC, Iv M, Gupta N, et al. Imaging spectrum of CNS coccidioidomycosis: prevalence and significance of concurrent brain and spinal disease. AJR Am J Roentgenol 2013;200(6):1334–46.
57. BUSS WC, GIBSON TE, GIFFORD MA. Coccidioidomycosis of the meninges. Calif Med 1950;72(3): 167–9.
58. Sobel RA, Ellis WG, Nielsen SL, et al. Central nervous system coccidioidomycosis: a clinicopathologic study of treatment with and without amphotericin B. Hum Pathol 1984;15(10):980–95.
59. Mischel PS, Vinters HV. Coccidioidomycosis of the central nervous system: neuropathological and vasculopathic manifestations and clinical correlates. Clin Infect Dis 1995;20(2):400–5.
60. Erly WK, Bellon RJ, Seeger JF, et al. MR imaging of acute coccidioidal meningitis. AJNR Am J Neuroradiol 1999;20(3):509–14.
61. Erly WK, Labadie E, Williams PL, et al. Disseminated coccidioidomycosis complicated by vasculitis: a cause of fatal subarachnoid hemorrhage in two cases. AJNR Am J Neuroradiol 1999;20(9):1605–8.
62. Zalduondo FM, Provenzale JM, Hulette C, et al. Meningitis, vasculitis, and cerebritis caused by CNS histoplasmosis: radiologic-pathologic correlation. AJR Am J Roentgenol 1996;166(1):194–6.
63. Crete RN, Gallmann W, Karis JP, et al. Spinal Coccidioidomycosis: MR Imaging Findings in 41 Patients. AJNR Am J Neuroradiol 2018;39(11):2148–53.
64. Bariola JR, Perry P, Pappas PG, et al. Blastomycosis of the central nervous system: a multicenter review of diagnosis and treatment in the modern era. Clin Infect Dis 2010;50(6):797–804.

Infectious Diseases of the Brain and Spine
Parasitic and Other Atypical Transmissible Diseases

Dhairya A. Lakhani, MD, Francis Deng, MD, Doris D.M. Lin, MD, PhD*

KEYWORDS

- Atypical CNS infections • Parasitic CNS infections • Atypical transmissible CNS infections
- Prion diseases • Creutzfeldt-Jakob disease

KEY POINTS

- Neurocysticercosis progresses through multiple stages, starting from a cyst containing a scolex, development of surrounding inflammatory reaction, and termination as a calcified nodule.
- Neurotoxoplasmosis results in mass-like lesions with targetoid or ring enhancement that mimic lymphoma in immunocompromised patients, for whom empiric treatment may prove diagnostic and therapeutic.
- Cerebral echinococcosis (neurohydatidosis) mostly appears as a solitary cyst in the brain parenchyma without enhancement or edema, but the associated mass effect can cause elevated intracranial pressure.
- Neuroschistosomiasis incites granulomatous inflammation in the brain or spinal cord, with the latter having a predilection for the conus medullaris.
- Creutzfeldt-Jakob disease typically manifests as nonenhancing DWI hyperintensity in the cerebral cortex and deep gray nuclei.

INTRODUCTION

Parasitic infections of the central nervous system (CNS) are broadly classified into two categories: unicellular protozoa and multicellular helminths (metazoan). Protozoal infections encompass toxoplasmosis, malaria, and amebiasis, whereas helminths consist of six parasitic taxa: flatworms (Platyhelminthes), tapeworms (cestodes), trematodes (flukes), roundworms (nematodes), acanthocephalans, and crustaceans. Cysticercosis and echinococcosis belong to the cestodes taxon, whereas schistosomiasis falls under Platyhelminth.[1,2] In the United States, the most common parasitic infections that lead to CNS manifestations are cysticercosis, echinococcosis, and toxoplasmosis. Less common parasitic infections include amebiasis, malaria, and schistosomiasis.[3]

Prion diseases are rare transmissible diseases that cause rapidly progressive spongiform encephalopathies, and are classified as acquired, hereditary, or sporadic types. Sporadic type is most common, whereas acquired type is extremely rare.

In this article, we provide an in-depth review of atypical infections in the brain and spine caused by parasitic and prion diseases using case examples.

PROTOZOAL INFECTIONS

Toxoplasmosis

Toxoplasmosis is caused by *Toxoplasma gondii*, an intracellular protozoan that is found worldwide.

FUNDING: None.
Division of Neuroradiology, Russell H. Morgan Department of Radiology and Radiological Science, Johns Hopkins University School of Medicine, Baltimore, MD, USA
* Corresponding author.
E-mail address: ddmlin@jhmi.edu

Magn Reson Imaging Clin N Am 32 (2024) 347–361
https://doi.org/10.1016/j.mric.2024.02.002
1064-9689/24/

It is the most common opportunistic infection affecting the CNS in patients with AIDS and a CD4 count of less than 100 cells/μL.[4]

Cat is the definitive host, where the protozoa multiply in the intestinal mucosa and release oocysts in feces. Oocysts can survive for up to a year in moist soil.[4] Intermediate hosts, including humans and poultry animals, get infected by the consumption of oocysts through contaminated vegetables or direct contact with cat feces. In the intermediate hosts, parasites transform into rapidly multiplying tachyzoites in the intestine and hematogenously disseminate. In the end organ, the parasites transform into the final stage of tissue cyst containing bradyzoites. *Toxoplasma* cysts can occur in any tissue but are most common in the brain, retina, skeletal muscle, and cardiac muscle, ultimately reaching the brain and muscles transforming into the final stage of tissue cyst/bradyzoites.[4] Human hosts can also be infected by ingesting undercooked meat contaminated with this tissue cyst.

Multifocal abscesses (**Fig. 1**) with a predilection for the basal ganglia are the most common manifestation of CNS toxoplasmosis (**Table 1**). Solitary lesions are reported in about one-third of the cases. Most lesions show ring-like enhancement patterns. Although only present in 30% of the cases, the "eccentric target sign," defined as an eccentric enhancing nodule along the lesion margin,[4] is pathognomonic for toxoplasmosis. The concentric target sign is also reported in cases of cerebral toxoplasmosis, in which there are a series of concentric rings of alternating T2 hyperintense and hypointense/isointense signal characteristics.[5]

As opposed to a well-defined enhancing wall in bacterial abscess with homogenous diffusion restriction, *Toxoplasma* abscesses have poorly defined peripheral enhancement and faint peripheral diffusion restriction, believed to reflect a poor host response to the infection.[4]

In patients with HIV presenting with a brain mass lesion, a common clinical challenge is distinguishing CNS lymphoma from toxoplasma abscess (**Fig. 2**). Both have peripheral enhancement and peripheral restricted diffusion. On dynamic susceptibility contrast perfusion imaging, lymphoma has higher relative cerebral blood volume than toxoplasmosis. On MR spectroscopy, toxoplasmosis lesions typically have decreased levels of choline, whereas lymphoma generally has elevated choline levels.[6] On fluorodeoxyglucose PET, lymphoma has higher uptake, whereas toxoplasmosis has decreased activity compared with contralateral normal brain.[7] When toxoplasmosis is suspected, an empirical trial of antitoxoplasma therapy for 2 to 3 weeks may prove to be definitive. The decreased size of the lesion is considered to be sufficiently confirmatory to continue therapy and imaging surveillance until resolution. Stable or increasing size of the lesion may be indicative of an alternate diagnosis, especially CNS lymphoma, and a brain biopsy may be necessary.[4,8]

It is important to note that calcification in acquired toxoplasmosis is uncommon, although it may be seen after therapy. However, calcification

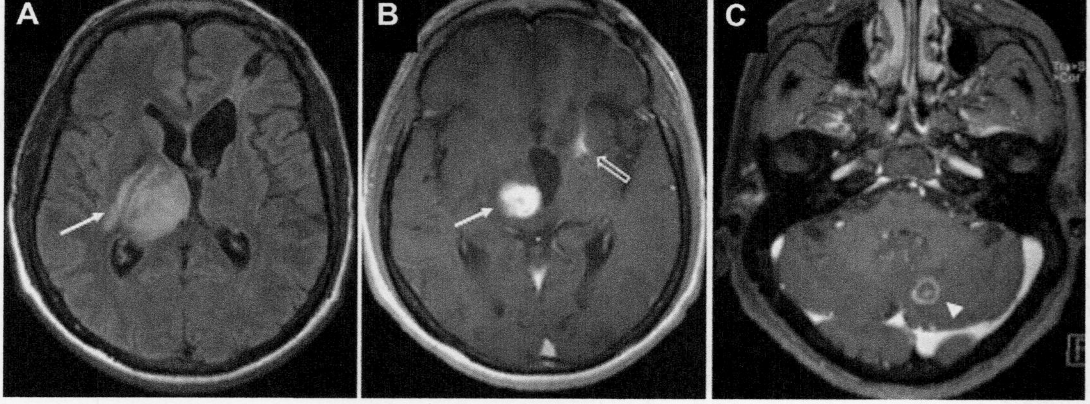

Fig. 1. CNS toxoplasmosis. Axial FLAIR (*A*) and axial T1 postcontrast (*B, C*) in a 45-year-old man with HIV/AIDS (noncompliant with highly active antiretroviral therapy) and previous toxoplasmosis encephalopathy who presented with altered mental status. Multifocal lesions: solidly enhancing in right thalamus with associated mass-effect and surrounding edema (*arrow*), targetoid in the left cerebellum (*arrowhead*), and flame-shaped enhancement (*block arrow*) around the left frontal encephalomalacia at prior biopsy site. There was improvement on imaging following 3 weeks of empiric toxoplasmosis therapy, confirming the diagnosis.

Table 1
Imaging features characteristic of certain infectious etiologies

	Finding	MR Imaging Appearance
Parasitic infections		
Toxoplasmosis	Multifocal abscesses with a predilection for the deep gray nuclei.	Ring-like enhancement, no central restricted diffusion (unlike pyogenic abscess) but may show peripheral or mixed diffusion restriction. "Eccentric target sign" is pathognomonic.
Neurocysticercosis	Variable depending on stages (see **Table 2**) and location. Vesicular stage has a simple cyst containing a live larvum.	Simple cyst with scolex, giving the appearance of a "target" or "dot in a hole," counts as an absolute criterion needed for diagnosis of neurocysticercosis.
Echinococcosis	Three-layered hydatid cysts; the outer pericyst formed by host immune cells. Cyst fluid contents: proteins, glucose, ions, lipids, and polysaccharides. Multiple daughter vesicles contain scolices and grow into daughter cysts.	Solitary (most common), or multiple clustered daughter cysts. Intraparenchymal, well-defined oval or round cystic mass following CSF signal, without enhancement, edema, or calcification. The outer pericyst may show a characteristic faint T2-hypointense rim because of fibrotic change.
Prion disease		
Creutzfeldt-Jakob disease	Spongiform encephalitis, rapidly progressive and fatal. Alteration of prion protein (PrP^{C}) to abnormal folded protein (PrP^{Sc}), which self-propagates by autocatalyzing the reconfiguration of normal PrP^{C}.	DWI and T2/FLAIR hyperintensity in the cortex ("cortical ribbon sign") and basal ganglia, diffuse or focal, symmetric or asymmetric. T2/FLAIR and DWI hyperintensity in the dorsomedial thalami (double hockey stick sign) and posterior thalami (pulvinar sign) most sensitive in the variant CJD.

is common in congenital toxoplasmosis.[9] Moreover, the disease may be transmitted transplacentally, which can have devastating effects on the fetal brain because maternal antibodies passed to the child are limited by the blood-brain barrier. Seizures, microcephaly, and chorioretinitis are noted in most cases.[4]

Malaria

Malaria is the most common parasitic disease worldwide, although fatal cases are mostly restricted to sub-Saharan Africa.[10] In the United States, from 2000 to 2014, there were 22,029 malaria-related hospitalizations (4.88 per 1 million population) and 4823 severe malaria cases.[11] Cerebral malaria is almost exclusively caused by protozoan parasite *Plasmodium falciparum*, transmitted by female *Anopheles* mosquitos, which flourish in stagnant water. During a blood meal, a *Plasmodium*-infected mosquito inoculates sporozoites into the human host. Sporozoites infect liver cells, mature, and release merozoites that multiply in erythrocytes. Blood-stage parasites are responsible for the clinical manifestations of malaria, such as fever. Cerebral malaria is thought to be caused by the sequestration of infected erythrocytes in the microcirculation. Cerebral malaria is associated with a mortality rate of 15% to 25% even when appropriate treatment is given.[10]

Cerebral malaria can present with a wide range of MR imaging findings, that includes T2/FLAIR hyperintensities in the white matter, deep gray nuclei, and corpus callosum[12–14]; hemorrhagic and nonhemorrhagic infarctions[13,15]; and petechial microhemorrhages at the gray matter–white matter junctions and deep white matter (**Fig. 3**).[13] In serious cases of cerebral malaria, MR imaging would show diffuse cerebral edema, vasogenic and cytotoxic in origin. It is caused by an increase in cerebral blood volume because of the sequestration of parasitized erythrocytes and compensatory

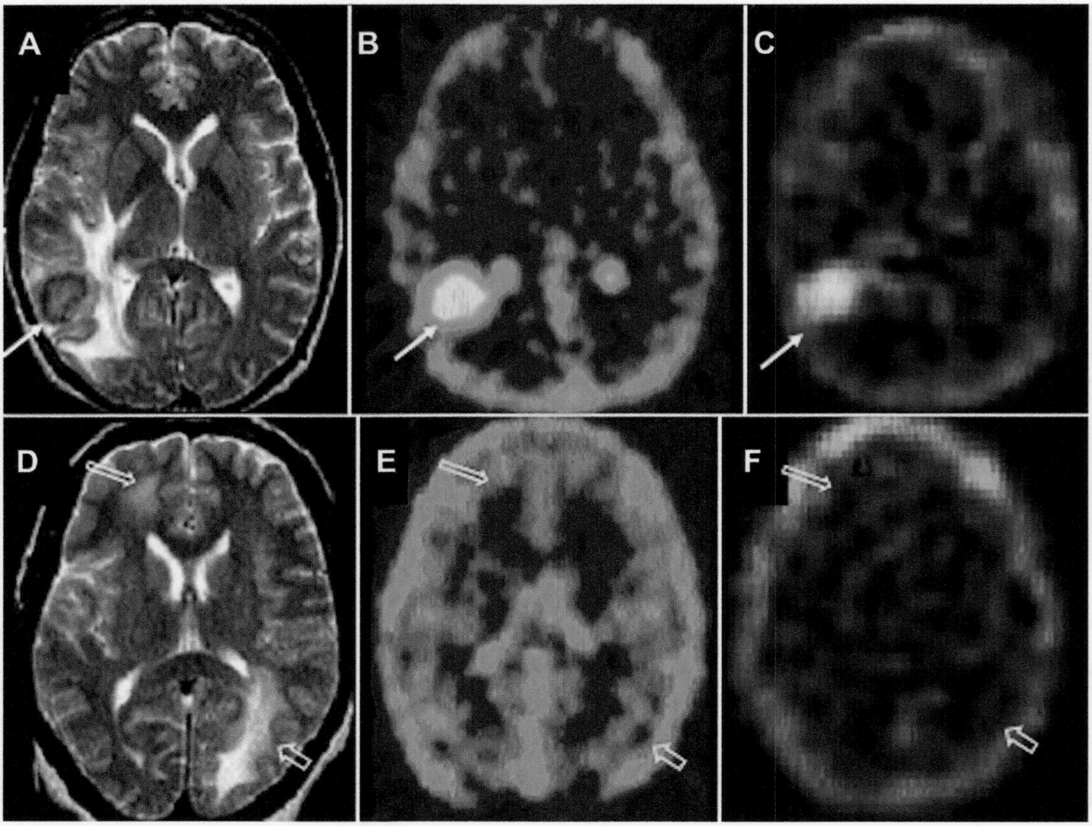

Fig. 2. Distinguishing toxoplasmosis from lymphoma in two different patients with HIV/AIDS. Axial T2 (*A*) shows a hyperintense mass with peripheral hypointensity in the right parietal lobe, corresponding to increased radiotracer uptake on ^{11}C-Thymidine (*B*) and ^{201}Thallium single-photon emission computed tomography (*C*) scans, consistent with a CNS lymphoma with increased metabolism (*arrows*). Axial T2 (*D*) shows right frontal and left parieto-occipital hyperintensity with underlying masses, corresponding to no abnormal increased radiotracer uptake on either ^{11}C-Thymidine (*E*) or ^{201}Thallium single-photon emission computed tomography (*F*), indicating an infectious/inflammatory cause (*block arrows*).

vasodilation, damage to cerebral capillary endothelium, and cerebral microvascular occlusion.[10]

Amebic Infections

Amebae are free-living protozoa that are widespread in water and soil worldwide.[16] Humans are frequently exposed to amebae, but the occurrence of the disease is rare. Although rare, amebic infections are virulent and have high mortality rates.[17] Neurologic manifestations of amebic infection come in two flavors: primary amebic meningoencephalitis (caused by *Naegleria fowleri*) and granulomatous amebic encephalitis (caused by *Acanthamoeba* spp; *Balamuthia mandrillaris*; and, in only one case to date, *Sappinia pedata*).[18] Primary amebic meningoencephalitis has no predilection for immunocompromised patients, whereas granulomatous amebic encephalitis usually affects immunocompromised patients, but rare cases in immunocompetent hosts have been reported.[17,19–22]

N fowleri, often called the "brain-eating ameba," is transmitted through the olfactory mucosa of the nasal cavity; most cases reported recent swimming or diving activities in freshwater. The other amebae can also be transmitted via the nasal route, in addition to via cutaneous lesions or inhalation of airborne cysts into the lower respiratory tract with subsequent hematogenous spread to the brain and other organs.

Primary amebic meningoencephalitis is clinically indistinguishable from acute bacterial meningitis, presenting with headache, fever, nausea, and vomiting. Incubation periods average 5 days from exposure to clinical presentation. Two-thirds of the cases would have rapid decline and death within 1 week of symptom onset, so fewer than one-third of patients in the United States have been diagnosed with primary amebic

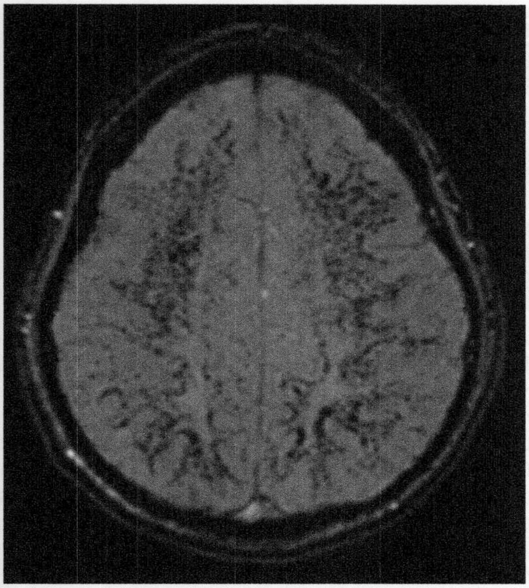

Fig. 3. Cerebral malaria. Axial susceptibility-weighted imaging demonstrates innumerable microhemorrhages at the corticomedullary junction and deep white matter of the bilateral cerebral hemispheres. (Image courtesy of Surjith Vattoth, MD.)

meningoencephalitis before death.[18] In extremely rare occasions, spinal cord involvement has been reported.[23]

Imaging findings of primary amebic meningoencephalitis are nonspecific. Early in the disease course, computed tomography and MR imaging may be normal, with the subsequent appearance of brain edema and basilar meningeal enhancement.[24] Hydrocephalus and basal ganglia infarcts have also been reported.[18] The nonspecific imaging features necessitate a high index of clinical suspicion to suggest the diagnosis before death.[24]

Granulomatous amebic encephalitis is a subacute or chronic CNS infection that presents with weeks to months of worsening headaches, fever, personality or cognitive changes, and/or focal neurologic deficits, progressing to seizures or depressed level of consciousness.[17,19–22] Despite aggressive therapy, death is common within 7 to 10 days after onset of illness.[25,26]

Granulomatous amebic encephalitis often manifests as multifocal parenchymal mass-like lesions (**Fig. 4**). These lesions represent focal edema, trophozoites, cysts, along with chronic granulomatous inflammatory cells. Leptomeningitis may accompany the parenchymal lesions.[27]

On MR imaging, these parenchymal lesions demonstrate T2 hyperintense signal and linear or superficial gyriform enhancement, which possibly represents a combination of enhancement in the overlying inflamed meninges covered with exudates and the actual enhancement of the underlying cortex. In rare occasions, granulomatous amebic encephalitis may present as multiple punctate foci of enhancement throughout the cerebral and cerebellar hemispheres. A few cases have shown evidence of intralesional hemorrhage and necrosis, which may relate to necrotizing angiitis that has been histopathologically described in severe granulomatous amebic encephalitis cases. The overall appearance is similar to that seen in other encephalitides and acute disseminated encephalomyelitis.[28] Case reports of granulomatous amebic encephalitis manifesting as a solitary mass-like lesion, hemorrhagic infarction, ring-enhancing lesions, and interhemispheric cyst have also been described.[19,24,29,30]

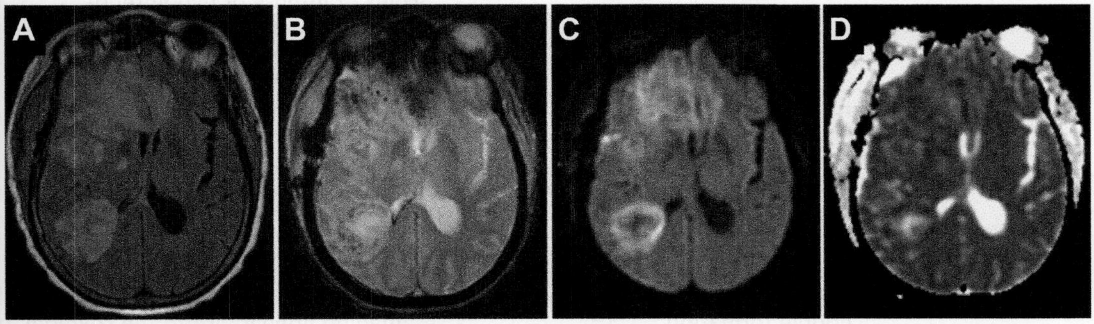

Fig. 4. Cerebral amebiasis. Axial FLAIR (*A*), axial T2*GRE (*B*), axial DWI trace (*C*), and axial ADC map (*D*) in a 59-year-old woman originally from Nigeria presenting with 2 weeks of headaches and found to have parenchymal enhancing masses thought to be glioblastoma. Resected mass was found to be amebic infection (concerning for *Naegleria fowleri* or *Entamoeba histolytica*) with pathology showing diffuse acute and chronic inflammation with a perivascular and leptomeningeal predominance. She was also found to be HIV positive. Images show multifocal FLAIR hyperintense masses, largest in the right frontal lobe with extension to the left frontal lobe. The masses have punctuate susceptibility suggesting microhemorrhages, and demonstrate peripheral restricted diffusion with centrally facilitated diffusion. Note right frontal craniotomy changes with scalp swelling.

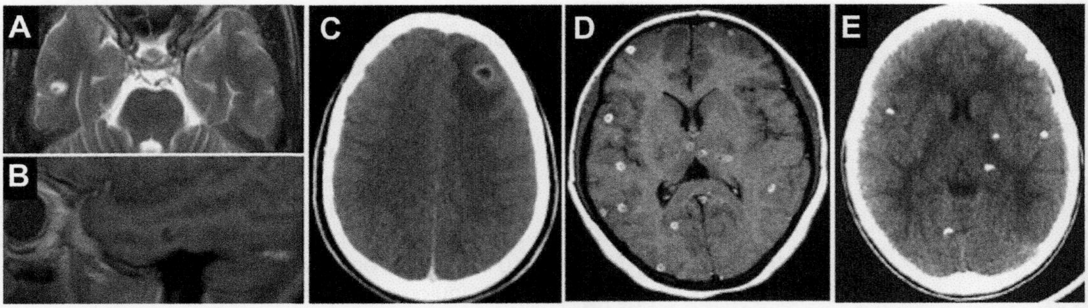

Fig. 5. Four stages of neurocysticercosis. Vesicular stage: Axial T2 (*A*) and sagittal T1 postcontrast (*B*) show a thin-walled circumscribed cyst with a mural nodule (scolex) in the right temporal lobe, without edema or cyst wall enhancement. Colloidal stage: Axial CT with contrast (*C*) shows thickened cyst wall with enhancement and prominent surrounding vasogenic edema caused by inflammatory response. Granular nodular: Axial T1 postcontrast (*D*) shows small, retracted cysts with thickened capsules and persistent edema and enhancement in a targetoid appearance. Nodular calcified: Axial unenhanced head CT (*E*) shows multiple calcified nodules. There is no contrast enhancement or edema at this stage. Note that only the vesicular stage, with evidence of cystic lesions containing scolex on CT or MR imaging, fulfills the absolute criteria for diagnosis of neurocysticercosis.

METAZOAL INFECTIONS

Cestodes

Neurocysticercosis

Neurocysticercosis is caused by encysted larvae of the tapeworm *Taenia solium*. Fecal-oral transmission of eggs is followed by the hatching of embryos that migrate through the intestinal mucosa into the circulation and lodge in the capillaries of the brain, where they develop into larvae called cysticerci. The cysts are protected from the host's immune system by the blood-brain barrier, and hence no inflammatory response is present as long as the cyst wall remains intact. However, when the parasite dies because of therapy or by a natural process, an inflammatory response with perilesional edema ensues, followed by calcification.[31]

Table 2
Stages of neurocysticercosis and their MR imaging characteristics

	Pathogenesis	MR Imaging Findings
Vesicular stage	Live larvum with thin glycoprotein-rich capsule, no inflammation.	Cyst with mural nodular enhancement (scolex), giving the appearance of a "target" or "dot in a hole." 5- to 20-mm cyst, following CSF signal with a thin imperceptible wall. Scolex isointense or hypointense relative to white matter on T1, and isointense to hyperintense on T2. No surrounding edema.
Colloidal stage	Larvum dies, capsule thickens, and larvum releases metabolites. Cyst wall disruption results in an intense inflammatory reaction to the unprotected parasite.	Cyst contents may be T1 and T2 hyperintense, reflecting proteinaceous contents. Cyst wall is thick, irregular, and enhances, with marked pericystic edema.
Granular nodular stage	The cyst retracts, capsule thickens, scolex calcifies. Granulomatous nodule formation.	Resembling a granuloma with decreased fluid content. Similar imaging appearance to the colloidal phase with persistent edema and thick enhancement.
Calcified nodular	Inactive stage. No live cysticerci, but parasite antigen may still be present. Nodule calcifies. Any residual edema or enhancement resolves during this stage.	Calcified nodules are hypointense on T1 and T2, and best depicted on susceptibility-weighted imaging. 2–10 mm in diameter. No edema or enhancement.

Neurocysticercosis is the most common parasitic disease of the CNS and the most common cause of acquired epilepsy.[32] Cysticercosis is endemic in most developing countries and closely associated with domestic pig raising. Immigration and travel have resulted in an increasing number of cases in developed countries. Incidental calcified granulomas are found in 10% to 20% of the general population in endemic settings.[33]

Neurocysticercosis is classified by location into intraparenchymal and extraparenchymal forms. In addition to the brain and spinal cord, cysticerci commonly develop in the subcutaneous tissues, muscles, and eyes.

Intraparenchymal neurocysticercosis stages of larvae development (**Fig. 5**) are well established (**Table 2**).[34] The vesicular stage is characterized by a 5- to 20-mm thin-walled cyst with no enhancement and no surrounding edema. On imaging, the presence of the scolex in the cyst appears as a "target" or "dot in a hole."[31] The vesicular colloidal or colloidal stage is characterized by the death of the scolex from either the natural processes or from therapy. Cyst wall disruption in this stage results in an intense inflammatory reaction to the unprotected parasite and clinical manifestation of diffuse encephalitis.[31] Cysts may be hyperintense on T1- and T2-weighted images, reflecting proteinaceous contents. The cyst wall is thicker than in the vesicular stage, and there is marked pericystic edema (**Fig. 6**) as reflected by surrounding enhancement and T2 signal changes.[31,35] The appearance is not specific to neurocysticercosis and may be mimicked by a neoplasm (**Fig. 7**). The granular nodular stage is characterized by cyst retraction and granulomatous nodule formation with surrounding gliosis. This phase has a similar imaging appearance of the cyst to the vesicular colloidal phase but has less edema and thicker enhancement.[31,34] The last phase is called calcified nodular, which is characterized by the calcification of this nodule. This is the nonactive stage of neurocysticercosis and any residual edema or enhancement resolves during this stage. The nodule is hypointense on T1 and T2,[31] and best depicted on susceptibility-weighted imaging. It is common to have multiple lesions at different stages.

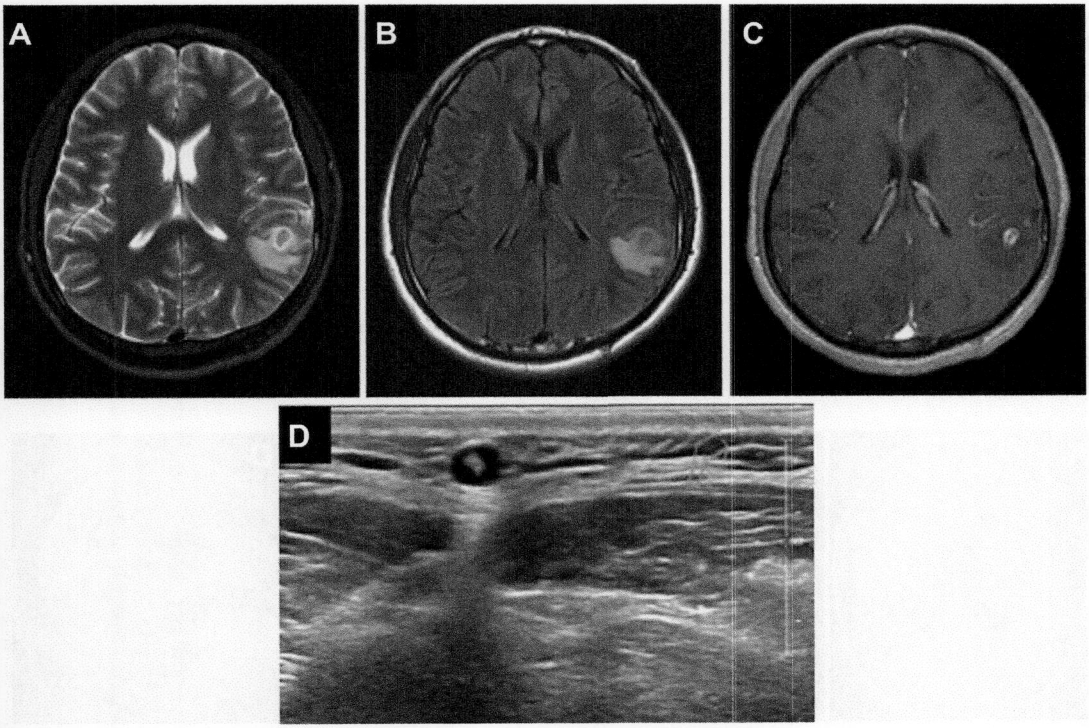

Fig. 6. A 23-year-old man presenting with first-time seizure. Axial T2 (*A*), axial FLAIR (*B*), axial T1 postcontrast (*C*) images show a left parietal subcentimeter intermediate signal lesion with peripheral enhancement and surrounding vasogenic edema. Similar lesion in the cerebellar vermis (not shown). These findings are nonspecific and could represent an infectious or neoplastic cause. Ultrasound of the nape of neck (*D*) corresponding to a palpable abnormality shows a well circumscribed, thin-walled cyst containing a nodule in the subcutaneous tissue, allowing a final diagnosis of cysticercosis in the brain (colloidal stage).

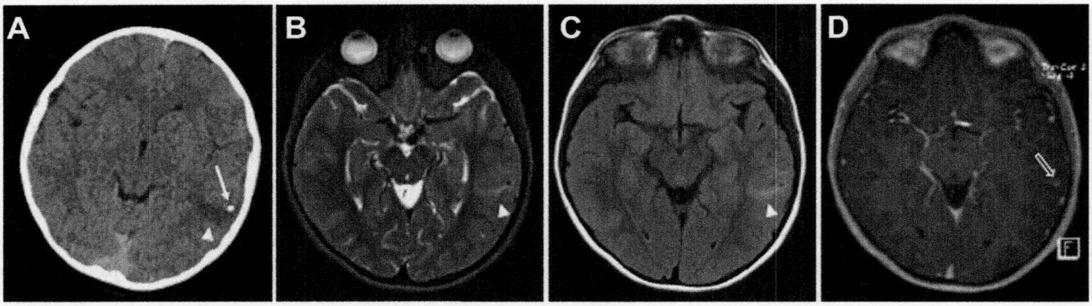

Fig. 7. Low grade glioneuronal tumor mimicking neurocysticercosis. Axial unenhanced head CT (*A*), axial T2 (*B*), axial FLAIR (*C*), axial T1 postcontrast (*D*) images in a 10-year-old girl presenting with first-time seizure. CT shows a punctate calcification (*arrow*) in the left temporal cortical region, with surrounding edema (*arrowheads*). MR imaging demonstrates peripheral enhancement (*block arrow*). Resected tissue reveals low-grade glioneuronal proliferation.

Extraparenchymal neurocysticercosis includes subarachnoid-cisternal and intraventricular locations, and can be large and multicystic clustered (so called "racemose"). Space-occupying lesions in subarachnoid space can result in hydrocephalus.[31] Intraventricular neurocysticercosis (**Figs. 8** and **9**) most commonly affects the fourth ventricle, followed by lateral ventricles, third ventricle, and aqueduct. Isolated ventricular neurocysticercosis has been reported in one-third of cases. It often presents with hydrocephalus and ventriculitis caused by ependymal inflammatory response or adhesions caused by prior ventricular infestation.[31]

Spinal neurocysticercosis (**Fig. 10**) is a result of cerebrospinal fluid (CSF) dissemination of the larvae throughout the craniospinal subarachnoid space. Spine involvement is almost always associated with concomitant intracranial involvement. Spinal neurocysticercosis is extremely rare, which might be explained by the relatively larger size of the cyst compared with the cervical CSF space.[31]

Echinococcosis

CNS cystic echinococcosis is caused by *Echinococcus granulosus* infestation. It is also known as hydatid disease or neurohydatidosis. Cystic echinococcosis is endemic in many sheep- and cattle-raising countries.[36] Dogs and other carnivores are the definitive hosts, whereas sheep, goats, and swine are the intermediate hosts. The adult worm attaches to the small intestine mucosa of the definitive host by hooklets and releases eggs in the feces. The intermediate host (mostly poultry animals) ingests these eggs. Once ingested in the duodenum of the host, the eggs lose their protective chitinous layer, and the embryo (also referred to as oncosphere) is released. The oncosphere passes through the intestinal wall into the portal and systemic circulation, developing into mature cysts within the end-organ. The lifecycle is complete when the definitive host eats the viscera of the infected intermediate host. Humans get infected by eating undercooked meat from intermediate hosts or egg-contaminated water or

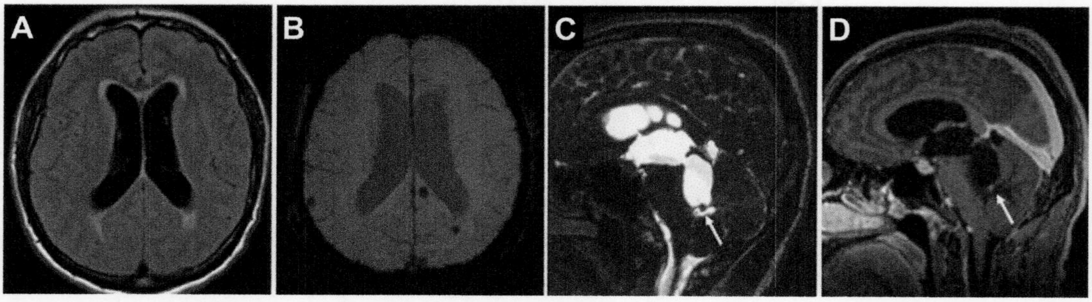

Fig. 8. A 38-year-old Spanish-speaking man presenting with 2 months of headaches followed by nausea and vomiting. (*A*) Axial FLAIR image shows moderate obstructive hydrocephalus with interstitial edema. (*B*) Susceptibility-weighted imaging shows multifocal calcifications also demonstrated on initial head CT. (*C*) Sagittal CISS shows a cystic lesion expanding the fourth ventricle with a small nodule (*arrows*) in its caudal aspect, which shows contrast enhancement in *D*. The combination of multifocal nonspecific calcified granulomas and more specific intraventricular cyst with a mural nodule allowed a clinical diagnosis of neurocysticercosis.

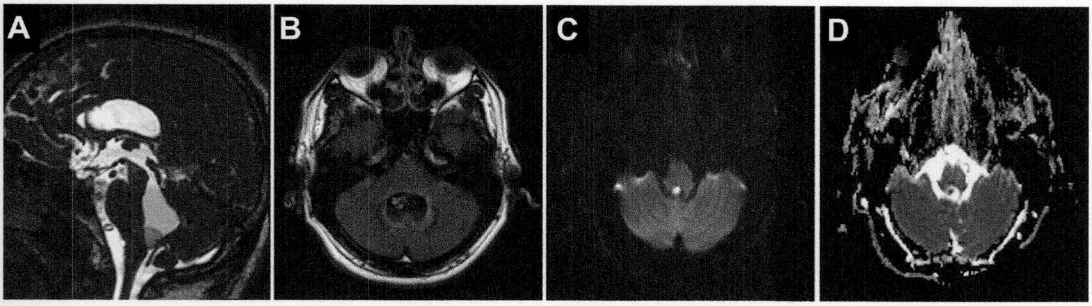

Fig. 9. Intraventricular neurocysticercosis in a 44-year-old man from Mexico with waxing waning headaches and dizziness for 2 months. (*A*) Sagittal CISS shows a cystic lesion expanding the fourth ventricle, containing an intermediate signal nodule in the caudal aspect. Note that the cyst has a T2 hyperintense signal slightly different from the ventricular and cisternal CSF. (*B*) Axial FLAIR shows expanded fourth ventricle with adjacent interstitial edema, and a nodule within the cyst. DWI trace (*C*) and ADC map (*D*) show a small area of restricted diffusion within the nodule, a feature often seen in scolex.

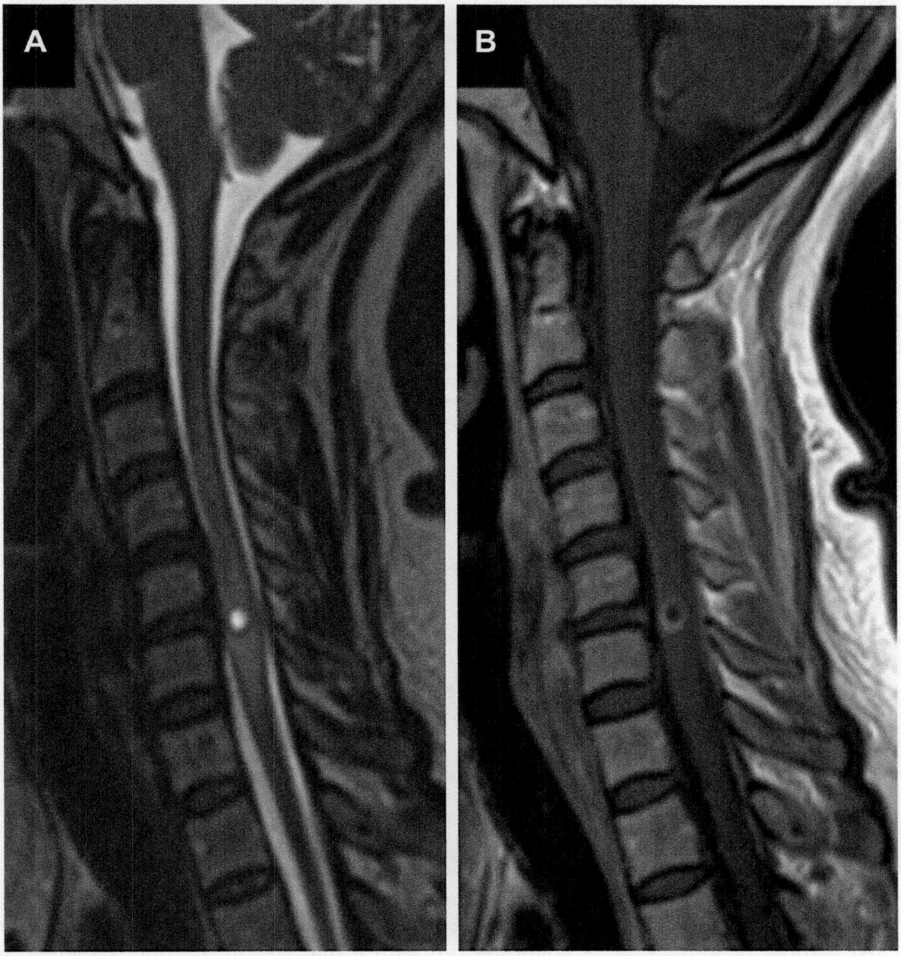

Fig. 10. Spinal intramedullary neurocysticercosis. Sagittal T2 (*A*) and sagittal postcontrast T1 (*B*) illustrate a well-circumscribed intramedullary cystic mass with thick enhancing capsule, slightly expanding the C5-6 cord and associated with surrounding edema. Findings are consistent with a colloidal stage of cysticercosis as the larva dies and incites inflammatory changes.

vegetables.[37] The viable parasite eggs subsequently penetrate the mucosa, reaching the liver (75%), lungs (15%), and CNS (2%) via hematogenous dissemination.[38] In the target end organs, they transform into mature cysts.

The hydatid cyst has three layers: (1) the outer pericyst, composed of host inflammatory cells that form a dense and fibrous protective layer; (2) the middle laminated membrane, which is an acellular membrane that allows passage of nutrients; and (3) the inner germinal layer, where the scolices (larvae) and the laminated membrane are produced. The middle laminated membrane and the inner germinal layer form the true wall of the cyst and are referred to as the endocyst. The outer layer is referred to as the ectocyst.[37] Daughter vesicles are small spherules that contain scolices, which are attached by a pedicle to the germinal layer of the mother cyst and resemble a bunch of grapes. Daughter vesicles may grow into daughter cysts and may extend through the wall of the mother cyst. Cyst fluid contains proteins, glucose, ions, lipids, and polysaccharides. The fluid is antigenic and may contain scolices and hooklets. When vesicles rupture within the cyst, scolices pass into the cyst fluid and form a white sediment known as hydatid sand.[37]

CNS cystic echinococcosis most often occurs as a simple-appearing cyst in the cerebral

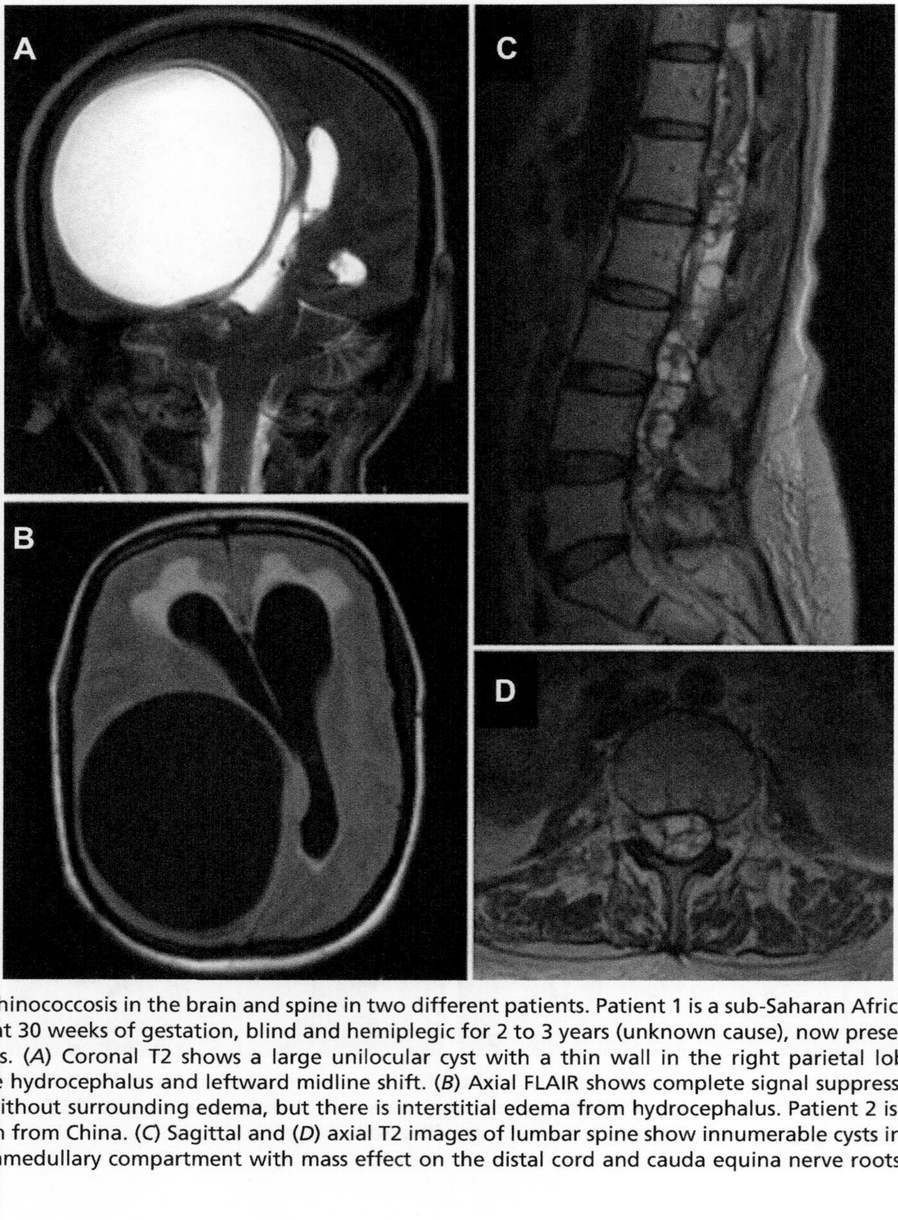

Fig. 11. Echinococcosis in the brain and spine in two different patients. Patient 1 is a sub-Saharan African woman pregnant at 30 weeks of gestation, blind and hemiplegic for 2 to 3 years (unknown cause), now presenting with convulsions. (*A*) Coronal T2 shows a large unilocular cyst with a thin wall in the right parietal lobe causing obstructive hydrocephalus and leftward midline shift. (*B*) Axial FLAIR shows complete signal suppression within the cyst, without surrounding edema, but there is interstitial edema from hydrocephalus. Patient 2 is a 32-year-old woman from China. (*C*) Sagittal and (*D*) axial T2 images of lumbar spine show innumerable cysts in the intradural extramedullary compartment with mass effect on the distal cord and cauda equina nerve roots.

hemispheres (**Fig. 11**). Rarely, cysts have been reported in the cerebellar hemispheres and may involve the dura, subarachnoid space, ventricular system, brainstem, and spinal canal.[38–42] Most of the cysts are solitary; few cases report multiple cysts, sometimes caused by rupture of a prior single cyst.[36] These cysts are well-defined, oval or round collections in the brain parenchyma, isointense to CSF without associated enhancement, edema, or calcification.[36,39] Occasionally, a faint halo of T2 hypointensity is present, which is believed to represent the fibrotic pericyst.[39] This layer may demonstrate calcification.[37]

Platyhelminths

Schistosomiasis

Schistosomiasis is caused by trematodes (a type of flatworm called flukes) of the genus *Schistosoma*. Five species are known to infect humans, three of which cause almost all reported cases of neuroschistosomiasis: *Sappinia mansoni*, *Sappinia haematobium*, and *Sappinia japonicum*. Schistosomiasis is a major public health hazard in developing countries. More than 200 million people in Africa, Asia, and South America are infected.[43] Different species have different geographic predilections: *S haematobium* and *S mansoni* are both found in Africa and the Middle East; *S mansoni* is also endemic in parts of Brazil, Venezuela, and the Caribbean; and *S japonicum* occurs in China and Southeast Asia.[44] Almost all reported cases of CNS schistosomiasis are caused by *S mansoni*, *S haematobium*, or *S japonicum*.[45]

Infected freshwater snails shed cercariae (larvae) into the water. The larvae penetrate the skin of the human host and then the adult worms enter the circulatory system. Complications result from the chronic granulomatous reaction to aberrant adult worm migration and egg deposition in end organs, such as the intestines, liver, urinary tract, and CNS.[46] Cerebral involvement in the form of acute encephalitis of the cortex, subcortical white matter, basal ganglia, or internal capsule is the most common manifestation of neuroschistosomiasis from *S japonicum*.[47] Spinal cord involvement in the form of acute transverse myelitis and subacute myeloradiculopathy is the most common manifestation of neuroschistosomiasis from *S mansoni* or *S haematobium*.

Cerebral schistosomiasis at computed tomography typically shows mass lesions (granulomas) with surrounding edema and variable contrast enhancement. MR imaging would depict small nodular or "silt-like" enhancements scattered or clustered at the cortical or subcortical areas (**Fig. 12**).[45] Sanelli and colleagues[48] reported an "arborized" enhancement pattern with a central linear enhancement that, when present, may be specific for schistosomiasis. Spinal schistosomiasis typically reveals edema and patchy contrast enhancement of the spinal cord, most often at the conus medullaris. Long-standing cases may result in cord atrophy.[45] In cerebral and spinal locations, it is difficult to differentiate granulomatous inflammation from neoplasms.[49,50]

In addition to the findings related to granulomatous lesions, the presence of bilateral symmetric T1 hyperintensity of the globus pallidi and substantia nigra (reflecting manganese deposition) have been reported as a sequala of portosystemic shunting in hepatic schistosomiasis (even in the absence of liver dysfunction).[51]

The presence of eggs in the stool or a positive serology provides only supportive evidence of neuroschistosomiasis. Definitive diagnosis requires histopathologic confirmation of *Schistosoma* eggs and granulomas.

OTHER TRANSMISSIBLE DISEASES

Creutzfeldt-Jakob Disease

Creutzfeldt-Jakob disease (CJD) is a human prion disease. It represents a heterogeneous group of rapidly progressive neurodegenerative diseases that are always fatal, usually within 1 year of onset. Fortunately, all prion diseases remain rare, at an

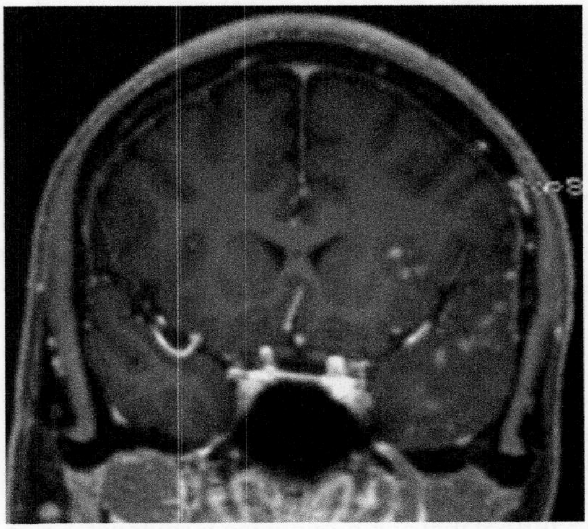

Fig. 12. Cerebral schistosomiasis. Coronal postcontrast T1 shows characteristic cluster of small nodular enhancement in the cortical and subcortical regions of the left temporal and frontal lobes, with surrounding edema most notable in the left temporal lobe. The diagnosis was confirmed on biopsy. (Image courtesy of Surjith Vattoth, MD.)

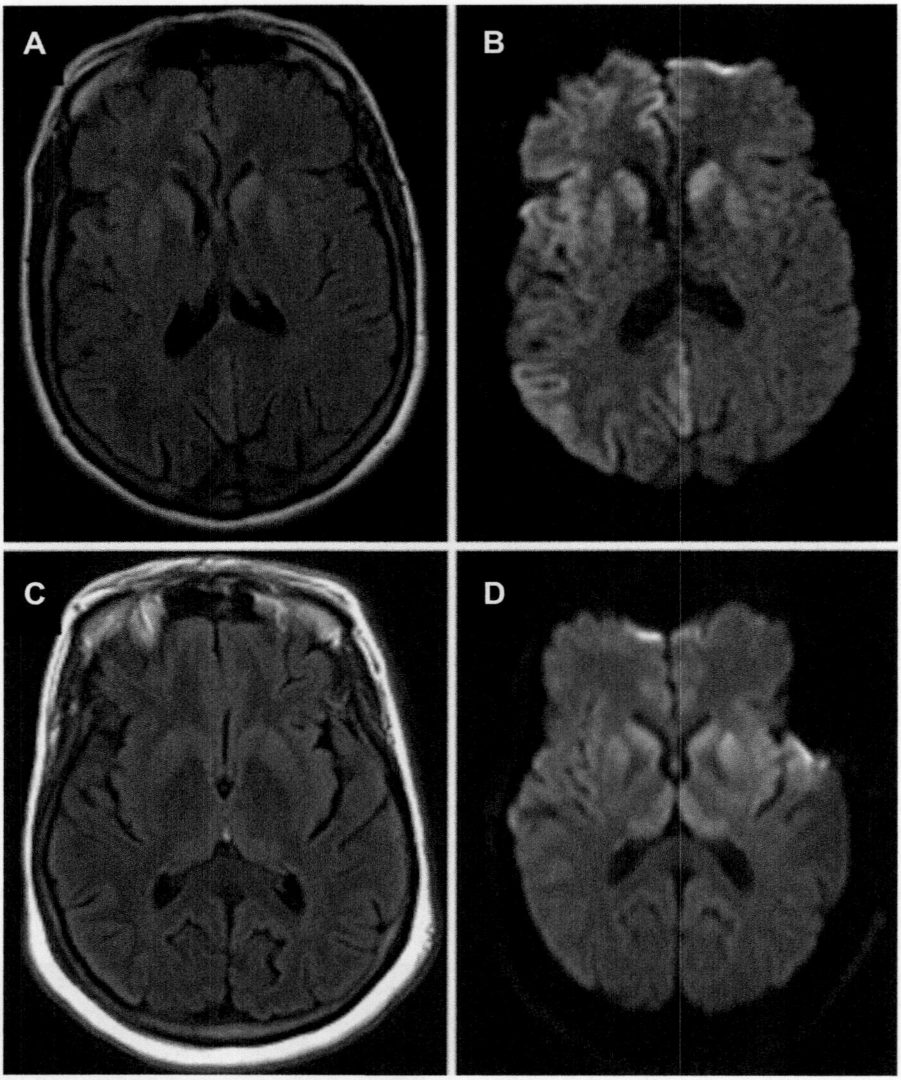

Fig. 13. CJD in two different patients in different forms. Patient 1 is a 58-year-old woman with profound cognitive decline, mood swings, fatigue, and insomnia. (*A*) Axial FLAIR and (*B*) axial DWI trace images show abnormal hyperintensity involving bilateral corpus striatum and right cortical ribbons, often described in "sporadic type." Patient 2 is a 68-year-old woman with rapidly progressive dementia. (*C*) Axial FLAIR and (*D*) axial DWI trace images show abnormal hyperintensity involving bilateral caudate and putamina and bilateral thalami in a hockey stick configuration, described in "variant type."

incidence around one case per 1 million people per year.[52] Prion disease results from the alteration of prion protein (PrP^{C}), normally present and most abundant in the brain, to an abnormally folded protein (PrP^{Sc}) that self-propagates by autocatalyzing the reconfiguration of normal PrP^{C}.

Depending on the pathogenesis, prion diseases are classified as acquired, hereditary, or sporadic. The largest group of prion diseases is idiopathic, accounting for 85% of the cases, and is generally referred to as sporadic. Hereditary prion disease is the second most common subtype, accounting for 10% to 15% of cases. It is further categorized according to their distinctive clinical and pathologic features, and includes genetic CJD, Gerstmann-Sträussler-Scheinker syndrome, and fatal familial insomnia. The acquired diseases are extremely rare and are further subclassified into kuru, iatrogenic CJD, and variant CJD. Kuru was isolated in a small tribe in New Guinea because of ritual cannibalism and has become almost extinct after the nterruption of this practice. Iatrogenic transmis-ion has been described from various medical rocedures that used infected human tissues. 'ariant CJD, or the human form of bovine spongi-orm encephalopathy ("mad cow disease"), is ransmitted from infected beef to humans.[52]

The classic presentation includes rapidly pro-ressive dementia with the presence of myoc-onus, visual or cerebellar signs, pyramidal/ xtrapyramidal signs, and akinetic mutism.[53]

Diffusion-weighted imaging (DWI) changes can recede the clinical onset, even in unsuspected ases with unremarkable/atypical electroen-ephalogram and CSF examination, making this echnique the cornerstone to support early diag-osis (see **Table 1**). Although there is a wide ange of radiologic patterns, "typical" findings of arly stage CJD consist of diffuse or focal, sym-netric or asymmetric DWI and T2/FLAIR hyperin-ensity involving the cortex and basal ganglia Fig. 13). Involvement of the peri-Rolandic area nd cerebellum is less common but has been eported.

The physicochemical basis for DWI abnormal-ies remains unclear. Histopathologic studies ave shown vacuolization of the neurophil, astro-liosis, and, in a few subtypes, amyloid deposition.)WI abnormalities may be attributed to diffusion estriction related to compartmentalization within acuoles or alternatively deposition of prion pro-ein. As the disease progresses, there is an in-rease in the degree and extent of T2/FLAIR and)WI hyperintensity in subcortical gray matter re-ions, which reflects the degree of spongiform egeneration. Signal changes in the cortex may uctuate with disease progression. Normal DWI ignal in advanced disease has been attributed o neuronal loss and atrophy.[52]

Atypical findings include T2/FLAIR and DWI hanges in the peri-Rolandic cortex, dorsomedial halami (double hockey stick sign) (see **Fig. 13**), osterior thalami (pulvinar area), and cerebellum. 'he "pulvinar" and double hockey stick signs ave been reported as the most sensitive radio-ogic markers for variant CJD but are not patho-nomonic for variant CJD and have also been eported in the more common sporadic CJD. ilateral basal ganglia T1 hyperintensity without)WI changes has also been reported in some ases, which is characterized by prion protein eposition in this area. Although putamen has n even higher prion protein content, the T1-hortening effects of protein in this area are pre-umed to be canceled out by the coexistent igh degree of spongiform degeneration, leading o an overall T1 relaxation time longer than that of he globus pallidus.[52]

SUMMARY

On neuroimaging atypical infections caused by parasites and prion diseases may resemble other infections, and neoplasms, metabolic or immune-mediated processes, or other noninfectious inflammatory conditions. Clinical history and presentation are important guiding differential diagnoses. Imaging plays a pivotal role in assessing the infection's extent, identifying complications, and potentially indicating the specific type of infection when characteristic features are present.

CLINICS CARE POINTS

- In patients with HIV, CNS lymphoma and toxoplasma abscess are challenging to differentiate; both have peripheral enhancement and peripheral restricted diffusion. When toxoplasmosis is suspected, an empirical trial of antitoxoplasma therapy for several weeks is considered sufficiently confirmatory. MR perfusion, MR spectroscopy, and fluorodeoxyglucose PET have been used with varying success.
- There are four stages of neurocysticercosis, and only the vesicular stage would have the characteristic cystic lesions containing scolex on computed tomography or MR imaging that fulfills the absolute criteria for diagnosis of neurocysticercosis.
- A few imaging characteristics can aid in distinguishing certain unusual infectious agents. For instance, the presence of an eccentric target sign could be indicative of cerebral toxoplasmosis, the presence of a mother cyst containing internal daughter cysts might suggest echinococcosis, and an arborized enhancement with a central linear enhancement may be specific for schistosomiasis.
- Creutzfeldt-Jakob disease is characterized by rapidly progressive dementia with the presence of myoclonus, visual or cerebellar signs, pyramidal/extrapyramidal signs, and akinetic mutism. MR imaging may show DWI hyperintensity in the cerebral cortex and deep gray nuclei.

DISCLOSURE

None

REFERENCES

1. Pittella JE. Pathology of CNS parasitic infections. Handb Clin Neurol 2013;114:65–88.

2. Jayakumar PN, Chandrashekar HS, Ellika S. Imaging of parasitic infections of the central nervous system. Handb Clin Neurol 2013;114:37–64.
3. Shih RY, Koeller KK. Bacterial, fungal, and parasitic infections of the central nervous system: radiologic-pathologic correlation and historical perspectives. Radiographics 2015;35(4):1141–69.
4. Ramsey RG, Gean AD. Neuroimaging of AIDS. I. Central nervous system toxoplasmosis. Neuroimaging Clin N Am 1997;7(2):171–86.
5. Mahadevan A, Ramalingaiah AH, Parthasarathy S, et al. Neuropathological correlate of the "concentric target sign" in MRI of HIV-associated cerebral toxoplasmosis. J Magn Reson Imaging 2013;38(2): 488–95.
6. Chinn RJ, Wilkinson ID, Hall-Craggs MA, et al. Toxoplasmosis and primary central nervous system lymphoma in HIV infection: diagnosis with MR spectroscopy. Radiology 1995;197(3):649–54.
7. Marcus C, Feizi P, Hogg J, et al. Imaging in differentiating cerebral toxoplasmosis and primary CNS lymphoma with special focus on FDG PET/CT. AJR Am J Roentgenol 2021;216(1):157–64.
8. Koeller KK, Smirniotopoulos JG, Jones RV. Primary central nervous system lymphoma: radiologic-pathologic correlation. Radiographics 1997;17(6): 1497–526.
9. Lee GT, Antelo F, Mlikotic AA. Best cases from the AFIP: cerebral toxoplasmosis. Radiographics 2009; 29(4):1200–5.
10. Mohanty S, Taylor TE, Kampondeni S, et al. Magnetic resonance imaging during life: the key to unlock cerebral malaria pathogenesis? Malar J 2014; 13:276.
11. Khuu D, Eberhard ML, Bristow BN, et al. Malaria-related hospitalizations in the United States, 2000-2014. Am J Trop Med Hyg 2017;97(1):213–21.
12. Potchen MJ, Kampondeni SD, Seydel KB, et al. Acute brain MRI findings in 120 Malawian children with cerebral malaria: new insights into an ancient disease. AJNR Am J Neuroradiol 2012;33(9):1740–6.
13. Gupta S, Patel K. Case series: MRI features in cerebral malaria. Indian J Radiol Imaging 2008;18(3): 224–6.
14. Yadav P, Sharma R, Kumar S, et al. Magnetic resonance features of cerebral malaria. Acta Radiol 2008;49(5):566–9.
15. Millan JM, San Millan JM, Muñoz M, et al. CNS complications in acute malaria: MR findings. AJNR Am J Neuroradiol 1993;14(2):493–4.
16. Martinez AJ, Visvesvara GS. Free-living, amphizoic and opportunistic amebas. Brain Pathol 1997;7(1): 583–98.
17. Alkhunaizi AM, Dawamneh MF, Banda RW, et al. Acanthamoeba encephalitis in a patient with systemic lupus treated with rituximab. Diagn Microbiol Infect Dis 2013;75(2):192–4.
18. Berger JR. Amebic infections of the central nervous system. J Neurovirol 2022;28(4–6):467–72.
19. Ranjan R, Handa A, Choudhary A, et al. Acanthamoeba infection in an interhemispheric ependymal cyst: a case report. Surg Neurol 2009;72(2):185–9.
20. Lackner P, Beer R, Broessner G, et al. Acute granulomatous acanthamoeba encephalitis in an immunocompetent patient. Neurocrit Care 2010;12(1): 91–4.
21. Booton GC, Visvesvara GS, Byers TJ, et al. Identification and distribution of *Acanthamoeba* species genotypes associated with nonkeratitis infections. J Clin Microbiol 2005;43(4):1689–93.
22. Martinez AJ. Infection of the central nervous system due to *Acanthamoeba*. Rev Infect Dis 1991; 13(Suppl 5):S399–402.
23. Viriyavejakul P, Rochanawutanon M, Sirinavin S. *Naegleria* meningomyeloencephalitis. Southeast Asian J Trop Med Public Health 1997;28(1):237–40.
24. Singh P, Kochhar R, Vashishta RK, et al. Amebic meningoencephalitis: spectrum of imaging findings. AJNR Am J Neuroradiol 2006;27(6):1217–21.
25. Güémez A, García E. Primary amoebic meningoencephalitis by. Biomolecules 2021;11(9). https://doi.org/10.3390/biom11091320.
26. Garcia HH. Parasitic infections of the nervous system. Continuum 2021;27(4):943–62.
27. Ma P, Visvesvara GS, Martinez AJ, et al. *Naegleria* and *Acanthamoeba* infections: review. Rev Infect Dis 1990;12(3):490–513.
28. Combs FJ, Erly WK, Valentino CM, et al. Best cases from the AFIP: *Balamuthia mandrillaris* amebic meningoencephalitis. Radiographics 2011;31(1): 31–5.
29. Schumacher DJ, Tien RD, Lane K. Neuroimaging findings in rare amebic infections of the central nervous system. AJNR Am J Neuroradiol 1995;16(4 Suppl):930–5.
30. Mayer PL, Larkin JA, Hennessy JM. Amebic encephalitis. Surg Neurol Int 2011;2:50.
31. Kimura-Hayama ET, Higuera JA, Corona-Cedillo R, et al. Neurocysticercosis: radiologic-pathologic correlation. Radiographics 2010;30(6):1705–19.
32. Wallin MT, Kurtzke JF. Neurocysticercosis in the United States: review of an important emerging infection. Neurology 2004;63(9):1559–64.
33. Del Brutto OH, Santibáñez R, Idrovo L, et al. Epilepsy and neurocysticercosis in Atahualpa: a door-to-door survey in rural coastal Ecuador. Epilepsia 2005;46(4):583–7.
34. Noujaim SE, Rossi MD, Rao SK, et al. CT and MR imaging of neurocysticercosis. AJR Am J Roentgenol 1999;173(6):1485–90.
35. Sotelo J, Guerrero V, Rubio F. Neurocysticercosis: a new classification based on active and inactive forms. A study of 753 cases. Arch Intern Med 1985;145(3):442–5.

36. Coates R, von Sinner W, Rahm B. MR imaging of an intracerebral hydatid cyst. AJNR Am J Neuroradiol 1990;11(6):1249–50.
37. Pedrosa I, Saíz A, Arrazola J, et al. Hydatid disease: radiologic and pathologic features and complications. Radiographics 2000;20(3):795–817.
38. Kantzanou M, Karalexi MA, Vassalos CM, et al. Central nervous system cystic echinococcosis: a systematic review. Germs 2022;12(2):283–91.
39. Rumboldt Z, Jednacak H, Talan-Hranilović J, et al. Unusual appearance of a cisternal hydatid cyst. AJNR Am J Neuroradiol 2003;24(1):112–4.
40. Ba'assiri A, Haddad FS. Primary extradural intracranial hydatid disease: CT appearance. AJNR Am J Neuroradiol 1984;5(4):474–5.
41. Mascalchi M, Ragazzoni A, Dal Pozzo G. Pontine hydatid cyst in association with an acoustic neurinoma: MR appearance in an unusual case. AJNR Am J Neuroradiol 1991;12(1):78–9.
42. Jena A, Tripathi RP, Jain AK. Primary spinal echinococcosis causing paraplegia: case report with MR and pathologic correlation. AJNR Am J Neuroradiol 1991;12(3):560.
43. Steinmann P, Keiser J, Bos R, et al. Schistosomiasis and water resources development: systematic review, meta-analysis, and estimates of people at risk. Lancet Infect Dis 2006;6(7):411–25.
44. Colley DG, Bustinduy AL, Secor WE, et al. Human schistosomiasis. Lancet 2014;383(9936):2253–64.
45. Lu CY, Zhao S, Wei Y. Cerebral schistosomiasis: MRI features with pathological correlation. Acta Radiol 2021;62(5):646–52.
46. Betting LE, Pirani C, de Souza Queiroz L, et al. Seizures and cerebral schistosomiasis. Arch Neurol 2005;62(6):1008–10.
47. Ross AG, McManus DP, Farrar J, et al. Neuroschistosomiasis. J Neurol 2012;259(1):22–32.
48. Sanelli PC, Lev MH, Gonzalez RG, et al. Unique linear and nodular MR enhancement pattern in schistosomiasis of the central nervous system: report of three patients. AJR Am J Roentgenol 2001;177(6):1471–4.
49. Wu K, Zhao HY, Shu K, et al. Encephalic. Front Neurol 2022;13:990998.
50. Jobanputra K, Raj K, Yu F, et al. Intramedullary neurocysticercosis mimicking cord tumor. J Clin Imaging Sci 2020;10:7.
51. Manzella A, Borba-Filho P, Brandt CT, et al. Brain magnetic resonance imaging findings in young patients with hepatosplenic schistosomiasis mansoni without overt symptoms. Am J Trop Med Hyg 2012;86(6):982–7.
52. Fragoso DC, Gonçalves Filho AL, Pacheco FT, et al. Imaging of Creutzfeldt-Jakob disease: imaging patterns and their differential diagnosis. Radiographics 2017;37(1):234–57.
53. Zerr I, Kallenberg K, Summers DM, et al. Updated clinical diagnostic criteria for sporadic Creutzfeldt-Jakob disease. Brain 2009;132(Pt 10):2659–68.

Multiple Sclerosis
Clinical Update and Clinically-Oriented Radiologic Reporting

Phuong Nguyen, MD[a], Torge Rempe, MD, PhD[b],
Reza Forghani, MD, PhD[a,c,d,e,*]

KEYWORDS

• Multiple sclerosis • McDonald criteria • MAGNIMS • MR imaging protocols • Central vein sign
• Paramagnetic rim lesion • Optic neuritis • Gadolinium-based contrast agents

KEY POINTS

- Imaging is an integral part of establishing hallmarks of multiple sclerosis (MS) diagnosis, including dissemination in space and time of demyelination, as well as monitoring disease status in MS patients on treatment.
- Findings on MR imaging of the brain and spine are incorporated in multiple revisions of the McDonald diagnosis criteria and are extensively discussed in consensus guidelines by the Magnetic Resonance Imaging in MS (MAGNIMS).
- Standardized MR protocols have been proposed by Consortium of Multiple Sclerosis Centers (CMSC) and discussed in 2021 Magnetic Resonance Imaging in Multiple Sclerosis (MAGNIMS) - Consortium of Multiple Sclerosis Centres (CMSC) - North American Imaging in Multiple Sclerosis Cooperative (NAIMS) international consensus recommendations.
- Emerging imaging findings in MS, including cortical lesions, central vein sign, and paramagnetic rim lesions are increasingly recognized and are topics of interests for future revisions of consensus guidelines.
- Data regarding the potential adverse effect of gadolinium-based contrast agents call for its judicious use in routine imaging to monitor disease status.

INTRODUCTION: MULTIPLE SCLEROSIS—BRIEF CLINICAL OVERVIEW AND UPDATES

Multiple sclerosis (MS) is a chronic inflammatory disease of the central nervous system. It affects 2.8 million people worldwide, with a global incidence of 2.1 per 100,000 persons/year.[1] It is commonly diagnosed in younger patient population and is more prevalent in females.[1] Though the precise pathogenesis of MS remains unclear and is likely multifactorial, MS is characterized by myelin destruction of the brain and spinal cord.[2,3] The pathologic hallmark of MS is the formation of plaques reflecting foci of inflammation, demyelination, and axonal destruction. These are macroscopically visible on modern MR imaging and aid in the diagnosis of MS by imaging.

[a] Department of Radiology, University of Florida College of Medicine, 1600 SW Archer Road, Gainesville, FL 32610-0374, USA; [b] Department of Neurology, University of Florida College of Medicine, Norman Fixel Institute for Neurological Diseases, 3009 SW Williston Road, Gainesville, FL 32608, USA; [c] Division of Movement Disorders, Department of Neurology, University of Florida College of Medicine, Norman Fixel Institute for Neurological Diseases, 3009 SW Williston Road, Gainesville, FL 32608, USA; [d] Division of Medical Physics, University of Florida College of Medicine, 1600 SW Archer Road, Gainesville, FL 32610-0374, USA; [e] Radiomics and Augmented Intelligence Laboratory (RAIL), Department of Radiology and the Norman Fixel Institute for Neurological Diseases, University of Florida College of Medicine, Room 221.1, 3011 SW Williston Road, Gainesville, FL 32608, USA
* Corresponding author. 1600 Southwest Archer Road, Gainesville, FL 32610-0374.
E-mail address: r.forghani@ufl.edu

Magn Reson Imaging Clin N Am 32 (2024) 363–374
https://doi.org/10.1016/j.mric.2024.01.001
1064-9689/24/

MS is a heterogenous clinical entity with many clinical subtypes reflecting various clinical courses. Traditional subtypes of MS include relapsing-remitting (RRMS), secondary progressive (SPMS), primary progressive (PPMS), and progressive relapsing (PRMS), though this classification does not adequately reflect the complexity of the disease.[4] At the time of presentation, MS patients exhibit symptoms related to acute demyelination in the brain and spine, including unilateral painful vision loss, weakness, and sensory deficits, as well as brain stem and cerebellar dysfunctions.[5] The diagnosis of MS is based on a combination of clinical assessment, laboratory findings, neurophysiological testing, and radiological imaging. It is centered around the establishment of dissemination in space (DIS) and dissemination in time (DIT) of demyelinating events, as specified by the McDonald criteria.[6] Multiple revisions of MS diagnostic criteria reflect continuously expanding knowledge of the disease and rapidly evolving technology available for disease assessment.

Though MS is not curable, there has been ongoing advancement in disease-modifying therapies (DMTs) to slow disease progression. Primarily acting by immunomodulatory and -immunosuppressive mechanisms, current DMTs include different classes of injectable, intravenous, and oral agents, including interferon beta, monoclonal antibodies, and small molecules.[7] Additionally, treatment strategies other than medication-induced immunosuppression have been proposed and are being studied. These include immune ablation and autologous hematopoietic stem cell transplantation, promotion of remyelination and myelin protection, etc.[5,8] With many effective treatment options available and in development, management of MS focuses on slowing or eliminating disease progression,[5] in which disease activity monitoring, especially with imaging, is essential.

OVERVIEW OF MR IMAGING IN DIAGNOSIS AND MONITORING OF MULTIPLE SCLEROSIS

Imaging plays an integral part in establishing the diagnosis of MS, differentiating it from many mimickers, as well as monitoring its activity. Findings on MR imaging of the brain and spinal cord have been incorporated into the McDonald criteria for MS since its initial version in 2001.[9] Multiple iterations of the diagnostic criteria as well as recommendations and guidelines put forth by various groups of multidisciplinary experts maintain the indispensable role of MR imaging in evaluating MS patients. These are revised frequently to keep up with the rapidly evolving knowledge of MS-related imaging findings as well as rapidly expanding novel array of imaging techniques.

The McDonald criteria play a central role in MS diagnosis and underscore the ability of MR imaging of the brain and spinal cord to complement clinical and paraclinical data. The criteria focus on 2 main features of the disease, that are dissemination in space (DIS) and dissemination in time (DIT) of demyelinating events. These features can often be established by imaging and aid the MS diagnosis in the appropriate clinical settings. DIS is supported by the presence of 1 or more T2-weighted hyperintense lesions in at least 2 out of 4 topographic areas of the brain, that are periventricular, cortical/juxtacortical, infratentorial, and spinal cord[6,10] (**Fig. 1**). DIS refers to the simultaneous presence of asymptomatic gadolinium-enhancing and non-enhancing lesions at any time; or at least 1 new lesion (enhancing or non-enhancing) on follow-up imaging.[10]

In the latest revision of the McDonald criteria issued in 2017, MR imaging of the brain is recommended in all patients with clinical presentation concerning for MS and MR imaging of the spinal cord when myelopathy is suspected clinically. The 2017 McDonald criteria attempted to simplify the diagnostic criteria in previous iterations and incorporated guidelines from other expert groups. Major changes in this version include allowing *cerebrospinal fluid* oligoclonal band to substitute DIT on initial and follow-up imaging, inclusion of symptomatic lesions in the brain stem and spinal cord in the determination of DIS and DIT, and inclusion of cortical lesions as juxtacortical equivalent.[6] This revision was found to shorten time to diagnosis while performing with similar accuracy, higher sensitivity, and lower specificity as compared to the 2010 McDonald criteria.[11–16]

The 2015 consensus guidelines from the Magnetic Resonance Imaging in MS (MAGNIMS) expert group specifically address the role of MR imaging in MS.[17] Applicable to brain MR imaging, these guidelines advocate increasing the number of lesions needed to define periventricular involvement, inclusion of optic nerve findings, and combining symptomatic and asymptomatic lesions in MS diagnostic criteria. For imaging of the spine, they recommended whole spinal cord imaging to aid to the establishment of DIS in patients with spinal cord symptoms or patients without spinal cord symptoms who do not adequately demonstrate DIS on MR imaging brain. The value of spinal cord MR imaging in establishing DIT without new symptoms localizing to the spinal cord is however low.[18]

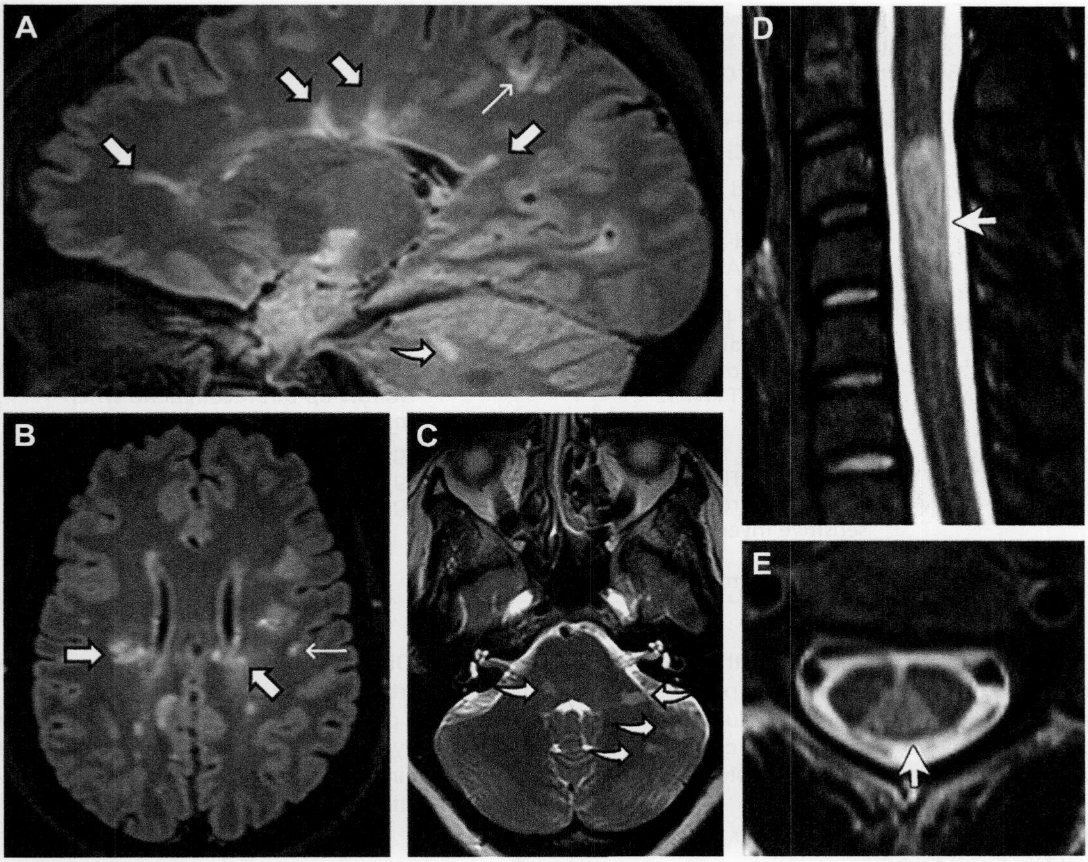

Fig. 1. Multiple sclerosis demyelinating lesions in topographic distribution included in McDonald criteria: periventricular lesions (*thick straight arrows*), juxtacortical lesions (*thin straight arrows*), infratentorial lesions (*curved arrows*), and spinal cord lesions (*arrowhead*) shown on sagittal and axial 3D T2 fluid-attenuated inversion recovery (FLAIR) (*A, B*), axial T2 TSE (*C*) of the brain, and sagittal STIR (*D*) and axial T2 TSE (*E*) of the cervical spine.

MR IMAGING PROTOCOLS IN MULTIPLE SCLEROSIS

The 2016 recommendations from the Consortium of Multiple Sclerosis Centers (CMSC)[19] propose guidelines for standardized MR imaging protocols (**Table 1**). For diagnosis and routine follow-up of MS patient, the proposed protocol for MR imaging of the brain includes 5 core sequences. Lesion detection is mainly achieved with a sagittal T2-weighted fluid-attenuated inversion recovery (FLAIR) and T2-weighted imaging (axial 2D spin-echo or 3D sequence), for better detection of corpus callosum lesions and posterior fossa lesions, respectively. A post-contrast T1-weighted sequence (axial spin echo or 3D techniques) is included to evaluate for lesion enhancement reflecting active inflammation. Additionally, other pathology such as ischemia and treatment-related complications such as progressive multifocal leukoencephalopathy (PML) can be evaluated on axial diffusion-weighted imaging (DWI). Volumetric analysis can be performed on anatomic pre-contrast 3D IR-prepared T1-weighted spoiled gradient echo sequence. For MR imaging of the spinal cord, it is recommended that cervical cord at a minimum should be imaged. The sagittal T2-weighted sequence is used for lesion detection with confirmation on at least 1 sagittal short Tl inversion recovery (STIR), proton attenuation or T1 phase-sensitive inversion recovery (PSIR), and axial T2 weighted image (WI) or post-contrast T1-weighted imaging (T1WI).

The MAGNIMS-CMSC-NAIMS 2021 international consensus recommendations[20] capture the 2015 MAGNIMS and 2016 CMSC guidelines, as well as the 2017 McDonald criteria, and expand on the use MR imaging in patients with MS. Regarding standardized magnetic resonance MR protocol, it mostly agrees with the

Table 1
Summary of standardized MR imaging protocols for multiple sclerosis patients proposed by the Consortium of Multiple Sclerosis Centers and MAGNIMS-CMSC-NAIMS 2021 guidelines

	Consortium of Multiple Sclerosis Centers (CMSC) 2016	MAGNIMS-CMSC-NAIMS 2021
Brain protocol	3D IR-prepared T1 gradient echo 3D Sagittal T2W FLAIR *or* 2D axial and sagittal fluid-attenuated inversion recovery (FLAIR) 3D T2WI *or* 2D axial PD or T2WI FSE 3D FLASH (FFE [Fast Field Echo]/SPGR [spoiled gradient recalled]) post-gadolinium *or* 2D axial post-gadolinium T1WI SE 2D axial DWI	3D T1W sequence is optional 3D Sagittal T2W FLAIR *or* 2D axial and sagittal FLAIR Axial T2WI FSE (Fast Spin Echo)/TSE (Turbo Spin Echo) Axial or 3D sagittal T1WI post-gadolinium *DWI is optional in diagnosis and follow-up but recommend when monitoring for PML*
Spine protocol	Sagittal T2W Sagittal short TI inversion recovery (STIR), PD (Proton Density), or phase-sensitive inversion recovery (PSIR) Axial T2/T2* Axial post-contrast T1	Sagittal T2W Sagittal STIR, PD, or PSIR Sagittal T1 post-contrast

2016 CMSC recommendations, though it considers DWI and pre-contrast IR-prepared T1W sequences optional for brain evaluation at diagnosis; and favors sagittal post-contrast T1WI over axial spinal imaging (see **Table 1**).

UPDATES ON BRAIN MR IMAGING IN MULTIPLE SCLEROSIS

Periventricular Lesions

Amongst topographic brain white matter areas considered in DIS, periventricular lesions (PVLs) are less specific to MS. Periventricular T2 hyperintensity capping along the frontal and occipital horns is commonly seen on 2D FLAIR in healthy adults, with occipital horn capping more prominent on 3T imaging.[21] PVLs are also seen in other etiologies other than demyelination. The total number and volume of PVLs in RRMS patients have been shown to be no different than in patient with ischemic stroke.[22] Compared to patients with migraine disorder, the number and volume of PVLs along the lateral ventricle body and posterior horns are higher in RRMS patients, but those of PVLs along the anterior and temporal horns show no difference.[22] Thus, as highlighted in the 2016 MAGNIMS guideline, there are currently considerations to increase the minimum number of lesions required to establish periventricular involvement from 1 to 3. In young patients with typical symptoms of MS, applying this change to the 2010 McDonald criteria results in a decrease in its sensitivity, with an increase in specificity of DIS criteria, though the overall specificity when combined DIS and DIT remains the same.[23] In a larger cohort with wider age range (16–60 years), this change demonstrates a very modest increase in specificity in DIS criteria at the expense of a larger drop in sensitivity.[18] Thus, it is not currently adopted in the 2017 McDonald criteria.

Cortical Lesions

The common presence of cortical lesions (CLs) in MS patients has been widely accepted in neuropathological studies.[24] Histologically, they reflect 3 patterns of demyelination: leukocortical, intracortical, and subpial.[25] With evolving modern imaging technologies, identification of CLs on MR imaging is becoming increasingly recognized in MS. These are not reported in migraine and NMO (neuromyelitis optica) and are rare in healthy adults.[17] Clinically CLs are associated with clinical disability in MS patients.[26–29]

Many of these CLs are however not visualized on standard 1.5 T and 3.0 T MR imaging available for clinical use, and poor contrast of these lesions compared to gray matter signal makes it more challenging to identify on conventional MR imaging sequences[24] (**Fig. 2**). A comparative study with immunohistochemistry demonstrated that only 3% to 5% of intracortical lesions and 22% to 41% of leukocortical lesions are detected on postmortem T2 spin-echo and 3D FLAIR, compared to 63% to 71% of white matter lesions.[30] Compared to 3T MR imaging, 7T MR imaging detects more CLs,[31,32] with more than twice the number of CLs detected on FLAIR and T2*[33]; as well as greater accumulation

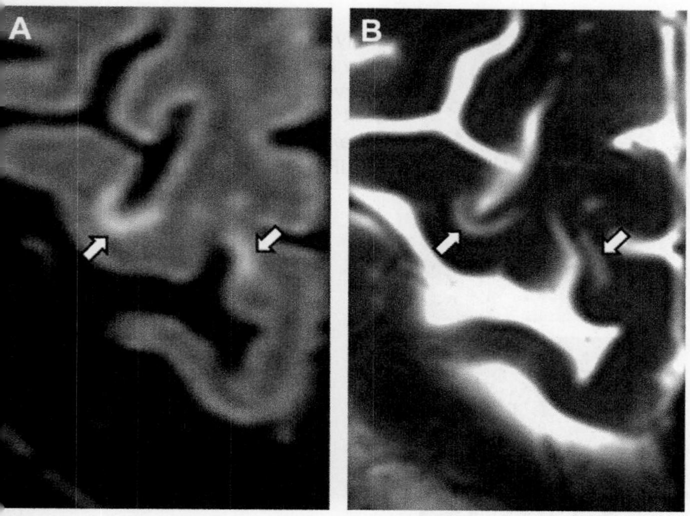

Fig. 2. Cortical demyelinating lesions (*arrows*) in an MS patient shown on axial 3D T2 FLAIR (*A*) and T2 TSE (*B*) images.

ate.[28] Advanced MR imaging sequences, such as ouble inversion recovery, phase-sensitive inversion ecovery, and magnetization-prepared rapid radient echo, further increase CL detection rate at arious field strengths.[29,34–36]

As there is currently a growing interest in CLs, 017 McDonald criteria expanded the juxtacortical esion classification to include cortical lesions.[6] However, identification and reporting of CLs on MR imaging is subject to limited availability of dvanced MR imaging sequences, lack of standardized parameters, and variable terminology.[17]

ptic Nerve Findings

ptic neuritis (ON) is one of the common clinical nanifestations of MS. It is the presenting symptom in 15% to 20% of MS patients and occurs at ome point during the course of the disease in 0% to 70% of patients.[37,38] While it can occur n isolation as a monophasic disease, patients vith optic neuritis have an approximately 50% sk of developing MS within 15 years after onset, nd this risk is associated with the presence of esions on brain MR imaging.[39,40] However, ompared to other symptoms of clinically isolated yndrome, optic neuritis implies a favorable prognosis with lower rates of developing MS.[40] Additionally, autoimmune-mediated optic neuritis can lso be present in other disorders such as neuromyelitis optica spectrum disorder (NMOSD) and nyelin oligodendrocyte glycoprotein antibody-ssociated disease (MOGAD). Distinguishing MS-associated ON from that seen in other disorders based on MR imaging findings is difficult, hough shorter segment optic nerve inflammation nd unilateral involvement are found more frequently in MS.[41,42] For a greater discussion of MR imaging findings in NMOSD and MOGAD, the reader is referred to a separate article dedicated to this topic in this issue.

MAGNIMS 2016 advocates for inclusion of MR imaging findings of optic nerve inflammation in DIS criteria.[17] In symptomatic patients, inclusion of optic nerve findings in DIS criteria increases sensitivity and decreases specificity of 2017 McDonald criteria, though it does not change its performance when applied to asymptomatic patients.[43] This is not currently adopted in 2017 McDonald criteria due to insufficient data.[6] Thus, optic nerve MR imaging is not recommended routinely in clinically typical ON, but can be considered to evaluate for alternative etiologies of optic neuropathy.

Central Vein Sign

The central vein sign (CVS) on MR imaging has been well documented in patients with MS. It denotes the presence of linear venular susceptibility artifact within MS lesions (**Fig. 3**) and is thought to reflect the hallmark perivenular inflammation histologically. It is reported in 41% to 92% of MS patients.[44–47] Amongst topographic areas of MS lesions, a large portion of lesions with CVS are in the periventricularly distributed lesions (41% on T2* echo planar imaging [EPI],[48] 55% on susceptibility weighted imaging [SWI][45]). CVS is present in 68% of new lesions on 3-year follow-up.[49] The ability to detect CVS however depends on field strength (higher at ultra-high-field 7T[46,50]) and on specific susceptibility-sensitive sequences. The proportion of white matter lesions with CVS is found to be statistically higher in MS compared to cerebral small

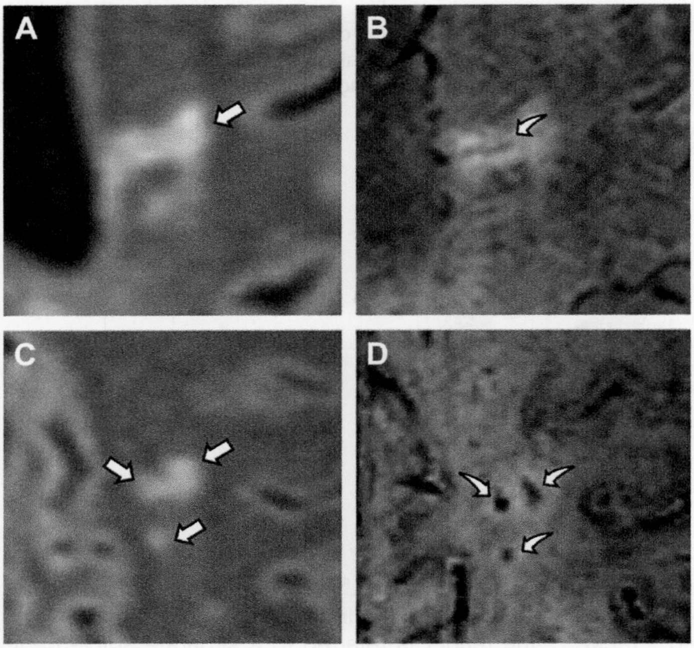

Fig. 3. Central veins seen longitudinally as a hypointense line (*curved arrow* in *B*) and in cross section as dots (*curved arrows* in *D*) on axial SWI, present within demyelinating lesions (*straight arrows*) shown on 3D T2 FLAIR (*A and C*).

vessel disease,[45] NMOSD,[44,47] and inflammatory vasculopathy, including antiphospholipid syndrome, systemic lupus, Behcet, Primary angiitis of the central nervous system,[48] as well as migraine.[51] There have been efforts to establish a threshold proportion of CVS-positive lesions for MS diagnosis. A threshold of about 40% provides high specificity of 84% to 100% and high sensitivity of 46% to 100% to MS versus other non-MS diagnoses.[52] However, the proportion of CVS-positive lesions has been reported to decrease with age and vascular risk factors such as hypertension, diabetes, and obesity and smoking,[53] complicating threshold setting. Due to rapidly evolving evidence regarding CVS and its role in diagnosing and differentiating MS from other etiologies, a consensus statement from the North American Imaging in Multiple Sclerosis Cooperative attempted to standardize the use CVS.[54] It proposed a standardized radiographic definition of a central vein on T2*-weighted images, which include thin hypointense line or small dot in morphology identified in 2 orthogonal planes, small (<2 mm) in diameter, central in position, and run partially or completely through the lesion.

Paramagnetic Rim Lesions

The paramagnetic rim lesions (PRLs) in MS have been increasingly recognized in the last decade. They describe chronic non-enhancing white matter lesions with a peripheral rim of susceptibility due to paramagnetism (**Fig. 4**). Histologically the paramagnetic rim correlates with iron-laden macrophages at the edge of smoldering or chronic active lesions.[52] They account for about 10% of MS lesions and are present in about 41% of MS patients.[55] Clinically PRLs are associated with poor prognosis, including greater severity, increased risk of relapse and progression, worse cognitive recovery, and disability.[56–59] Larger size and higher T1 time are features of enhancing MS lesions that evolve into PRLs.[60] PRLs themselves demonstrate higher T1 time compared to non-PRLs, reflecting a higher degree of demyelination and cell loss.[57] Though PRLs are mostly reported on studies at 7T MR imaging, they can be identified at similar rate with 1.5 T and 3T MR imaging with comparable interobserver agreement.[61] Identification of 1 or more PRLs has a 93% to 100% specificity for MS and CIS diagnosis with low sensitivity of 19% to 52%.[62,63] Being a relatively new finding, PRLs have not been incorporated into MS diagnostic criteria. However, due to their diagnostic and prognostic potentials, PRLs are gaining interests in the field and, together with CVS, should be considered ancillary findings and reported in MR imaging examination in patients with suspected demyelinating diseases.

UPDATES ON SPINE MR IMAGING IN MULTIPLE SCLEROSIS

As included in the McDonald criteria, lesions in the spinal cord can contribute to DIS and DIT.[6,10] MR

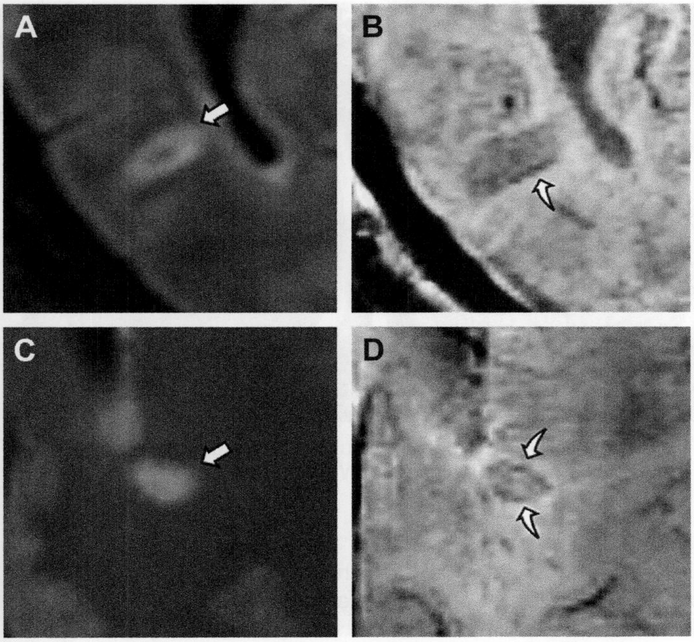

Fig. 4. Paramagnetic rims seen as peripheral hypointense line (*curved arrows*) on axial SWI (*B and D*) surrounding demyelinating lesions (*straight arrows*) shown on 3D T2 FLAIR (*A and C*).

imaging of spinal cord also allows for evaluation of alternative etiologies of spinal cord symptoms. Therefore, imaging of the spinal cord is an integral part of MS evaluation and diagnosis. While the 2015 MAGNIMS consensus guidelines only recommend MR imaging of the spinal cord in patients with signs and symptoms localizing to the spinal cord or when DIS is not fulfilled by brain MR imaging findings,[17] spinal cord imaging is frequently included in initial MS work-up in clinical practice given the relatively high rate of asymptomatic spinal cord lesions (approximately 27% in patients with clinically isolated syndrome).[64] Furthermore, spinal cord MR imaging can aid in prognostication as spinal cord lesions on baseline MR imaging signify a higher MS risk in clinically isolated syndrome and a higher risk for development of MS-related disability and secondary progressive MS.[65–67]

Current guidelines do not recommend spinal cord MR imaging in routine MS monitoring. However, asymptomatic spinal cord lesions are observed in 15% to 31% of clinically stable patients.[68–70] While new spinal cord lesions are associated with increased risk of relapse and worsened disability,[71] the presence of asymptomatic spinal cord lesions is not associated with increased relapse, disease progression,[68] or time to disability development,[72] but correlates with new brain or spinal cord lesions.[68] Thus, the specific role of spinal cord MR imaging in patients without spinal cord symptoms for disease monitoring and prognostication remains a topic of ongoing discussion.

THE USE OF GADOLINIUM IN MONITORING PATIENTS WITH MULTIPLE SCLEROSIS

Gadolinium enhancement in MS lesions (**Fig. 5**) reflects early phase of inflammation, representing distribution of gadolinium in MS lesions through disrupted blood-brain-barrier and glymphatic system.[73] Therefore, besides aiding in evaluation of non-MS etiologies, the use of gadolinium-based contrast agent (GBCA) in the initial MR imaging examination helps identify lesions with active inflammation and establish DIT. Thus, there is little controversy regarding the use of gadolinium in the diagnosis of MS on MR imaging. However, the routine use of GBCA on follow-up MR imaging is the subject of debate. Early data suggested that GBCA increased sensitivity in detecting disease progression on imaging.[74] However, this benefit is under scrutiny given advancement in spatial and contrast resolution in modern imaging techniques. On follow-up imaging, though a small proportion (approximately 2%–5%) of enhancing lesions can be missed on non-contrast imaging, it does not affect overall assessment of disease status.[75] In a small study of 33 MR imaging examinations, all patients with enhancing lesions also demonstrated disease progression on non-contrast imaging.[76]

The diminishing benefits of GBCA in lesion detection are also weighed against growing

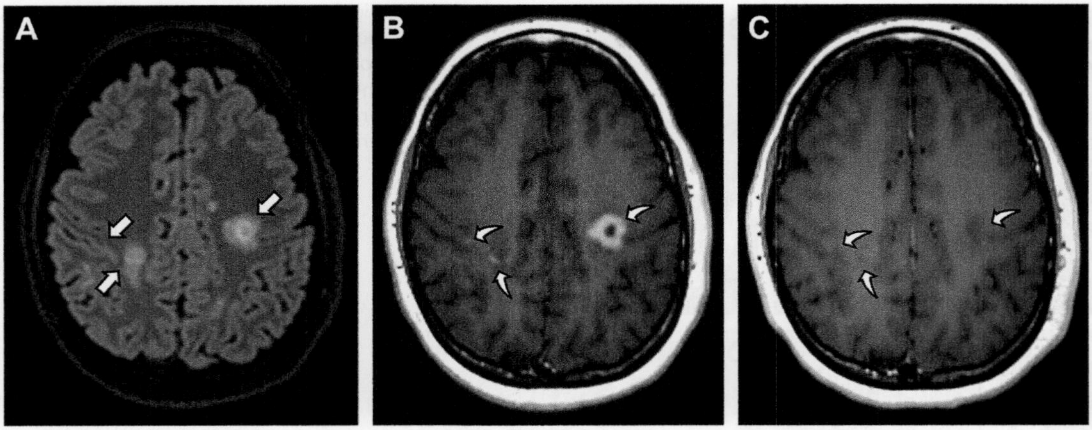

Fig. 5. Demyelinating lesions (*straight arrows*) on 3D T2 FLAIR (*A*) demonstrating gadolinium contrast enhancement (*curved arrows*) on 3D post-contrast T1W images (*B*). Post-contrast T1W images obtained 12 weeks after starting on therapy showing resolution of enhancement (*C*).

considerations of GBCA's adverse effects. There is the potential association of nephrogenic systemic fibrosis (NSF), a rare but potentially lethal condition in patients with renal impairment, with the use of GBCA, particularly with nonionic linear class, and with higher than standard GBCA doses.[77] However, it should be noted that with changes in clinical practice that include avoiding multiple high-dose GBCA injections in patients with renal impairment and introduction of novel GBCAs, NSF has nearly been eliminated.[78] In patients with chronic kidney disease stages 4 and 5 (eGFR < 30 mL/min/1.73 m2), ACR (American College of Radiology) group-I GBCAs are contraindicated and only ACR group-II GBCAs should be used.[79] Nonetheless, if there is not a true added value, a case may be made for not using GBCA for MS surveillance, especially in patients with renal impairment. In addition, there has been a growing evidence of gadolinium deposition in the globus pallidus and dentate nucleus[80] since its first description in 2014.[81] While its clinical significance remains uncertain,[80] its presence raises the question of judicious use of GBCA in multiple routine follow-up MR imaging examinations in MS patients. Whether or not GBCA is necessary for follow-up in MS patients is an on-going debate, as its proponents advocate for its role in evaluating treatment complications such as PML and immune reconstitution inflammatory syndrome (IRIS) or identify additionally ancillary findings of active disease such as leptomeningeal inflammation.[82,83]

Table 2
Recommendation for minimum[a] essential information to be included in clinically-oriented reporting of brain MR imaging studies for patient with suspected or known diagnosis of multiple sclerosis

	Initial Evaluation	Follow-up
Brain	1. Description of lesion distribution, divided into 4 topographic areas (a) periventricular; (b) cortical/juxtacortical; (c) infratentorial; and (d) spinal cord (if spine imaging was performed). 2. Description of non-enhancing and enhancing lesions (if contrast-enhanced sequences were performed) Strongly consider: 3. Evaluation of lesions with central vein sign 4. Evaluation of paramagnetic rim lesions 5. Evaluation of lesions with restricted diffusion	1. Description and comparison of new lesions on T2/FLAIR sequence 2. Description and comparison of non-enhancing and enhancing lesions (if contrast-enhanced sequences were performed) Strongly consider: 3. Evaluation of paramagnetic rim lesions 4. Evaluation of lesions with restricted diffusion

[a] This table recommends the minimal suggested information pertaining to MS and does not preclude a broader evaluation, including standard evaluation performed on brain MR imaging or evaluation of other lesions and ancillary findings.

SEGMENTATION TOOLS

Segmentation tools for volumetric assessment of the brain and the mean upper cervical spinal cord area with the determination of annual volume loss rates have become a common radiographic research metric for progressive MS trials and are now commercially available. However, the use of such segmentation tools is not yet recommended for routine use in clinical practice given significant noise and a high degree of variability across scanners and segmentation tools.

SUMMARY AND RECOMMENDATIONS FOR RADIOLOGY REPORTING

This article summarizes the important role of magnetic resonance (MR) imaging in MS diagnosis and disease monitoring as part of many diagnostic criteria and consensus guidelines, and efforts to standardize imaging protocols. In **Table 2**, the authors provide recommendations on minimum criteria that should be included in radiologic reports of brain MR imaging scans for patients suspected or known to have MS. Emerging radiologic features seen in patients with MS which can potentially play a role in the future are also highlighted. Finally, the authors conclude the article with a discussion of the use of GBCA in disease monitoring. In the context of this article, several key pieces of information should be considered in radiology reporting of imaging studies for MS. Distribution of demyelinating lesions should be summarized according to regions of the central nervous system included in the McDonald criteria (ie, periventricular, juxtacortical/cortical, infratentorial, and spinal cord) to facilitate assessment of dissemination in space. The number of lesions should be reported as single or multiple, particularly in the periventricular region. The presence of contrast enhancing and/or non-enhancing lesions needs to be reported to help distinguish dissemination in time or lack thereof. Ancillary findings of demyelinating lesions in MS, such as central veins and paramagnetic rims, should be assessed and commented on. For surveillance radiological examinations of MS patients who are on treatment, identification of new lesions is crucial. Finally, as new data are being produced, judicious use of GBCA should be considered in surveillance examination, particularly in patients with impaired renal function.

DISCLOSURE

R. Forghani has or has recently had a research collaboration/grant and has acted as consultant and/or speaker for Nuance Communications Inc., Canon Medical Systems Inc., and GE Healthcare. R. Forghani is also a co-investigator on a National Institutes of Health STTR grant subaward and a co-principal investigator on a National Science Foundation grant.

REFERENCES

1. Walton C, King R, Rechtman L, et al. Rising prevalence of multiple sclerosis worldwide: Insights from the Atlas of MS, third edition. Mult Scler 2020; 26(14):1816–21.
2. Lemus HN, Warrington AE, Rodriguez M. Multiple sclerosis: mechanisms of disease and strategies for myelin and axonal repair. Neurol Clin 2018; 36(1):1–11.
3. Garg N, Smith TW. An update on immunopathogenesis, diagnosis, and treatment of multiple sclerosis. Brain Behav 2015;5(9):e00362.
4. Oh J, Vidal-Jordana A, Montalban X. Multiple sclerosis: clinical aspects. Curr Opin Neurol 2018;31(6): 752–9.
5. Reich DS, Lucchinetti CF, Calabresi PA. Multiple sclerosis. N Engl J Med 2018;378(2):169–80.
6. Thompson AJ, Banwell BL, Barkhof F, et al. Diagnosis of multiple sclerosis: 2017 revisions of the McDonald criteria. Lancet Neurol 2018;17(2):162–73.
7. Tintore M, Vidal-Jordana A, Sastre-Garriga J. Treatment of multiple sclerosis - success from bench to bedside. Nat Rev Neurol 2019;15(1):53–8.
8. Gholamzad M, Ebtekar M, Ardestani MS, et al. A comprehensive review on the treatment approaches of multiple sclerosis: currently and in the future. Inflamm Res 2019;68(1):25–38.
9. McDonald WI, Compston A, Edan G, et al. Recommended diagnostic criteria for multiple sclerosis: guidelines from the International Panel on the diagnosis of multiple sclerosis. Ann Neurol 2001;50(1): 121–7.
10. Polman CH, Reingold SC, Banwell B, et al. Diagnostic criteria for multiple sclerosis: 2010 revisions to the McDonald criteria. Ann Neurol 2011;69(2): 292–302.
11. van der Vuurst de Vries RM, Mescheriakova JY, Wong YYM, et al. Application of the 2017 revised mcdonald criteria for multiple sclerosis to patients with a typical clinically isolated syndrome. JAMA Neurol 2018;75(11):1392–8.
12. Gaetani L, Prosperini L, Mancini A, et al. 2017 revisions of McDonald criteria shorten the time to diagnosis of multiple sclerosis in clinically isolated syndromes. J Neurol 2018;265(11):2684–7.
13. Filippi M, Preziosa P, Meani A, et al. Performance of the 2017 and 2010 revised mcdonald criteria in predicting MS diagnosis after a clinically isolated syndrome: A MAGNIMS study. Neurology 2022;98(1): e1–14.

14. Habek M, Pavičić T, Ruška B, et al. Establishing the diagnosis of multiple sclerosis in Croatian patients with clinically isolated syndrome: 2010 versus 2017 McDonald criteria. Mult Scler Relat Disord 2018;25: 99–103.
15. Hyun JW, Kim W, Huh SY, et al. Application of the 2017 McDonald diagnostic criteria for multiple sclerosis in Korean patients with clinically isolated syndrome. Mult Scler 2019;25(11):1488–95.
16. Lee DH, Peschke M, Utz KS, et al. Diagnostic value of the 2017 McDonald criteria in patients with a first demyelinating event suggestive of relapsing-remitting multiple sclerosis. Eur J Neurol 2019;26(3): 540–5.
17. Filippi M, Rocca MA, Ciccarelli O, et al. MRI criteria for the diagnosis of multiple sclerosis: MAGNIMS consensus guidelines. Lancet Neurol 2016;15(3): 292–303.
18. Filippi M, Preziosa P, Meani A, et al. Prediction of a multiple sclerosis diagnosis in patients with clinically isolated syndrome using the 2016 MAGNIMS and 2010 McDonald criteria: a retrospective study. Lancet Neurol 2018;17(2):133–42.
19. Traboulsee A, Simon JH, Stone L, et al. Revised recommendations of the consortium of MS centers task force for a standardized MRI protocol and clinical guidelines for the diagnosis and follow-up of multiple sclerosis. AJNR Am J Neuroradiol 2016;37(3): 394–401.
20. Wattjes MP, Ciccarelli O, Reich DS, et al. 2021 MAGNIMS-CMSC-NAIMS consensus recommendations on the use of MRI in patients with multiple sclerosis. Lancet Neurol 2021;20(8):653–70.
21. Neema M, Guss ZD, Stankiewicz JM, et al. Normal findings on brain fluid-attenuated inversion recovery MR images at 3T. AJNR Am J Neuroradiol 2009; 30(5):911–6.
22. Casini G, Yurashevich M, Vanga R, et al. Are periventricular lesions specific for multiple sclerosis? J Neurol Neurophysiol 2013;4(2):150.
23. Brownlee WJ, Miszkiel KA, Altmann DR, et al. Periventricular lesions and MS diagnostic criteria in young adults with typical clinically isolated syndromes. Mult Scler 2017;23(7):1031–4.
24. Calabrese M, Filippi M, Gallo P. Cortical lesions in multiple sclerosis. Nat Rev Neurol 2010;6(8): 438–44.
25. Peterson JW, Bö L, Mörk S, et al. Transected neurites, apoptotic neurons, and reduced inflammation in cortical multiple sclerosis lesions. Ann Neurol 2001;50(3):389–400.
26. Calabrese M, Rocca MA, Atzori M, et al. Cortical lesions in primary progressive multiple sclerosis: a 2-year longitudinal MR study. Neurology 2009;72(15): 1330–6.
27. Calabrese M, Rocca MA, Atzori M, et al. A 3-year magnetic resonance imaging study of cortical lesions in relapse-onset multiple sclerosis. Ann Neurol 2010;67(3):376–83.
28. Treaba CA, Granberg TE, Sormani MP, et al. Longitudinal characterization of cortical lesion development and evolution in multiple sclerosis with 7.0-T MRI. Radiology 2019;291(3):740–9.
29. Beck ES, Maranzano J, Luciano NJ, et al. Cortical lesion hotspots and association of subpial lesions with disability in multiple sclerosis. Mult Scler. Aug 2022;28(9):1351–63.
30. Geurts JJ, Bö L, Pouwels PJ, et al. Cortical lesions in multiple sclerosis: combined postmortem MR imaging and histopathology. AJNR Am J Neuroradiol 2005;26(3):572–7.
31. Madsen MAJ, Wiggermann V, Bramow S, et al. Imaging cortical multiple sclerosis lesions with ultra-high field MRI. Neuroimage Clin 2021;32:102847.
32. Maranzano J, Dadar M, Rudko DA, et al. Comparison of multiple sclerosis cortical lesion types detected by multicontrast 3T and 7T MRI. AJNR Am J Neuroradiol 2019;40(7):1162–9.
33. Kilsdonk ID, Jonkman LE, Klaver R, et al. Increased cortical grey matter lesion detection in multiple sclerosis with 7 T MRI: a post-mortem verification study. Brain 2016;139(Pt 5):1472–81.
34. Bouman PM, Steenwijk MD, Pouwels PJW, et al. Histopathology-validated recommendations for cortical lesion imaging in multiple sclerosis. Brain 2020; 143(10):2988–97.
35. Geurts JJ, Pouwels PJ, Uitdehaag BM, et al. Intracortical lesions in multiple sclerosis: improved detection with 3D double inversion-recovery MR imaging. Radiology 2005;236(1):254–60.
36. Seewann A, Kooi EJ, Roosendaal SD, et al. Postmortem verification of MS cortical lesion detection with 3D DIR. Neurology 2012;78(5):302–8.
37. Balcer LJ. Clinical practice. Optic neuritis. N Engl J Med 2006;354(12):1273–80.
38. Toosy AT, Mason DF, Miller DH. Optic neuritis. Lancet Neurol 2014;13(1):83–99.
39. Group ONS. Multiple sclerosis risk after optic neuritis: final optic neuritis treatment trial follow-up. Arch Neurol 2008;65(6):727–32.
40. Tintore M, Rovira À, Río J, et al. Defining high, medium and low impact prognostic factors for developing multiple sclerosis. Brain 2015;138(Pt 7): 1863–74.
41. Darakdjian M, Chaves H, Hernandez J, et al. MRI pattern in acute optic neuritis: Comparing multiple sclerosis, NMO and MOGAD. NeuroRadiol J 2023; 36(3):267–72.
42. Mealy MA, Whetstone A, Orman G, et al. Longitudinally extensive optic neuritis as an MRI biomarker distinguishes neuromyelitis optica from multiple sclerosis. J Neurol Sci 2015;355(1–2):59–63.
43. Brownlee WJ, Miszkiel KA, Tur C, et al. Inclusion of optic nerve involvement in dissemination in space

criteria for multiple sclerosis. Neurology 2018; 91(12):e1130–4.
44. Cortese R, Prados Carrasco F, Tur C, et al. Differentiating multiple sclerosis from AQP4-neuromyelitis optica spectrum disorder and MOG-antibody disease with imaging. Neurology 2023;100(3):e308–23.
45. Sparacia G, Agnello F, Gambino A, et al. Multiple sclerosis: high prevalence of the 'central vein' sign in white matter lesions on susceptibility-weighted images. NeuroRadiol J 2018;31(4):356–61.
46. Tallantyre EC, Morgan PS, Dixon JE, et al. A comparison of 3T and 7T in the detection of small parenchymal veins within MS lesions. Invest Radiol 2009;44(9):491–4.
47. Sinnecker T, Dörr J, Pfueller CF, et al. Distinct lesion morphology at 7-T MRI differentiates neuromyelitis optica from multiple sclerosis. Neurology 2012; 79(7):708–14.
48. Maggi P, Absinta M, Grammatico M, et al. Central vein sign differentiates Multiple Sclerosis from central nervous system inflammatory vasculopathies. Ann Neurol 2018;83(2):283–94.
49. Al-Louzi O, Letchuman V, Manukyan S, et al. Central vein sign profile of newly developing lesions in multiple sclerosis: a 3-year longitudinal study. Neurol Neuroimmunol Neuroinflamm 2022;9(2).
50. Kollia K, Maderwald S, Putzki N, et al. First clinical study on ultra-high-field MR imaging in patients with multiple sclerosis: comparison of 1.5T and 7T. AJNR Am J Neuroradiol 2009;30(4):699–702.
51. Solomon AJ, Schindler MK, Howard DB, et al. "Central vessel sign" on 3T FLAIR* MRI for the differentiation of multiple sclerosis from migraine. Ann Clin Transl Neurol 2016;3(2):82–7.
52. Martire MS, Moiola L, Rocca MA, et al. What is the potential of paramagnetic rim lesions as diagnostic indicators in multiple sclerosis? Expert Rev Neurother 2022;22(10):829–37.
53. Guisset F, Lolli V, Bugli C, et al. The central vein sign in multiple sclerosis patients with vascular comorbidities. Mult Scler 2021;27(7):1057–65.
54. Sati P, Oh J, Constable RT, et al. The central vein sign and its clinical evaluation for the diagnosis of multiple sclerosis: a consensus statement from the North American Imaging in Multiple Sclerosis Cooperative. Nat Rev Neurol 2016;12(12):714–22.
55. Ng Kee Kwong KC, Mollison D, Meijboom R, et al. Rim lesions are demonstrated in early relapsing-remitting multiple sclerosis using 3 T-based susceptibility-weighted imaging in a multi-institutional setting. Neuroradiology 2022;64(1):109–17.
56. Reeves JA, Weinstock Z, Zivadinov R, et al. Paramagnetic rim lesions are associated with greater incidence of relapse and worse cognitive recovery following relapse. Mult Scler 2023;29(8):1033–8.
57. Choi S, Lake S, Harrison DM. Evaluation of the Blood-Brain Barrier, Demyelination, and Neurodegeneration in Paramagnetic Rim Lesions in Multiple Sclerosis on 7 Tesla MRI. J Magn Reson Imaging 2024;59(3): 941–51.
58. Harrison DM, Li X, Liu H, et al. Lesion heterogeneity on high-field susceptibility MRI is associated with multiple sclerosis severity. AJNR Am J Neuroradiol 2016;37(8):1447–53.
59. Hemond CC, Baek J, Ionete C, et al. Paramagnetic rim lesions are associated with pathogenic CSF profiles and worse clinical status in multiple sclerosis: A retrospective cross-sectional study. Mult Scler 2022; 28(13):2046–56.
60. Clark KA, Manning AR, Chen L, et al. Early magnetic resonance imaging features of new paramagnetic rim lesions in multiple sclerosis. Ann Neurol 2023; 94(4):736–44.
61. Hemond CC, Reich DS, Dundamadappa SK. Paramagnetic rim lesions in multiple sclerosis: comparison of visualization at 1.5-T and 3-T MRI. AJR Am J Roentgenol 2022;219(1):120–31.
62. Maggi P, Sati P, Nair G, et al. Paramagnetic rim lesions are specific to multiple sclerosis: an international multicenter 3t mri study. Ann Neurol 2020; 88(5):1034–42.
63. Meaton I, Altokhis A, Allen CM, et al. Paramagnetic rims are a promising diagnostic imaging biomarker in multiple sclerosis. Mult Scler 2022;28(14): 2212–20.
64. O'Riordan JI, Losseff NA, Phatouros C, et al. Asymptomatic spinal cord lesions in clinically isolated optic nerve, brain stem, and spinal cord syndromes suggestive of demyelination. J Neurol Neurosurg Psychiatry 1998;64(3):353–7.
65. Arrambide G, Rovira A, Sastre-Garriga J, et al. Spinal cord lesions: A modest contributor to diagnosis in clinically isolated syndromes but a relevant prognostic factor. Mult Scler 2018;24(3):301–12.
66. Brownlee WJ, Altmann DR, Alves Da Mota P, et al. Association of asymptomatic spinal cord lesions and atrophy with disability 5 years after a clinically isolated syndrome. Mult Scler 2017;23(5):665–74.
67. Brownlee WJ, Altmann DR, Prados F, et al. Early imaging predictors of long-term outcomes in relapse-onset multiple sclerosis. Brain 2019;142(8):2276–87.
68. Ostini C, Bovis F, Disanto G, et al. Recurrence and prognostic value of asymptomatic spinal cord lesions in multiple sclerosis. J Clin Med 2021;10(3).
69. Granella F, Tsantes E, Graziuso S, et al. Spinal cord lesions are frequently asymptomatic in relapsing-remitting multiple sclerosis: a retrospective MRI survey. J Neurol 2019;266(12):3031–7.
70. Zecca C, Disanto G, Sormani MP, et al. Relevance of asymptomatic spinal MRI lesions in patients with multiple sclerosis. Mult Scler 2016;22(6):782–91.
71. Ruggieri S, Prosperini L, Petracca M, et al. The added value of spinal cord lesions to disability accrual in multiple sclerosis. J Neurol 2023;270(10):4995–5003.

72. Dekker I, Sombekke MH, Witte BI, et al. Asymptomatic spinal cord lesions do not predict the time to disability in patients with early multiple sclerosis. Mult Scler 2018;24(4):481–90.
73. Saade C, Bou-Fakhredin R, Yousem DM, et al. Gadolinium and multiple sclerosis: vessels, barriers of the brain, and glymphatics. AJNR Am J Neuroradiol 2018;39(12):2168–76.
74. Miller DH, Barkhof F, Nauta JJ. Gadolinium enhancement increases the sensitivity of MRI in detecting disease activity in multiple sclerosis. Brain 1993; 116(Pt 5):1077–94.
75. Eichinger P, Schön S, Pongratz V, et al. Accuracy of unenhanced MRI in the detection of new brain lesions in multiple sclerosis. Radiology 2019;291(2): 429–35.
76. Mattay RR, Davtyan K, Bilello M, et al. Do all patients with multiple sclerosis benefit from the use of contrast on serial follow-up mr imaging? a retrospective analysis. AJNR Am J Neuroradiol 2018;39(11): 2001–6.
77. Prince MR, Zhang HL, Roditi GH, et al. Risk factors for NSF: a literature review. J Magn Reson Imag 2009;30(6):1298–308.
78. Forghani R. Adverse effects of gadolinium-based contrast agents: changes in practice patterns. Top Magn Reson Imag 2016;25(4):163–9.
79. Gallo-Bernal S, Patino-Jaramillo N, Calixto CA, et al. Nephrogenic systemic fibrosis in patients with chronic kidney disease after the use of gadolinium-based contrast agents: a review for the cardiovascular imager. Diagnostics 2022;12(8).
80. Gulani V, Calamante F, Shellock FG, et al. Gadolinium deposition in the brain: summary of evidence and recommendations. Lancet Neurol 2017;16(7): 564–70.
81. Kanda T, Ishii K, Kawaguchi H, et al. High signal intensity in the dentate nucleus and globus pallidus on unenhanced T1-weighted MR images: relationship with increasing cumulative dose of a gadolinium-based contrast material. Radiology 2014;270(3): 834–41.
82. Granziera C, Reich DS. Gadolinium should always be used to assess disease activity in MS - Yes. Mult Scler 2020;26(7):765–6.
83. Okar SV, Reich DS. Routine gadolinium use for MRI follow-up of multiple sclerosis: point-the role of leptomeningeal enhancement. AJR Am J Roentgenol 2022;219(1):24–5.

Basic Science of Neuroinflammation and Involvement of the Inflammatory Response in Disorders of the Nervous System

epideh Parsi, PhD[a], Cindy Zhu[a], Negin Jalali Motlagh, MD[a], Daeki Kim[a],
nrico G. Küllenberg, MD[a], Hyung-Hwan Kim, PhD[a],
ebecca L. Gillani, MD, PhD[b], John W. Chen, MD, PhD[a,c,*]

KEYWORDS

• Neuroinflammation • Microglia • Astrocytes • Macrophages • Neutrophils • Lymphocytes
• Molecular imaging

KEY POINTS

- Neuroinflammation is a key immune response in the central nervous system (CNS) observed in many neurologic diseases.
- The CNS is separated from the periphery by the blood–brain barrier (BBB) that creates an immune-privileged site with its own unique immune cells and immune response.
- BBB compromise causes an influx of peripheral immune cells and factors that interact with resident immune cells in the CNS.
- Neuroinflammation can exert damaging as well as beneficial effects depending on the context.

NTRODUCTION

nflammation plays a key role in highly prevalent iseases, including many cardiovascular, neuroogic, and rheumatological diseases. Although an ppropriate immune response can be beneficial nd protective, aberrant activation of this response ecruits excessive proinflammatory cells to cause amage (**Fig. 1**). Neuroinflammation is inflammaon within the central nervous system (CNS). ecause the CNS is separated from the periphery by the blood–brain barrier (BBB) that creates an immune-privileged site, it has its own unique immune cells and immune response. Moreover, neuroinflammation can compromise the BBB causing an influx of peripheral immune cells and factors. This article will provide a broad overview of neuroinflammation and describe its unique aspects. Key immune cells and factors in mediating neuroinflammation will be introduced followed by a discussion of neuroinflammation in different neurologic diseases.

[a] Institute for Innovation in Imaging, Neurovascular Research Unit, Center for Systems Biology, Massachusetts General Hospital, Harvard Medical School, Boston, MA, USA; [b] Department of Neurology, Neuroimmunology and Neuro-Infectious Diseases Division, Massachusetts Institute for Neurodegenerative Disease, Massachusetts General Hospital, Harvard Medical School, Boston, MA, USA; [c] Division of Neuroradiology, Department of Radiology, Massachusetts General Hospital, Harvard Medical School, Boston, MA, USA
* Corresponding author. 10-114 CNY-149 13th Street, Charlestown, MA 02129.
E-mail address: jwchen@mgh.harvard.edu

Magn Reson Imaging Clin N Am 32 (2024) 375–384
https://doi.org/10.1016/j.mric.2024.01.003
1064-9689/24/

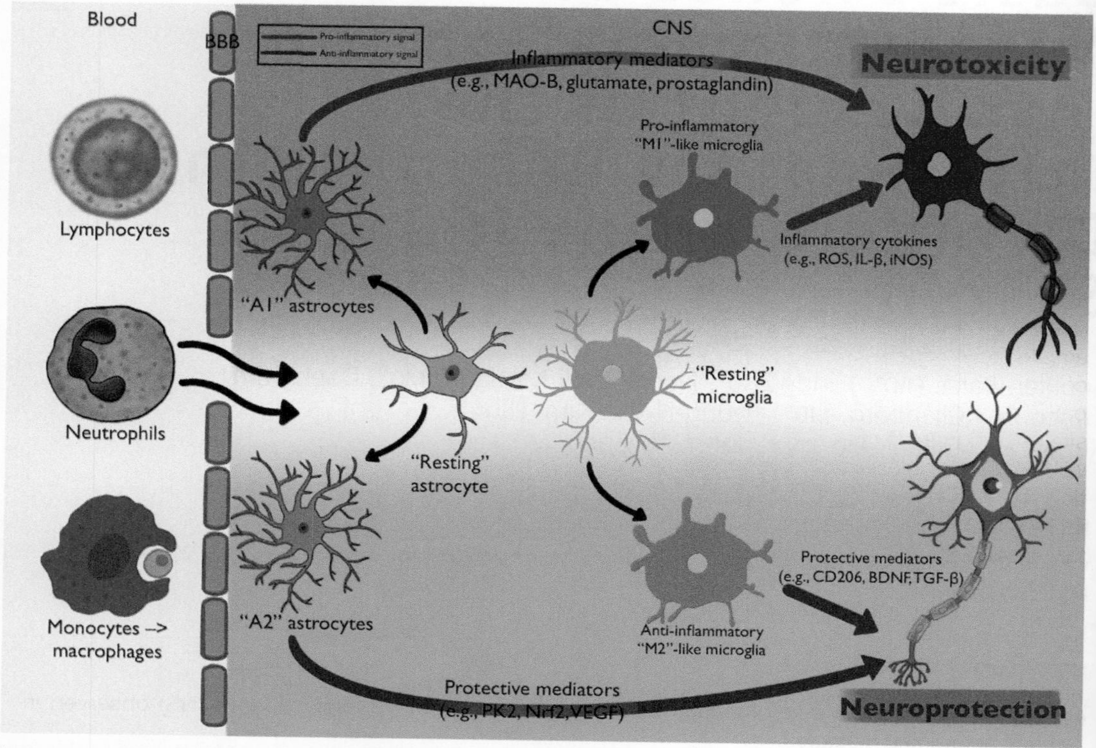

Fig. 1. Neuroinflammation. When the BBB is compromised, peripheral immune cells infiltrate into the CNS and interact with microglia and astrocytes. Depending on the stimuli, the resultant response can be either detrimental or protective to the CNS.

KEY PLAYERS IN NEUROINFLAMMATION

Neutrophils

Neutrophils form 50% to 70% of leukocytes and play a central role in neuroinflammation. As one of the major defenses, neutrophils are quickly activated in the bloodstream and are the first peripheral leukocytes to respond to stimuli. Neutrophils at the injured site will attempt to eliminate pathogens and initiate an inflammatory cascade to repair the damaged tissue. Neutrophils phagocytose pathogens to form a phagosome that undergoes lysosomal degradation to destroy the pathogen's cell walls and proteins. After ingesting a pathogen, a neutrophil produces reactive oxygen species (ROS) such as superoxide (O_2^-), hypochlorite (HOCl), hydrogen peroxide (H_2O_2), hydroxyl radicals, and nitric oxide (NO).[1] Neutrophils also secrete myeloperoxidase (MPO), an enzyme that produces HOCl and other reactive species. MPO is also involved in the formation of neutrophil extracellular traps (NETs), which limit pathogens from multiplying by entrapping bacteria, viruses, and fungi.[2] However, NETs can also cause a proinflammatory responses and lead to tissue damage via long-term production of proteolytic enzymes. Formation of NETs can eventually lead to apoptosis, known as NETosis.

The BBB serves as a significant immunologic defense from foreign pathogens and toxic molecules. However, with injury and resultant neuroinflammation, the BBB can become compromised allowing peripheral immune cells to infiltrate into the CNS. The infiltration of neutrophils has been related to brain damage due to the appearance of proinflammatory cytokines, ROS, and NETs release. However, not all neutrophils are proinflammatory. Recently, other neutrophil phenotypes have been described that have roles in tissue repair, tumor killing, and immune regulation.[3] This has implications in therapy because strategies that indiscriminately deplete or inhibit neutrophils may not always be beneficial.

Macrophages

Activated macrophages regulate inflammatory responses and have diverse phenotypes and functions, allowing macrophage to change fluidly into different states depending on its environment.[4] An M1/M2 classification has been described from in vitro observations. Macrophages (M0) can be "classically" stimulated with proinflammatory mediators, that is, lipopolysaccharide (LPS) and interferon gamma (IFNγ), to adopt an aggressive (M1) phenotype. Conversely, cells "alternatively" stimulated with anti-inflammatory cytokines (ie, interleukin [IL]-4 and IL-13) will adopt an M2 phenotype, which is thought to have restorative and immunomodulating functions. When inflammation initially occurs, macrophages can polarize into M1-like phenotypes and generate proinflammatory cytokines and chemokines such as tumor necrosis factor (TNF), IL-1β, and IL-12.[5] These macrophages will amplify inflammation by generating large amounts of proinflammatory cytokines and ROS to remove pathogens or foreign molecules from the injured site, although prolonged M1 macrophage activity will result in tissue damage and chronic inflammation. M2-like phenotypes are thought to be anti-inflammatory and reduces inflammation to enable tissue repair by secreting anti-inflammatory cytokines, chemokines, and growth factors such as IL-10, transforming growth factor beta, and chemokine ligand 18 (CCL18).[6] Underscoring the complexity and diversity of macrophages, the M2 phenotype has been found to have subsets known as M2a, M2b, M2c, and M2d. M2a amplifies cell growth and tissue repair, M2b plays a central role in inflammation, M2c is important for phagocytosis, and M2d stimulates tumor progression.[7] Beyond the M1/M2 phenotypes, other phenotypes are starting to be described, primarily based on advanced techniques such as RNAseq.[8]

Lymphocytes

Lymphocytes are classified into B cells, T cells, and natural killer (NK) cells. The T cells and B cells participate in acquired or antigen-specific immune responses. B cells can turn into plasmacytes to produce antibodies. Although humoral immunity depends on B cells, cell immunity depends on T cells.[9] T cells play major roles in adaptive immune response to tissue damage and infection. They are able to clone highly polymorphic antigen receptors that allow them to detect protein-based antigens.[10] On recognition of protein-associated antigens, T cells will undergo clonal amplification and progressively obtain the ability to react to stimuli. Major types of T cells are CD4+ (helper T cells) and CD8+ (cytotoxic T cells).[11] T-cell receptors and their related receptors, such as CD3 and CD4, form a complex between the major histocompatibility complex-II receptor and the target antigen. CD4+ cells generate cytokines to start an immune reaction and activate T-cell-associated humoral immunity. Once activated, CD8+ cells migrate to its target antigen to eventually kill it. Regulatory T cells (Tregs) can help manage immune tolerance and suppress extreme inflammation, playing a protective role. Conversely, effector T cells such as Th1 and Th17 cells can play a part in neuroinflammation and tissue damage. NK cells play a versatile role by serving as a rapid defense mechanism against neural damage and helping immune modulation within the CNS.

Microglia

Microglia, originating from the yolk sac,[12] are the primary immune cells of the CNS, constituting 5% to 10% of the adult brain cell population. They are the resident macrophages in the CNS and first responders to insults.[13] These cells have highly motile processes allowing them to scan their environment constantly. The 3 primary functions of microglia are as follows: (1) surveying their environments for any changes using their sensomes, which encode various proteins to allow microglia to sense endogenous ligands and microbes[14]; (2) physiologic housekeeping, which includes migrating to sites of injury,[15] synapse pruning and remodeling,[16] myelin homeostasis,[17] and interacting with astrocytes[18]; and (3) protecting the organism against harmful stimuli, which include pathogen-associated molecular patterns and damage-associated molecular patterns recognized by the various receptors expressed on microglia, including toll-like receptors, nuclear oligomerization domain-like receptors, and more (**Fig. 2**).[19] As the immune cells of the CNS, microglia protect the brain from harmful antigens, such as apoptotic cells, microbes, protein aggregates, and lipoprotein particles.

Microglia are also capable of contributing to oxidative stress and have a role in producing ROS that lead to tissue damage when produced in excess. These phagocytes can mediate respiratory burst to produce powerful microbicidal agents downstream of the initial superoxide production.[20] Activated microglia produce nitric oxide (NO) via inducible nitric oxide synthase (iNOS), and the release of NO leads to neuronal cell death by inhibiting neurons from undergoing cellular respiration.[21] Contributing to oxidative stress is MPO.[22] Normal brain microglia rarely express MPO[23,24] but activated microglia are positive for MPO.[25] Elevated MPO activity can be detrimental to tissues and is implicated in many diseases.[26] In vivo MPO activity can be imaged by molecular imaging agents for MR imaging[27–31] and PET.[32]

Astrocytes

Astrocytes are the brain's most common glial cells and help regulate neuronal activity and maintain

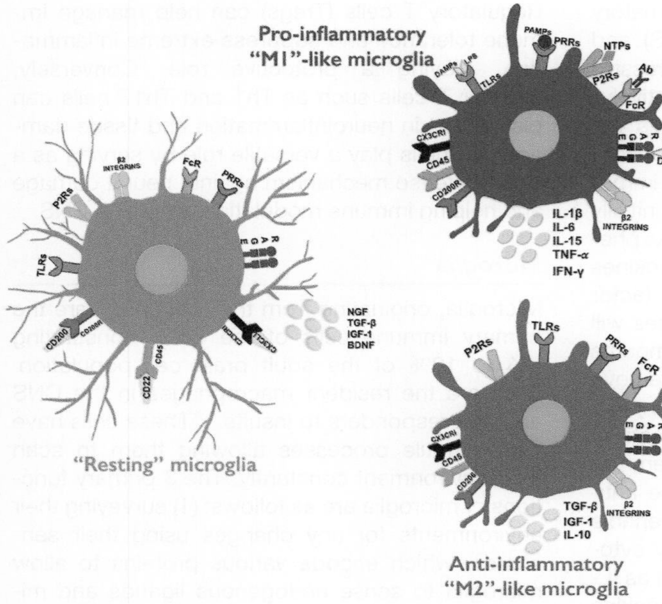

Fig. 2. Microglia. Under normal physiologic circumstances, "resting" microglia are ramified, consisting of many receptors. Receptor and cytokine interactions maintain the ramified state. On activation, microglia can shift toward an ameboid "M1" phenotype that upregulates a proinflammatory response. Activated microglial cells can also shift to the M2-phenotype that is more reparative and anti-inflammatory.

brain homeostasis. They regulate blood flow; maintain BBB integrity; supply energy metabolites to neurons; modulate synaptic activity; monitor the secretion of neurotrophins; remove dead cells from their surrounding environment; manage the extracellular balance of ions, fluids, and neurotransmitters; and form scars in response to brain injury or damage.[13] Furthermore, astrocytes can phagocytose protein aggregates such as amyloid plaques.[33] In contrast to microglia, astrocytes tend to engulf distal processes and diffuse neuritic debris.[34]

Astrocytes respond to insults by a process called reactive astrogliosis. Activation of astrocytes changes its molecular expression and morphology such as increasing the number and size of astrocytes expressing glial fibrillary acidic protein (GFAP).[35] When astrocytes are activated, they can take 1 of the 2 phenotypes: the A1-phenotype or A2-phenotype, which are neurotoxic or neuroprotective, respectively.[13] Many intercellular signaling molecules can also trigger reactive astrogliosis, for example, ROS, neurotransmitters, cytokines (fibroblast growth factor 2 [FGF2], IL-10, ciliary neutrophic factor [CNTF], IFNγ), and molecules associated with systemic metabolic toxicity.[36] Activated astrocytes become not only neurotoxic but also lose many of their vital functions pertinent to homeostasis and maintenance of neuronal health. A1-reactive astrocytes negatively affect synaptic activity by disassembling synapses and inducing the formation of fewer synapses. Additionally, A1 astrocytes almost completely lose their ability to phagocytose myelin debris from their environment. Other detrimental functions include production of neurotoxic levels of ROS,[37] releasing potentially excitotoxic glutamate,[38] and compromising the BBB via vascular endothelial growth factor production.[39]

Not all reactive astrocytes are detrimental. Astrocytes also contribute to normal physiologic inflammatory responses to protect the CNS. Some beneficial functions of reactive astrogliosis include uptake of glutamate,[40] protection against oxidative stress by producing glutathione,[41] degradation of β-amyloid plaques,[42] facilitating repair of the BBB,[43] and restricting the spread of inflammatory cells or infectious agents into healthy CNS parenchyma.[44]

Identification, Polarization, and Imaging

Macrophages and microglia

To differentiate macrophages from microglia, human and murine microglia specifically express TMEM119, by which they may be identified.[45] Among the putative M1-macrophages/microglia markers are iNOS, CD38, CD80, CD86, and formyl peptide receptor 2 (FPPR2) as well as proinflammatory cytokines such as TNF, IL-6, IL-12A, IL-23A, and IL-27. Putative markers of M2-macrophages/microglia are Arginase-1, CD206, CD163, resistin-like molecule alpha (RELMα), chitinase 3-like 3 (CHI3L3), arachidonate 15-lipoxygenase (ALOX15), early grwoth response 2 (EGR2), and cellular myc (c-MYC).[46] However, transcriptomic experiments suggest that the M1/M2 nomenclature falls short of the complexity of activation states in vivo. A study comparing homeostatic microglia to those in different diseases found 10 transcriptomic patterns during development, which reappeared under disease conditions, and 3 other distinct clusters associated with neurodegeneration, demyelination, and remyelination, hinting at a highly diverse inflammatory milieu.[47]

Molecular imaging studies aim to unravel some aspects of this convoluted network using established disease models to address different aspects of neuroinflammation. One example is imaging agents targeting MPO. Paramagnetic substrates that are activated and retained at sites of MPO allow for visualization of MPO activity with MR imaging.[27,31,48] Activated innate immune cells phagocytose and store Fe^{2+} which can be visualized by iron oxide nanoparticles.[49] MPO and iron oxide nanoparticle MR imaging have been used in combination to identify and map M1-dominant and M2-dominant lesions in the CNS (**Fig. 3**).[50] PET imaging requires significantly less agent to be detectable, which increases sensitivity. Imaging probes targeting the translocator protein (TSPO), which is expressed by activated microglia and to a lesser extent reactive macrophages and astrocytes, are widely used in the research setting.[51] A radioligand targeting MPO has been recently developed.[32] Targets for PET-agents beyond TSPO and MPO include endocannabinoid receptor CB2,[52] cyclooxygenase 1[53] and 2,[54] matrix metalloproteinases,[55] and P2RY12.[56]

Astrocytes

Even though GFAP has been commonly used to characterize reactive astrogliosis, many caveats exist. One of the main limitations includes regional differences within the brain regarding GFAP expression. Most importantly, GFAP does not allow for the differentiation between the A1-phenotype and A2-phenotype. Transcriptomic studies found 57 genes, such as C3 and guanine nucleotide-binding protein 2, that exhibited preferential expression in A1-astrocytes, as well as 150 genes, such as the S100 calcium-binding protein A10 (S100a10), that were preferentially expressed in A2-astrocytes.[57] Of these genes, the most used marker for A1-astrocytes is C3, whereas the most common markers for distinguishing A2-astrocytes include S100a10 and pentraxin-3.[58] Imaging astrocytes includes PET agents targeting monoamine oxidase B, acetate metabolism, and imidazoline$_2$ binding sites,[59] although none differentiate between the different phenotypes.

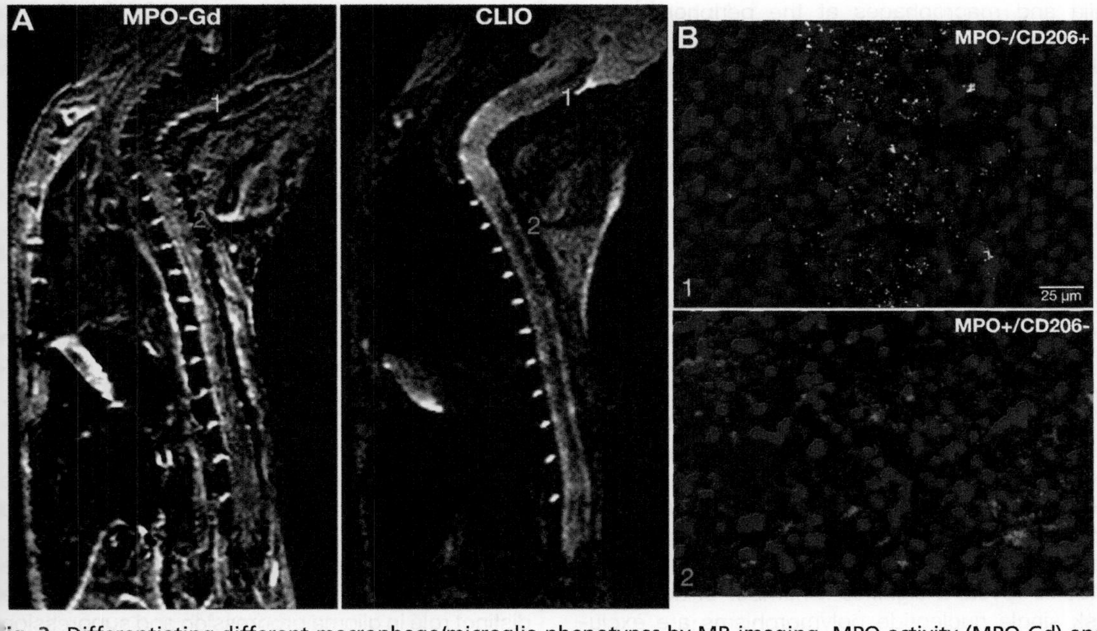

Fig. 3. Differentiating different macrophage/microglia phenotypes by MR imaging. MPO activity (MPO-Gd) and iron oxide nanoparticle (CLIO) MR imaging in a murine model of experimental autoimmune encephalomyelitis. In (A) MPO-Gd + lesions with matched CLIO + lesions (area 2) represent M1-like cells, corroborated by immunohistochemistry in (*B*) (*red* = MPO, *yellow* = CD206, *blue* = DAPI). Lesions that were CLIO + only without corresponding MPO-Gd + signal (area 1) represent M2-like phagocytes that expressed CD206 but virtually no MPO on immunohistochemistry. (*Modified from* Ref.[50])

NEUROINFLAMMATION IN DISEASES

Multiple Sclerosis

People living with MS (PwMS) develop neurodegeneration due to neuroinflammation throughout the brain and spinal cord, leading to accelerated atrophy. Neuroinflammation in MS results from a complex interplay of adaptive and innate immune cells.[60] Traditionally, MS has been viewed as a T-cell-mediated disease. Autoreactive $CD4^+$ and $CD8^+$ T cells migrate across the broken-down BBB and are present in active demyelinating lesions.[61] Dysregulated Tregs may also contribute to the development of autoreactivity in MS.[62]

Although T cells play a central role in MS neuroinflammation, the critical importance of B cells has recently been recognized. B cells act through interaction and antigen presentation to T cells, the release of inflammatory cytokines and chemokines, and the production of pathogenic antibodies.[63] PwMS have immune cell infiltrates and ectopic lymphoid follicles in the meninges.[64] Innate immune cells are also important in MS. Microglia and macrophages are abundant in active demyelinating lesions.[65] Active demyelinating lesions predominate early in the disease course but become less frequent later in the disease.[66] These later lesions slowly expand, called smoldering plaques, and have iron-containing microglia and macrophages at the periphery[67] that may play an important role in the gradual progression of disability in PwMS.[68]

Neurodegenerative Diseases

Alzheimer disease (AD) is the most frequent cause of dementia. A substantial unmet need exists to elucidate the mechanisms underlying AD and find robust noninvasive biomarkers to aid the diagnosis and earlier detection of AD but also the development and assessment of new therapeutic strategies. In AD, there are multiple potential triggers of inflammation, among which protein aggregates seem to be playing a pivotal role,[69] and cross talk of protein misfolding and inflammation are a constant part of the neurodegenerative processes.[70] Persistent activation of glial cells that compromises neuronal functionality can result from continuous exposure to an inflammatory stimulus or impairment of resolution.[71] Recent studies reveal a significant number of novel AD-risk single nucleotide polymorphisms are exclusively or dominantly expressed in microglia, emphasizing the critical roles these cells play in AD.[72] Different phenotypes of microglia have been found in AD, including activated response microglia, interferon-responsive microglia, human AD microglia,[73] disease-associated microglia,[74] microglial neurodegenerative,[75] and dark microglia.[76] Research is ongoing to elucidate the roles these different types of microglia play in AD and other neurodegenerative diseases.

Stroke

Stroke induces a complex cascade of changes dominated by the innate immune response, with activation of local microglia, influx of leukocytes into the brain, and production of ROS that elevate oxidative stress and contribute to stroke progression.[77] Whereas neutrophils become scarce after 3 days, activated microglia and macrophages are elevated within hours and can last for weeks to months after stroke.[29,78] Neutrophils arrive in the ischemic brain within 24 hours after stroke with macrophages peaking about 3 days after.[79] Proinflammatory molecules and cytokines such as TNF and IL-1β are elevated in the blood of patients. The levels of proinflammatory molecules and leukocytes correlate with outcomes after stroke.[80] Similarly, decreasing leukocyte recruitment and proinflammatory and oxidizing molecules, such as MPO, have decreased infarct size by 30% to 60%,[81] demonstrating that inflammation extends ischemic injury. Another example is Rho-associated kinase (ROCK), which is elevated in patients after stroke and is an independent predictor for recurrent stroke.[27,28] ROCK inhibition reduced neutrophil accumulation in the ischemic region and resulted in the reduction of infarction volume.[30,31]

Glioma

The tumor microenvironment in glioma is characterized by a complex interplay of various cell types including tumor cells, immune cells, and endothelial cells, along with the secretion of various proinflammatory and anti-inflammatory cytokines.[82] Glioma-associated macrophages/microglia (GAMs) can manipulate immune response and tumor development. M1-like GAMs exhibit an antitumor effect whereas M2-like GAMs have an immunosuppressive impact. The presence of macrophages in low-grade gliomas decreases survival, and they are more abundant in higher grade gliomas compared with microglia.[83] Similarly, tumor-infiltrated neutrophils can modulate other immune cells and promote tumor infiltration. T-lymphocytes also have a distinct role in glioma progression and suppression but at lower fractions than in brain metastasis.[84] T cells constitute 1% to 5% of total glioma cellular content. The percentages of both $CD4^+$ and $CD8^+$ tumor-infiltrating T cells increase with tumor grade.[85]

SUMMARY

Neuroinflammation is a complex interplay between different peripheral and central immune cells that can have damaging and beneficial effects depending on the context. Imaging of these cells and their functions is still at a relatively early stage and represents opportunities in imaging and clinical research to advance our knowledge and improve patient care.

DISCLOSURES

J.W. Chen has a financial interest in Silverier LLC, a company that founds biotech start-up companies, and its subsidiary, Einsenca, Inc., a company developing PET and MR imaging agents that target MPO. Dr J.W. Chen's interests were reviewed and are managed by Massachusetts General Hospital and Mass General Brigham in accordance with their conflict-of-interest policies. The other authors declare no conflict of interest.

FUNDING

NIH (R01NS103998, RF1AG075055), National Multiple Sclerosis Society.

REFERENCES

1. Healy LM, Perron G, Won S-Y, et al. MerTK is a functional regulator of myelin phagocytosis by human myeloid cells. J Immunol 2016;196(8):3375–84.
2. Hidalgo A, Libby P, Soehnlein O, et al. Neutrophil extracellular traps: from physiology to pathology. Cardiovasc Res 2022;118(13):2737–53. https://doi.org/10.1093/cvr/cvab329.
3. Hellebrekers P, Vrisekoop N, Koenderman L. Neutrophil phenotypes in health and disease. Eur J Clin Invest 2018;48(Suppl 2):e12943. https://doi.org/10.1111/eci.12943.
4. Butterfield TA, Best TM, Merrick MA. The dual roles of neutrophils and macrophages in inflammation: a critical balance between tissue damage and repair. J Athl Train 2006;41(4):457–65.
5. Yunna C, Mengru H, Lei W, et al. Macrophage M1/M2 polarization. Eur J Pharmacol 2020;877:173090.
6. Novak ML, Koh TJ. Macrophage phenotypes during tissue repair. J Leukoc Biol 2013;93(6):875–81.
7. Yao Y, Xu XH, Jin L. Macrophage Polarization in Physiological and Pathological Pregnancy. Front Immunol 2019;10:792.
8. Sreejit G, Fleetwood AJ, Murphy AJ, et al. Origins and diversity of macrophages in health and disease. Clin Transl Immunology 2020;9(12):e1222.
9. Cano R, Lopera H. Introduction to T and B lymphocytes. In: Anaya J, Shoenfeld Y, A R-V, editors. Autoimmunity: from bench to bedside. Bogota, CO: El Rosario University Press; 2013. p. 77–95. chap 5.
10. Fabbri M, Smart C, Pardi R. T lymphocytes. Int J Biochem Cell Biol 2003 2003;35(7):1004–8.
11. Bauer ME, Teixeira AL. Neuroinflammation in Mood Disorders: Role of Regulatory Immune Cells. Neuroimmunomodulation 2021;28(3):99–107.
12. Saijo K, Glass CK. Microglial cell origin and phenotypes in health and disease. Nat Rev Immunol 2011;11(11):775–87. https://doi.org/10.1038/nri3086.
13. Kwon HS, Koh S-H. Neuroinflammation in neurodegenerative disorders: the roles of microglia and astrocytes. Transl Neurodegener 2020;9:1–12.
14. Hickman SE, Kingery ND, Ohsumi TK, et al. The microglial sensome revealed by direct RNA sequencing. Nat Neurosci 2013;16(12):1896–905.
15. Sieger D, Moritz C, Ziegenhals T, et al. Long-range Ca2+ waves transmit brain-damage signals to microglia. Dev Cell 2012;22(6):1138–48.
16. Vasek MJ, Garber C, Dorsey D, et al. A complement–microglial axis drives synapse loss during virus-induced memory impairment. Nature 2016;534(7608):538–43.
17. Pluvinage JV, Haney MS, Smith BA, et al. CD22 blockade restores homeostatic microglial phagocytosis in ageing brains. Nature 2019;568(7751):187–92.
18. Rothhammer V, Borucki DM, Tjon EC, et al. Microglial control of astrocytes in response to microbial metabolites. Nature 2018;557(7707):724–8.
19. Stephenson J, Nutma E, van der Valk P, et al. Inflammation in CNS neurodegenerative diseases. Immunology 2018;154(2):204–19.
20. Thomas DC. The phagocyte respiratory burst: Historical perspectives and recent advances. Immunol Lett 2017;192:88–96.
21. Bal-Price A, Brown GC. Inflammatory neurodegeneration mediated by nitric oxide from activated glia-inhibiting neuronal respiration, causing glutamate release and excitotoxicity. J Neurosci 2001;21(17):6480–91.
22. Yap YW, Whiteman M, Cheung NS. Chlorinative stress: an under appreciated mediator of neurodegeneration? Cell Signal 2007;19(2):219–28.
23. Reynolds WF, Rhees J, Maciejewski D, et al. Myeloperoxidase polymorphism is associated with gender specific risk for Alzheimer's disease. Exp Neurol 1999;155(1):31–41.
24. Nagra RM, Becher B, Tourtellotte WW, et al. Immunohistochemical and genetic evidence of myeloperoxidase involvement in multiple sclerosis. J Neuroimmunol 1997;78(1–2):97–107.
25. Gellhaar S, Sunnemark D, Eriksson H, et al. Myeloperoxidase-immunoreactive cells are significantly increased in brain areas affected by neurodegeneration in Parkinson's and Alzheimer's disease. Cell Tissue Res 2017;369:445–54.

26. Pravalika K, Sarmah D, Kaur H, et al. Myeloperoxidase and neurological disorder: a crosstalk. ACS Chem Neurosci 2018;9(3):421–30.
27. Chen JW, Breckwoldt MO, Aikawa E, et al. Myeloperoxidase-targeted imaging of active inflammatory lesions in murine experimental autoimmune encephalomyelitis. Brain 2008;131(4):1123–33. https://doi.org/10.1093/brain/awn004.
28. Chen JW, Querol Sans M, Bogdanov A Jr, et al. Imaging of myeloperoxidase in mice by using novel amplifiable paramagnetic substrates. Radiology 2006;240(2):473–81. https://doi.org/10.1148/radiol.2402050994.
29. Breckwoldt MO, Chen JW, Stangenberg L, et al. Tracking the inflammatory response in stroke in vivo by sensing the enzyme myeloperoxidase. Proc Natl Acad Sci U S A 2008;105(47):18584–9. https://doi.org/10.1073/pnas.0803945105.
30. Wang C, Pulli B, Jalali Motlagh N, et al. A versatile imaging platform with fluorescence and CT imaging capabilities that detects myeloperoxidase activity and inflammation at different scales. Theranostics 2019; 9(25):7525–36. https://doi.org/10.7150/thno.36264.
31. Wang C, Cheng D, Jalali Motlagh N, et al. Highly Efficient Activatable MRI Probe to Sense Myeloperoxidase Activity. J Med Chem 2021;64(9):5874–85. https://doi.org/10.1021/acs.jmedchem.1c00038.
32. Wang C, Keliher E, Zeller MWG, et al. An activatable PET imaging radioprobe is a dynamic reporter of myeloperoxidase activity in vivo. Proc Natl Acad Sci USA 2019;116(24):11966–71. https://doi.org/10.1073/pnas.1818434116.
33. Fujita Y, Maeda T, Sato C, et al. Engulfment of Toxic Amyloid β-protein in Neurons and Astrocytes Mediated by MEGF10. Neuroscience 2020;443:1–7.
34. Damisah EC, Hill RA, Rai A, et al. Astrocytes and microglia play orchestrated roles and respect phagocytic territories during neuronal corpse removal in vivo. Sci Adv 2020;6(26):eaba3239.
35. Eddleston M, Mucke L. Molecular profile of reactive astrocytes—implications for their role in neurologic disease. Neuroscience 1993;54(1):15–36.
36. Sofroniew MV, Vinters HV. Astrocytes: biology and pathology. Acta Neuropathol 2010;119:7–35.
37. Šimić G, Lucassen PJ, Krsnik Ž, et al. nNOS expression in reactive astrocytes correlates with increased cell death related DNA damage in the hippocampus and entorhinal cortex in Alzheimer's disease. Exp Neurol 2000;165(1):12–26.
38. Talantova M, Sanz-Blasco S, Zhang X, et al. Aβ induces astrocytic glutamate release, extrasynaptic NMDA receptor activation, and synaptic loss. Proc Natl Acad Sci USA 2013;110(27):E2518–27.
39. Argaw AT, Gurfein BT, Zhang Y, et al. VEGF-mediated disruption of endothelial CLN-5 promotes blood-brain barrier breakdown. Proc Natl Acad Sci USA 2009;106(6):1977–82.
40. Mahmoud S, Gharagozloo M, Simard C, et al. Astrocytes maintain glutamate homeostasis in the CNS by controlling the balance between glutamate uptake and release. Cells 2019;8(2):184.
41. Franco R, Cidlowski J. Apoptosis and glutathione: beyond an antioxidant. Cell Death Differ 2009;16(10): 1303–14.
42. Li M-Z, Zheng L-J, Shen J, et al. SIRT1 facilitates amyloid beta peptide degradation by upregulating lysosome number in primary astrocytes. Neural regeneration research 2018;13(11):2005.
43. Heithoff BP, George KK, Phares AN, et al. Astrocytes are necessary for blood–brain barrier maintenance in the adult mouse brain. Glia 2021;69(2):436–72.
44. Toft-Hansen H, Füchtbauer L, Owens T. Inhibition of reactive astrocytosis in established experimental autoimmune encephalomyelitis favors infiltration by myeloid cells over T cells and enhances severity of disease. Glia 2011;59(1):166–76.
45. Bennett ML, Bennett FC, Liddelow SA, et al. New tools for studying microglia in the mouse and human CNS. Proc Natl Acad Sci USA 2016;113(12):E1738–46. https://doi.org/10.1073/pnas.1525528113.
46. Amici SA, Dong J, Guerau-de-Arellano M. Molecular Mechanisms Modulating the Phenotype of Macrophages and Microglia. Front Immunol 2017;8(NOV): 1–18. https://doi.org/10.3389/fimmu.2017.01520.
47. Jordão MJC, Sankowski R, Brendecke SM, et al. Single-cell profiling identifies myeloid cell subsets with distinct fates during neuroinflammation. Science 2019;363:6425. https://doi.org/10.1126/science.aat7554.
48. Li A, Wu Y, Pulli B, et al. Myeloperoxidase Molecular MRI Reveals Synergistic Combination Therapy in Murine Experimental Autoimmune Neuroinflammation. Radiology 2019;293(1):158–65. https://doi.org/10.1148/radiol.2019182492.
49. Kirschbaum K, Sonner JK, Zeller MW, et al. In vivo nanoparticle imaging of innate immune cells can serve as a marker of disease severity in a model of multiple sclerosis. Proc Natl Acad Sci U S A 2016; 113(46):13227–32. https://doi.org/10.1073/pnas.1609397113.
50. Wang J, Jalali Motlagh N, Wang C, et al. d-mannose suppresses oxidative response and blocks phagocytosis in experimental neuroinflammation. Proc Natl Acad Sci U S A 2021;(44):118. https://doi.org/10.1073/pnas.2107663118.
51. Alam MM, Lee J, Lee SY. Recent Progress in the Development of TSPO PET Ligands for Neuroinflammation Imaging in Neurological Diseases. Nuclear Medicine and Molecular Imaging 2017;51(4): 283–96. https://doi.org/10.1007/s13139-017-0475-8.
52. Evens N, Muccioli GG, Houbrechts N, et al. Synthesis and biological evaluation of carbon-11- and fluorine-18-labeled 2-oxoquinoline derivatives for type 2 cannabinoid receptor positron emission tomography

imaging. Nucl Med Biol 2009;36(4):455–65. https://doi.org/10.1016/j.nucmedbio.2009.01.009.

53. Shukuri M, Mawatari A, Takatani S, et al. Synthesis and Preclinical Evaluation of 18F-Labeled Ketoprofen Methyl Esters for Cyclooxygenase-1 Imaging in Neuroinflammation. Journal of nuclear medicine 2022; 63(11):1761–7. https://doi.org/10.2967/jnumed.121.263713.
54. de Vries EFJ, Doorduin J, Dierckx RA, et al. Evaluation of [11C]rofecoxib as PET tracer for cyclooxygenase 2 overexpression in rat models of inflammation. Nucl Med Biol 2008;35(1):35–42. https://doi.org/10.1016/j.nucmedbio.2007.07.015.
55. Gerwien H, Hermann S, Zhang X, et al. Imaging matrix metalloproteinase activity in multiple sclerosis as a specific marker of leukocyte penetration of the blood-brain barrier. Sci Transl Med 2016;8(364):1–13. https://doi.org/10.1126/scitranslmed.aaf8020.
56. Baez-Pagan CA, Martinez-Ortiz Y, Otero-Cruz JD, et al. Potential role of caveolin-1-positive domains in the regulation of the acetylcholine receptor's activatable pool: implications in the pathogenesis of a novel congenital myasthenic syndrome. Channels 2008; 2(3):180–90. https://doi.org/10.4161/chan.2.3.6155.
57. Zamanian JL, Xu L, Foo LC, et al. Genomic analysis of reactive astrogliosis. J Neurosci 2012;32(18):6391–410.
58. Lopez-Sanchez C, Poejo J, Garcia-Lopez V, et al. Kaempferol prevents the activation of complement C3 protein and the generation of reactive A1 astrocytes that mediate rat brain degeneration induced by 3-nitropropionic acid. Food Chem Toxicol 2022; 164:113017.
59. Liu Y, Jiang H, Qin X, et al. PET imaging of reactive astrocytes in neurological disorders. Eur J Nucl Med Mol Imag 2022;49(4):1275–87. https://doi.org/10.1007/s00259-021-05640-5.
60. Attfield KE, Jensen LT, Kaufmann M, et al. The immunology of multiple sclerosis. Nat Rev Immunol 2022; 22(12):734–50. https://doi.org/10.1038/s41577-022-00718-z.
61. Fransen NL, Hsiao C-C, Mvd P, et al. Tissue-resident memory T cells invade the brain parenchyma in multiple sclerosis white matter lesions. Brain 2020;143(6):1714–30. https://doi.org/10.1093/brain/awaa117.
62. Benallegue N, Nicol B, Lasselin J, et al. Patients With Severe Multiple Sclerosis Exhibit Functionally Altered CD8+ Regulatory T Cells. Neurology Neuroimmunology Neuroinflammation 2022;9(6):e200016. https://doi.org/10.1212/nxi.0000000000200016.
63. Comi G, Bar-Or A, Lassmann H, et al. Role of B Cells in Multiple Sclerosis and Related Disorders. Ann Neurol 2021;89(1):13–23. https://doi.org/10.1002/ana.25927.
64. Magliozzi R, Howell OW, Calabrese M, et al. Meningeal inflammation as a driver of cortical grey matter pathology and clinical progression in multiple sclerosis. Nat Rev Neurol 2023;19(8):461–76. https://doi.org/10.1038/s41582-023-00838-7.
65. Kuhlmann T, Ludwin S, Prat A, et al. An updated histological classification system for multiple sclerosis lesions. Acta Neuropathol 2017;133(1):13–24. https://doi.org/10.1007/s00401-016-1653-y.
66. Frischer JM, Weigand SD, Guo Y, et al. Clinical and pathological insights into the dynamic nature of the white matter multiple sclerosis plaque. Ann Neurol 2015;78(5):710–21. https://doi.org/10.1002/ana.24497.
67. Dal-Bianco A, Grabner G, Kronnerwetter C, et al. Slow expansion of multiple sclerosis iron rim lesions: pathology and 7 T magnetic resonance imaging. Acta Neuropathol 2017;133(1):25–42. https://doi.org/10.1007/s00401-016-1636-z.
68. Calvi A, Carrasco FP, Tur C, et al. Association of Slowly Expanding Lesions on MRI With Disability in People With Secondary Progressive Multiple Sclerosis. Neurology 2022;98(17):e1783–93. https://doi.org/10.1212/wnl.0000000000200144.
69. Michalska P, León R. When It Comes to an End: Oxidative Stress Crosstalk with Protein Aggregation and Neuroinflammation Induce Neurodegeneration. Antioxidants (Basel) 2020;9(8):740.
70. Forloni G, La Vitola P, Balducci C. Oligomeropathies, inflammation and prion protein binding. Front Neurosci 2022;16:82242.
71. Chamani S, Bianconi V, Tasbandi A, et al. Resolution of Inflammation in Neurodegenerative Diseases: The Role of Resolvins. Mediat Inflamm 2020. https://doi.org/10.1155/2020/3267172.
72. Wightman DP, Jansen IE, Savage JE, et al. A genome-wide association study with 1,126,563 individuals identifies new risk loci for Alzheimer's disease. Nat Genet 2021;53(9). https://doi.org/10.1038/s41588-021-00921-z.
73. Srinivasan K, Friedman BA, Etxeberria A, et al. Alzheimer's Patient Microglia Exhibit Enhanced Aging and Unique Transcriptional Activation. Cell Rep 2020; 31(13):107843. https://doi.org/10.1016/J.CELREP.2020.107843.
74. Rangaraju S, Dammer EB, Raza SA, et al. Identification and therapeutic modulation of a pro-inflammatory subset of disease-associated-microglia in Alzheimer's disease. Mol Neurodegener 2018; 13(1). https://doi.org/10.1186/s13024-018-0254-8.
75. Krasemann S, Madore C, Cialic R, et al. The TREM2-APOE Pathway Drives the Transcriptional Phenotype of Dysfunctional Microglia in Neurodegenerative Diseases. Immunity 2017;47(3):566–81.e9. https://doi.org/10.1016/j.immuni.2017.08.008.
76. Bisht K, Sharma KP, Lecours C, et al. Dark microglia: A new phenotype predominantly associated with pathological states. Glia 2016;64(5). https://doi.org/10.1002/glia.22966.
77. Rayasam A, Hsu M, Kijak JA, et al. Immune responses in stroke: how the immune system contributes to

damage and healing after stroke and how this knowledge could be translated to better cures? Immunology 2018;154(3):363–76. https://doi.org/10.1111/imm.12918.

78. Jin R, Yang G, Li G. Inflammatory mechanisms in ischemic stroke: role of inflammatory cells. J Leukoc Biol 2010;87(5):779–89. https://doi.org/10.1189/jlb.1109766.
79. Tarkowski E, Rosengren L, Blomstrand C, et al. Intrathecal release of pro- and anti-inflammatory cytokines during stroke. Clin Exp Immunol 1997;110(3):492–9.
80. Boehme AK, Esenwa C, Elkind MS. Stroke Risk Factors, Genetics, and Prevention. Circ Res 2017;120(3):472–95. https://doi.org/10.1161/CIRCRESAHA.116.308398.
81. Forghani R, Kim HJ, Wojtkiewicz GR, et al. Myeloperoxidase propagates damage and is a potential therapeutic target for subacute stroke. J Cerebr Blood Flow Metabol 2015;35(3):485–93. https://doi.org/10.1038/jcbfm.2014.222.
82. Anderson NM, Simon MC. The tumor microenvironment. Curr Biol 2020;30(16):R921–5. https://doi org/10.1016/j.cub.2020.06.081.
83. Venteicher AS, Tirosh I, Hebert C, et al. Decoupling genetics, lineages, and microenvironment in IDH-mutant gliomas by single-cell RNA-seq. Science 2017. https://doi.org/10.1126/science.aai8478.
84. Mitsdoerffer M, Aly L, Barz M, et al. The glioblastoma multiforme tumor site promotes the commitment of tumor-infiltrating lymphocytes to the T(H)17 lineage in humans. Proc Natl Acad Sci U S A 2022;119(34). https://doi.org/10.1073/pnas.2206208119. e2206208119.
85. Heimberger AB, Abou-Ghazal M, Reina-Ortiz C et al. Incidence and prognostic impact of FoxP3+ regulatory T cells in human gliomas. Clin Cancer Res 2008;14(16):5166–72. https://doi.org/10.1158/1078-0432.CCR-08-0320.

Printed and bound by CPI Group (UK) Ltd, Croydon, CR0 4YY
08/05/2025
01864749-0019